CURRENT HEPATOLOGY
VOLUME 14

CURRENT HEPATOLOGY ®

VOLUME 14

Edited by

Gary Gitnick, M.D.

Professor of Medicine
Chief, Division of Digestive Diseases
UCLA School of Medicine
Los Angeles, California

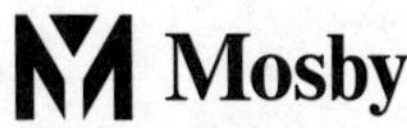

St. Louis Baltimore Berlin Boston Carlsbad Chicago London Madrid
Naples New York Philadelphia Sydney Tokyo Toronto

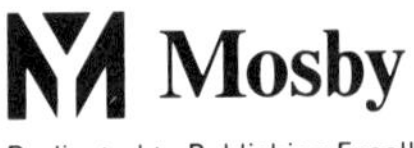

Dedicated to Publishing Excellence

Vice President and Publisher, Continuity Publishing: Kenneth H. Killion
Director, Editorial Development: Gretchen C. Murphy
Developmental Editor: Miranda Jackson
Project Manager: Denise Dungey
Project Supervisor: Maria Nevinger
Proofreading Supervisor: Barbara M. Kelly
Vice President, Professional Sales and Marketing: George M. Parker
Marketing and Circulation Manager: Barry J. Bowlus
Marketing Coordinator: Lynn Stevenson

Printed in the United States of America
Composition by The Clarinda Company
Printing/binding by The Maple Vail Book Manufacturing Group

Editorial Office:
Mosby–Year Book, Inc.
200 North LaSalle St.
Chicago, IL 60601

Mosby–Year Book, Inc.
11830 Westline Industrial Drive
St. Louis, Missouri 63146

International Standard Serial Number: 0198-8093
International Standard Book Number: 0-8151-3675-7

To my family who helped make this book possible: Cherna, Neil, Kim, Jill, Tracy, Jerry, Saranne, and Ann.

Contributors

Ashok K. Batta, Ph.D.
Associate Professor of Medicine
University of Medicine and Dentistry of New Jersey-New Jersey Medical
School
Newark, New Jersey

Harold O. Conn, M.D.
Professor Emeritus
Yale University School of Medicine
New Haven, Connecticut
Department of Veteran's Affairs Medical Center
West Haven, Connecticut

George J. Dawson, Ph.D.
Senior Virologist
Experimental Biology Research
Abbott Laboratories
North Chicago, Illinois

Geoffrey C. Farrell, M.D., F.R.A.C.P.
Professor in Hepatic Medicine
University of Sydney
Sydney, Australia
Head, Department of Gastroenterology and Hepatology
Westmead Hospital
Westmead, New South Wales, Australia

Jacob George, M.B., B.S., F.R.A.C.P.
Australian National Health and Medical Research Council Medical
  Postgraduate Research Scholar
Department of Medicine
University of Sydney
Sydney, Australia
Westmead Hospital
Westmead, New South Wales, Australia

Brian Ginzburg, M.D.
Clinical Instructor of Radiology
University of California, Los Angeles Medical Center
Los Angeles, California

Ronald L. Koretz, M.D.
Associate Chief
Division of Gastroenterology
Olive View Medical Center
Sylmar, California
Professor of Medicine
University of California School of Medicine
Los Angeles, California

Ruud A.F. Krom, M.D.
Professor of Surgery
Mayo Medical School
Consultant in General Surgery and Transplantation
Methodist Hospital
Rochester, Minnesota

Yeu-Tsu Margaret Lee, M.D.
Colonel, Medical Corps
United States Army
Chief, Surgical Oncology Section
Department of Surgery
Tripler Army Medical Center
Associate Clinical Professor in Surgery
John A. Burns School of Medicine
University of Hawaii
Honolulu, Hawaii
Clinical Associate Professor of Surgery
F. Edward School of Medicine
Uniformed Services University of Health Sciences
Bethesda, Maryland

Richard R. Lesniewski, Ph.D.
Associate Research Fellow
Experimental Biology Research
Abbott Laboratories
North Chicago, Illinois

Larry T. Mimms, Ph.D.
Associate Research Fellow
Experimental Biology Research
Abbott Laboratories
North Chicago, Illinois

Mikio Nishioka, M.D.
Professor of Medicine
Kagawa Medical College
Chief of Gastroenterology Service
Third Department of Medicine
Kawaga Medical School Hospital
Mikimachi, Kagawa-ken, Japan

Kunio Okuda, M.D., Ph.D.
Emeritus Professor
Department of Medicine
Chiba University School of Medicine
Chiba, Japan

Rudolf Preisig, M.D.
Professor of Medicine and Clinical Pharmacology
Department of Clinical Pharmacology
University of Berne, Inselspital
Berne, Switzerland

Nagesh Ragavendra, M.D.
Professor of Radiology
University of California, Los Angeles Medical Center
Los Angeles, California

Jorge Rakela, M.D.
Professor of Medicine
Mayo Medical School
Consultant, Mayo Clinic
Rochester, Minnesota

Gerald Salen, M.D.
Professor of Medicine
University of Medicine and Dentistry of New Jersey-
New Jersey Medical School
Newark, New Jersey
Gastrointestinal Research Laboratory
Veterans Administration Medical Center
East Orange, New Jersey

Dev Samarasinghe, M.B., Ch.B., F.R.A.C.P.
Australian National Health and Medical Research Council Medical
Postgraduate Research Scholar
Department of Medicine
University of Sydney
Sydney, Australia
Westmead Hospital
Westmead, New South Wales, Australia

G. Steven Tint, Ph.D.
Professor of Medicine
University of Medicine and Dentistry of New Jersey-
New Jersey Medical School
Newark, New Jersey
Gastrointestinal Research Laboratory
Veterans Administration Medical Center
East Orange, New Jersey

Jeffrey S. Weinstein, M.D.
Clinical Gastroenterology Fellow
Mayo Clinic
Rochester, Minnesota

Joseph Yee, M.D.
Associate Professor of Radiology
New York University Medical Center
New York, New York

Rowen K. Zetterman, M.D.
Professor, Department of Internal Medicine
University of Nebraska Medical Center and Liver Study Unit
Veteran Affairs Medical Center
Omaha, Nebraska

Preface

The study of diseases of the liver is an ever-changing science. The areas of research and clinical experience are continually expanding our knowledge. Rapid developments in hepatology have brought an increasing demand for authoritative, informative, and expert opinions to put the very latest achievements in perspective. This volume consists of literature reviews by experts in their respective fields who have agreed to review last year's literature and to present the reader with an overview of trends, interrelationships, evolving strategies, and new concepts. Each author has been asked to highlight those areas of basic and clinical hepatology in which the most progress has been made during the past year.

As has been our goal in previous volumes, this volume strives to integrate clinical and basic studies. The authors are not only clinicians but also basic scientists, surgeons, and radiologists. Each has been asked to avoid presenting an encyclopedic summary of all the literature published, but rather to concentrate on those areas that seem most important. Instead of a series of abstracts, the authors provide overviews that reveal the interrelationship of research activities throughout last year's literature, as well as revealing new trends and ideas. They have been asked to develop chapters that are easily readable and not ponderous. The most important goal of this book is to present to the reader an easily understood practical guide to evolving concepts based on the most important scientific articles published during the past year.

To avoid unnecessary bias, one or more peer reviewers, also established experts in their fields, have reviewed each chapter to ensure that the author has not brought undue emphasis to less significant research. This approach ensures that a wealth of new insights and new perspectives is brought to the review of the literature of liver disease.

I am indebted to the peer reviewers who worked with me in reviewing these chapters. Finally, I am deeply grateful to Susan Dashe who organized and efficiently compiled the chapters and presented this work to the publisher in sufficient time to keep this volume current.

Gary Gitnick, M.D.

Contents

Mosby Document Express

Copies of the full text of journal articles referenced in this book are available by calling Mosby Document Express, toll-free, at 1-800-55-MOSBY.

With Mosby Document Express, you have convenient 24-hour-a-day access to literally every journal reference within this book. In fact, through Mosby Document Express, virtually any medical or scientific article can be located and delivered by FAX, overnight delivery service, international airmail, electronic transmission of bitmapped images (via Internet), or regular mail. The average cost of a complete delivered copy of an article, including copyright clearance charges and first-class mail delivery, is $12.

For inquiries and pricing information, please call the toll-free number shown above.

CHAPTER 1

Acute Hepatitis: Single Papers, Two Reelers

Ronald L. Koretz, M.D.

Associate Chief, Division of Gastroenterology, Olive View Medical Center, Sylmar, California; Professor of Medicine, University of California, Los Angeles, California

If I were to ask you to picture a library in your mind, you would probably envision tables, chairs, shelves of books, and quiet. Since it becomes necessary for me to entertain myself in such places, I have to find soundless diversions. A number of nonmedical themes have interwoven themselves through most of these chapters in the past[1-14]; this year we will consider (but not hear) silent movies.

In this chapter we will look at the shorter films as we consider aspects of acute hepatitis and save the full-length movies for the discussion of chronic hepatitis (the next chapter, if I interpreted the director's [G.L. Gitnick, not D.W. Griffith] shooting schedule correctly). This chapter's cast will include considerations of the molecular biology of the hepatitis viruses, new information about the spread of hepatitis C and E, controversy about universal vaccination, and the longest appearance to date of a potential new star, the hepatitis A vaccine.

If you are ready, we can start the organ (liver, in this case) music and begin.

Current Hepatology®, vol. 14
© 1994, Mosby–Year Book, Inc.

ETIOLOGY

1929 was the year in which sound movies replaced silent ones. That year was better remembered for the beginning of the Great Depression. The herpes simplex virus (HSV) has long been recognized as causing severe hepatitis in patients with depressed immunity.[3-5, 8, 10, 11, 13] Four groups have recently described such cases.[15-18] Five Japanese authors reported a case of fulminant disease in an apparently healthy man.[19] In at least the immunosuppressed population, the liver disease may represent reactivation of a latent infection. Johnson et al. found HSV antibodies in pre–bone marrow transplant sera from all of their patients.[15] Concomitant mucocutaneous lesions were not always observed.[17-19] Acyclovir may or may not have helped.[15-17]

Brooks et al. saw a child with kwashiorkor who died of apparent pneumonia.[20] The postmortem examination, "begun 33 minutes after death" (permission having been "routinely obtained at admission"), demonstrated HSV hepatitis and pulmonary emboli of infected necrotic hepatocytes. It is unclear whether these emboli played a role in the demise of the patient or whether they were merely antemortem epiphenomena.

Herpesvirus-6 has been associated with fulminant hepatic failure (FHF).[13, 14] This year we learn of an infant girl who had a lingering subclinical hepatitis attributed to this virus.[21] The patient had a typical skin rash, as well as serologic confirmation of infection. However, the virus was never demonstrated in the liver tissue; could she have had a second hepatic process?

Icteric hepatitis (with more prominent elevations of the alkaline phosphatase level than are usually seen in typical viral infection) serologically attributed to cytomegalovirus (CMV) developed in a pregnant woman.[22] The illness resolved after her baby was born, and there was no apparent transmission of disease to the youngster.

Using polymerase chain reaction (PCR) assays, Chang et al. found CMV DNA in the liver tissue of 23 (out of 50) infants with neonatal hepatitis.[23] Identification of hepatic CMV DNA correlated (albeit not extremely well) with serologic evidence of CMV infection and/or the finding of CMV in the urine. In an editorial accompanying this paper, Persing and Rakela did caution readers about the potential technical problems of PCR assays.[24]

Adenovirus produced acute hepatitis in five (2%) pediatric patients with recent liver transplants.[25] The three who survived had had the immunosuppressive medications temporarily (10 to 12 days) stopped. The rotavirus was found in the liver of four children dying of various immunodeficiency syndromes[26]; although they all had diarrhea, none of them had any clinically important hepatic dysfunction.

A peculiar giant-cell hepatitis has attracted our attention in the past.[13, 14] Devaney et al. reviewed the pathologic material from 20 patients with "postinfantile giant-cell transformation."[27] Most were adults, and many had associated clinical and/or serologic features of an autoimmune disease. A number of concomitant histologic patterns were found, including acute hepatitis, chronic active hepatitis, cholestasis, and/or cirrhosis. The authors wondered whether these giant cells might not represent an unusual but nonspecific tissue reaction to injury.

In a chronic carrier of hepatitis B surface antigen (HBsAg) also infected with the human immunodeficiency virus (HIV) acute icteric hepatitis due to *Listeria monocytogenes* developed.[28] He had a characteristic biochemical picture, namely, high (40 to 50 times normal) elevations of the alanine aminotransferase (ALT) and aspartate aminotransferase (AST) concentrations. A liver biopsy demonstrated granulomas in addition to severe necroinflammatory disease. The patient recovered after receiving appropriate antibiotic therapy.

Psittacosis allegedly caused icteric hepatitis in three siblings.[29] However, these diagnoses were based solely on the demonstration of low-titer immunoglobulin M (IgM) antibodies in two siblings. The immunoglobulin G (IgG) antibody titers did not rise (if anything, they fell) over the subsequent months. Tests for IgM-specific antibody to hepatitis A (anti-HA) were not done. The father of these children did have psittacoccal pneumonia.

A 4-year-old girl with a clinical picture of acute hepatitis (and fever) underwent a liver biopsy, the results of which were histologically compatible with leishmaniasis, although the parasite was not seen.[30] After 40 days of fever, she was treated with antileishmanials and became afebrile within 48 hours.

What about noninfectious causes of hepatitis? Rex et al. saw two patients with postoperative hemorrhagic cardiac tamponade in whom ALT and AST elevations preceded overt manifestations of the pericardial problem.[31] Loeliger et al. saw one patient with eosinophilic fasciitis in whom icteric hepatitis developed subsequently[32]; the entire syndrome improved after the institution of steroid therapy. In this latter case, the authors failed to describe any evaluation for other causes of liver disease (e.g., viral serologic studies or exposure to potential hepatotoxins).

DIAGNOSTIC CONSIDERATIONS

As has been true in past years, this section will focus on the serologic tests for hepatitis A, B, and C. In passing, however, we have been reminded that the serum ALT level can be elevated in diseases of skeletal muscle.[33, 34]

Serology of Hepatitis A

Fred Ott's Sneeze, the first production of Thomas Edison's New Jersey studio, recorded an employee sneezing. Testing such secretions would avoid the need for venipuncture. Two groups demonstrated anti-HA in saliva.[35, 36] In one study, "oral" IgM–anti-HA was found in all patients who had positive sera.[35] In the other study, IgG–anti-HA was detected, albeit in lower titers, in 63 of 67 individuals who had this antibody in their blood; there were no false negatives in the 31 fully dentate (and younger) individuals. Using the serum specimen as the gold standard, there was one false positive (out of 47) oral specimen for IgM–anti-HA[35] and no false positive results (out of 24) for IgG–anti-HA.[36]

The Immigrant was a Charlie Chaplin movie (1917). Do hepatitis viruses migrate? Robertson et al. studied the nucleotide sequences of hepatitis A virus (HAV) strains recovered from different areas of the world.[37] Although they were able to demonstrate geographic localization to particular genotypes, there was heterogeneity in Japan and Western Europe, which raises the question of "strain importation." The relative lack of genetic variation suggests that this RNA virus is genetically more stable than other RNA viruses. Interestingly, many of the nucleotide substitutions would not translate into amino acid changes; if the nucleic acid sequence they studied is responsible for coding the antigen detected in the anti-HA assay, this would allow for a ubiquitous application of the test without concern for subtype variations.

Serology of Hepatitis B

Billy West was very good at imitating Charlie Chaplin's physical mannerisms, although he could not duplicate the emotional content. We are constantly encountering positive serologic test results that are also not the real thing. In past years we have discussed the issue of individuals with isolated antibody to hepatitis B core antigen (anti-HBc); hepatitis B vaccine challenges have suggested that the core antibody assay is usually a false positive.[10, 11, 38–40]

Other investigators addressed the issue of isolated anti-HBc positivity by looking for hepatitis B virus DNA (HBV-DNA).[41–43] In blood donors positive only for anti-HBc, HBV-DNA was rarely demonstrated[41]; HBV-DNA was seen frequently in such seropositive patients who had concomitant liver disease.[42, 43]

IgM-specific anti-HBc has been used to define patients with acute hepatitis B. However, it can be found in chronic disease, where its presence correlated with the degree of hepatic inflammation.[9–13, 44, 45]

Det Hemmelighedsfulde X ("The Mysterious X") was a 1913 Danish film that presaged the consternation we would have in trying to establish a role for the hepatitis B x antigen (HBxAg).[11–13] Blum et al. created a mutant HBV that did not produce HBxAg.[46] The fact that the mutant could grow in cell lines suggested that the protein was not essential for viral replication.

Secrets of Nature, a British documentary, may have alluded to the genetic secrets that modern molecular biology is attempting to unravel. Very sensitive techniques (e.g., PCR) detect the presence of nucleic acid sequences of various hepatitis viruses in serum and in tissue. My concerns in past years have revolved around the reliability of these assays with regard to both false positives and false negatives.[10–14]

Wirth et al., who described some of these findings twice,[47, 48] found HBV-DNA in the serum and liver of all of their HBsAg-positive children with chronic hepatitis as well as in carriers with normal aminotransferase levels. HBV-DNA has been found in the serum[11-14] and even in liver tissue[14] of such individuals before. Some investigators have found HBV-DNA (by PCR) in the serum of HBsAg-negative individuals, even those who have no HBV markers.[11-14] Three groups recently looked for HBV-DNA in liver tissue from such patients[43, 49, 50]; the data are summarized in Table 1. In those with hepatomas, HBV-DNA was almost always only demonstrated if the patient had serologic evidence of past exposure to HBV.[49, 50] On the other hand, most of the patients with non-B chronic hepatitis (no evidence of any HBV exposure) had HBV-DNA identified in their liver cells. Was this genetic material really there or is the test not specific?

Luo et al. looked at the hepatitis B vaccine response in more than 300 HBsAg-negative people.[51] In none of those in whom antibody to HBsAg (anti-HBs) developed was there serologic evidence of HBV-DNA. On the other hand, over half of the nonresponders were positive for HBV-DNA. In this relatively small sample, the PCR HBV-DNA assay was reliable in that there was a 100% positive predictive value for vaccine nonresponsiveness.

Hepatitis B e antigen (HBeAg) is used as a marker of viral replication; the presence of antibody to HBeAg (anti-HBe) is thought to represent a quiescent phase of viral infection. Some anti-HBe–positive patients are also positive for HBV-DNA, and genetic analysis of this DNA has often identified a "stop codon" in the precore region that prevents the production of HBeAg.[12-14] I have wondered how the host makes anti-HBe if there is no antigenic stimulus.[12, 13] Lyra et al. found the native HBV-DNA (no precore mutant) in the peripheral blood mononuclear cells (PBMCs) of four patients with the "pre-core mutation serologic profile" (i.e., anti-HBe and HBV-DNA positive).[52] They speculated that the PBMCs were a reservoir of the native virus. However, they did not do genetic analysis of the HBV-DNA in the serum to support the contention that a precore mutant strain was also infecting their patients.

TABLE 1.

HBV-DNA in the Liver of Hepatitis B Surface Antigen–Negative Patients

Study Reference	Patients*	Tissue Examined	B Antibody Status†	Frequency of HBV-DNA* Found
43	CH	Liver	−	15/21(71%)
49	HCC	Nonmalignant liver	+	8/15(53%)
			−	0/7 (0%)
50	HCC	HCC	+	3/9 (33%)
			−	1/2 (50%)

*CH = chronic hepatitis; HCC = hepatocellular carcinoma; HBV-DNA = hepatitis B virus deoxyribonucleic acid.
†+ = patients' sera positive for antibody to hepatitis B core antigen and/or hepatitis B surface antigen; − = patients' sera negative for these antibodies.

Serology of Hepatitis C

Mary Pickford's first movie, *Her First Biscuits,* was 6 minutes in length. The first-generation assay for antibody to hepatitis C (anti-HCV), which measured an antibody to a non-structural hepatitis C virus (HCV)-derived polypeptide known as C-100, did not remain out for much longer. We have seen wide-spread implementation of second-generation assays that detect antibodies to an HCV core protein as well as other nonstructural polypeptides.[14] Data supporting this supplantation are now appearing.

Like the first-generation assay, the commercial second-generation one is an enzyme immunoassay (EIA). In most series of patients, this test is positive more frequently.[14, 53–62] This may mean that the test is more sensitive or that it is plagued by more false positives. How can one tell the difference? This question has been addressed by using other "gold standards" to compare the results.

It has been widely accepted that the recombinant immunoblot assay (RIBA) is more specific than EIA in determining the presence of anti-HCV, although we have seen in past years[13, 14] that the RIBA result may not always agree with yet other gold standards. Two groups did use RIBA to make the argument that the second-generation EIA (EIA-2) is indeed more sensitive.[53, 59] (We will return to this subject shortly.)

Others have supported the claim that EIA-2 has improved sensitivity based on the results of PCR assays for HCV-RNA.[54, 55] This conclusion assumes that these molecular biological assays are very reliable. Two groups[56, 57] described patients who were positive for antibodies to four different HCV antigens but were HCV-RNA negative. Was HCV-RNA truly absent? On the other hand, three reports included patients who were negative for all of these second-generation anti-HCV assays but positive for HCV-RNA.[57, 63, 64] Are the second-generation assays still not detecting every HCV-infected person or does the HCV-RNA assay have associated false positives?

Two groups used, as their gold standard, the clinical scenario of the patient, namely, how often the EIA-2 suggested HCV infection in populations with non-A, non-B (NANB) hepatitis.[59, 60] In both reports, the EIA-2 was positive more often than the first-generation assay (EIA-1).

Curiously, occasionally the EIA-1 was positive when the EIA-2 was not.[58, 65] Nonetheless, it would appear that the EIA-2 is, in general, more sensitive than the EIA-1; one would hope that there has been no major loss of positive predictiveness. It would appear appropriate to begin using the EIA-2 as the standard test.

Appearances can still be deceiving. Rudolf Valentino was noted for his narrow-eyed glances that aroused the passions of his female fans. The look, however, may have been due to his severe myopia and his inability to get his leading lady into focus. Serologically speaking, the problem of the false positive anti-HCV assay has not gone away, especially in blood donors.[66]

As we have noted, RIBA has been proposed as a confirmatory assay. Since last year, seven more studies have attempted to validate this use of the second-generation RIBA (RIBA-2) by using PCR assays for HCV-RNA as the independent gold standard.[56, 67-72] The seven reports, summarized in Table 2, all had the same basic experimental design. Serum specimens that were positive by EIA-1 or EIA-2 were tested by RIBA-2 and PCR. With the PCR assay used as the gold standard, discordance (the frequency with which the PCR and RIBA assays disagreed) was calculated. Although one study[72] found remarkably low discordance, this rate was 10% or greater in all of the others. In blood donors there was less discordance if RIBA-2 indeterminant results were considered negative. These rates of disagreement with other gold standards are similar to those seen with the first-generation RIBA.[13, 14]

Serfaty et al. compared the results of RIBA-2 with the presence or absence of risk factors for hepatitis C exposure in anti-HCV–positive blood donors.[73] When compared with anti-HCV–negative controls, the RIBA-2–positive donors were more likely to have such risk factors whereas the RIBA-2–negative ones were not. However, almost 20% of the RIBA-2–positive donors had no risk factors.

Czaja et al. compared RIBA-positive and RIBA-negative anti-HCV–positive patients who were seen as part of the large chronic active hepatitis study at the Mayo Clinic.[74] Those who were RIBA negative were more likely to have lower titers of anti-HCV, have higher serum levels of immunoglobulins, and have the antibody disappear with immunosuppressive therapy. (In other words, the RIBA-negative group tended to behave more like they had an autoimmune rather than viral process.)

False positive anti-HCV assays have been described in hyperglobulinemic

TABLE 2.

Is the Second-Generation Recombinant Immunoblot Assay Confirmatory?

| | | PCR HCV-RNA* | | | | |
| | | Positive | | Negative | | |
Reference	Patient Population (N)	RIBA+	RIBA–	RIBA+	RIBA–	Discordance (%)
67	Pregnant women (26)	9†	1	9†	7	38
68	NANB* hepatitis (26)	11	2	2	11	15
59	Donors (70)	28†	0	20†	22	29
		24‡	4	3‡	39	10
69	Donors (179)	89†	0	43†	47	48
70	Donors (53)	20†	5	4†	24	17
		20‡	5	1‡	27	11
71	Donors (93)	49†	0	29†	15	31
		42‡	7	2‡	42	10
72	Donors (65)	6†	1	3	55	6
		5‡	2	0	58	3

*PCR HCV-RNA = hepatitis C virus ribonucleic acid assayed by polymerase chain reaction; + = positive; – = negative; RIBA = recombinant immunoblot assay; NANB = non-A, non-B.
†RIBA indeterminant considered positive.
‡RIBA indeterminant considered negative.

states.[13, 14] This may be the reason for the anti-HCV positivity in some alcoholics.[75, 76] Prolonged storage of sera (many years) may also result in nonspecific positive reactions.[77]

Hence, last year's observations[14] that the EIA-2 was more sensitive (albeit not 100%) than the EIA-1 and that the RIBA-2 was not perfect have been borne out with subsequent reports. We also noted then that the EIA-2 may become positive earlier in the course of the disease.[14] More recently, several groups of investigators have obtained serial specimens of blood from patients[60, 78–82] or chimpanzees[83, 84] exposed to HCV. Antibodies to the putative HCV core antigens do indeed usually arise before or at the same time as antibodies to C-100[78–80, 82]; the EIA-2 assay usually became positive before the EIA-1.[60, 81, 84] The only report not showing this phenomenon was one chimpanzee challenge study in which antibodies to C-100 and other nonstructural HCV antigens were observed first[83]; antibodies to HCV core antigen never developed in four of those eight animals.

What about using an IgM-specific assay for anti-HCV to make the diagnosis of acute hepatitis C? Preliminary data from several studies have suggested that this will be of little use. The IgG antibody usually arises at about the same time,[83, 85, 86] and IgM–anti-HCV can be found in chronic hepatitis C.[87–89]

We previously considered looking for anti-HA in saliva. We can now read a report in which anti-HCV was found in urine obtained at autopsy.[90] If the antibody is present during life, this would be another way to avoid venipuncture.

Andre Reed is generally given credit for being the first movie clown. His name is not well known because it was different in different countries. Hepatitis C virus may share this characteristic; it is reported to be genetically different in different regions of the world.[13, 14]

Still new variants are being described in China,[91, 92] France,[93, 94] Japan,[95] and Scotland.[96] Much of this work has been conducted in Japan where at least some portions of the genomes of different strains do maintain high degrees (>90%) of homology.[97–99]

There are implications from having a variety of strains. Genes encode amino acid sequences of protein products. If these proteins are the serologic immunogens and if there is limited or no cross-reactivity, we could need individual assay systems (although, in reality, this has not yet been a problem of major consequence). More importantly, we might need polyvalent (rather than monovalent) vaccines.

The situation may even be more complex. When investigators examined separate HCV-RNAs isolated from the same patients, genomic variations were observed.[100, 101] It is unclear at this time whether this represents separate infections by different strains of HCV, mutations that occur after an infection has been established, or technical problems with the nucleotide sequencing assay.

Although molecular biologists express great confidence in the accuracy of these various techniques, I must describe cautionary observations. Zaaijer et al. sent coded serum panels to 31 laboratories for HCV-RNA analysis by PCR; only 5 correctly broke the code, which raises concern about the reproducibility of this technique.[102] Within the same laboratory heparin and/or storage conditions can also reduce the amount of detectable HCV-RNA.[103, 104]

EPIDEMIOLOGIC ISSUES

Population Studies

A Corner in Wheat was an early D.W. Griffith short film. Neither it nor "herd immunity" refers to cows in whom sprue develops. Herd immunity relates to the degree of susceptibility to infection of a particular population group; it is the explanation for cyclic epidemics of hepatitis A. It may now be less important because of improvements in sanitation and the use of globulin prophylaxis.[105]

Like hepatitis A, hepatitis E is enterically transmitted. Fortunately it was not a problem in the United States during the silent movie era, or it could have become an occupational hazard of actors who were hit in the face by custard pies or other food.

Hepatitis E virus (HEV) has now been serologically identified as the cause of past waterborne NANB epidemics.[106–109] By using the recently developed antibody test against HEV (anti-HEV), the suspicions[14] that this virus is endemic in various parts of the Third World and is responsible for sporadic cases of NANB hepatitis have been validated (Table 3).[110–113] In Russia, 15 of 27 patients with acute non-A, non-B, non-C hepatitis were IgM–anti-HEV positive.[107] Even in the First World (Netherlands), 1% of blood donors were anti-HEV positive.[114] It should also be appreciated that many of the patients with acute hepatitis E (assuming that IgM–anti-HEV does identify this disease) had concomitant hepatitis A.[110, 113]

In the early days of movies, hopeful actors and actresses would do almost any-

TABLE 3.

Endemicity of Hepatitis E

Reference	Location	Number (%) of Admitted Acute Hepatitis Patients Positive for IgM–anti-HEV*	Background Anti-HEV Positivity Rate	
			Population	Frequency
110	Hong Kong	23/394 (6%)†	Relatives of hepatitis B carriers	57/355 (16%)
111	Ethiopia	36/110 (33%)‡	Soldiers	4/59 (7%)
112	Sudan§	23/39 (59%)	Hospital patients	3/39 (8%)
113	Egypt§	11/73 (15%)¶		

*Anti-HEV = antibody to hepatitis E virus; IgM = immunoglobulin M specific.
†Seventeen of 23 IgM–anti-HEV–positive cases had concomitant hepatitis A; the other 6 cases represented a third of the patients serologically proved to have non-A, non-B, non-C hepatitis.
‡Total anti-HEV (not IgM–anti-HEV) used to define hepatitis E.
§All pediatric patients.
¶Two of 11 IgM–anti-HEV–positive cases had concomitant hepatitis A.

thing to get into a picture. Now we find one investigator who voluntarily infected himself with a clarified stool specimen from a patient with hepatitis E.[115] Viremia developed on day 22 (postinoculation), anicteric hepatitis on day 30, and jaundice on day 38. The abnormal aminotransferase levels persisted for at least 3 months. The viremia disappeared by the time of the ALT peak. On day 41 anti-HEV appeared and persisted for at least 2 years. Virus particles were present in the stool from day 34 at least until the ALT peak (day 46); no further specimens were collected (because of the severe nausea, vomiting, and lack of food consumption).

Interpersonal Transmission

A number of Mack Sennett comedies had potential implications regarding the sexual transmission of hepatitis C. Consider, for example, *Cruel, Cruel Love, Twenty Minutes of Love, Her Trysting Place, The Rounders,* and *Those Love Pangs.*

Last year we tabulated the frequencies of anti-HCV positivity in the heterosexual partners of anti-HCV–positive individuals. Those rates were generally low, 6% or less (although higher in high-risk groups).[14] Subsequent reports[116–127] are summarized in Table 4. When the EIA-1 was used to screen these contacts,[116–122] the frequency of positivity was still low. With EIA-2 (or EIA-2 equivalent) screening,[123–125] the frequency of positivity appeared to be higher, 10% to 20%. Two studies suggested that anti-HCV positivity was more common in sexual contacts of patients with chronic hepatitis.[120, 125] This conclusion should be viewed

TABLE 4.

Anti-HCV Positivity in Heterosexual Contacts of Anti-HCV–Positive Patients

Reference	HCV Test Employed*	Frequency of Anti-HCV* Positivity (%)	
116	EIA-1	2/50	(4)†‡
117	EIA-1/RIBA	1/30	(3)
118	EIA-1	0/11	(0)
119	EIA-1	3/48	(6)†
120	EIA-1	11/164	(7)
121	EIA-1	3/29	(10)
122	EIA-1/RIBA	2/42	(5)‡
123	C-100/core	32/176	(18)
124	EIA-2	8/38	(21)
125	EIA-2	13/86	(15)†
126	PCR-RNA	0/3	(0)
127	PCR-RNA	12/37	(32%)

*EIA-1 = first-generation enzyme-linked immunoassay; EIA-2 = second-generation enzyme-linked immunoassay; RIBA = confirmed by recombinant immunoblot assay; PCR-RNA = polymerase chain reaction assay for HCV-associated RNA; anti-HCV = antibody to hepatitis C virus.
†False positive hepatitis C assay may be a problem.
‡Some of the contacts used intravenous drugs.

cautiously since the other index cases (no apparent liver disease) may have been more likely to have had false positive anti-HCV assays (and thus have no infection to transmit).

Comparisons of anti-HCV–seropositive and anti-HCV–seronegative individuals have identified epidemiologic risk factors.[14, 128, 129] Intravenous drug use or blood transfusions appear to be more important than heterosexual transmission. However, we should note that 6% of Japanese prostitutes who did not use drugs and who never received blood transfusions or tattoos (as compared to 1.5% of the general population) were anti-HCV positive.[130]

Among male homosexuals, the rate of anti-HCV positivity may be modestly higher than expected.[14, 131, 132] As with heterosexual transmission, other nonsexual factors are probably more important.[132]

What about finding HCV in other body fluids? Last year we noted two papers addressing this issue[14]; one found HCV-RNA in various fluids and the other did not. Several other investigators have joined the foray.[118, 133–136] All but one[136] of them found HCV-RNA in saliva, it has also been demonstrated in the salivary gland itself,[137] and HCV-RNA is[133] or is not[126, 136] in semen.

Nonsexual family contacts of anti-HCV–positive individuals are only at low risk of being anti-HCV positive themselves.[120, 125] However, Nishiguchi et al.[127] found HCV-RNA in the serum of 24% of the children of patients with chronic hepatitis C. (These same investigators reported the highest rate of HCV infection in Table 4, and I am worried that their assay may be detecting false positives.)

All on Account of the Milk was a two-reeler starring Blanche Sweet. With regard to HCV transmission from infected mothers, in the absence of an HIV infection the outcome for the neonate (development of anti-HCV) is generally sweet.[13, 14, 138, 139] However, when investigators look for HCV-RNA in such neonates, much higher frequencies of positive children are found.[13, 14, 140] The nucleotide sequences of the RNA in mothers and children are identical.[140, 141]

Let us briefly consider one aspect of the interpersonal transmission of hepatitis B. I have long been concerned about the replacement of selective screening of all pregnant women for HBsAg with universal screening.[10–14] Universal screening is, at the least, very expensive. There is a low HBsAg carrier rate in the private patient population (vs. women who attend public hospitals) and a low frequency of HBeAg positivity in non-Oriental female carriers. The sparse data available have failed to show that immunoprophylaxis even protects neonates of HBsAg-positive, HBeAg-negative women. Finally, compliance is never 100%.

Graham et al. found that the carrier rate in pregnant women in a rural population was only 0.1%[142]; this rate appeared to be 0.06% in the truly private patient population. Extrapolating the data of Kuller et al.,[143] I calculated that the HBsAg carrier rate in women without identifiable risk factors was approximately 0.01%! Hill et al. had to expend much effort (and resources) to achieve an 86% compliance rate for vaccinations, and even then most of the children did not receive the three doses at the recommended intervals.[144]

A Canadian study suggested that universal screening would result in an average expenditure of approximately $9000 to prevent one chronic carrier.[145] The authors appeared to assume that prophylaxis would be 90% effective in the HBeAg-negative situation; that the cost of the screening test was $8.50, the hepatitis B immune globulin (HBIG) $26.00, and the vaccine $45.00; and that compliance would be 100%. Even under this model, the cost of preventing one carrier in a native-born Canadian was over $125,000, compared with the cost for an Asian immigrant of $540. Although the actual figures may still be too low, the dramatic difference in the magnitude of the costs reflects the loss of economic efficiency when low-risk pregnant women are added to the screening lists.

There has been no dramatic reduction in the cost of the vaccine. Now public health officials are calling for adding routine vaccination to the burden of universal screening! We will consider this later.

Fomite Transmission

Watering the Gardener was the movies' first comedy. One might wonder what gardeners are now using to water, or otherwise contaminate, crops with HAV. Multifocal outbreaks of hepatitis A have been traced to commercially distributed lettuce[146] and frozen strawberries.[147] Oysters harvested in Florida caused hepatitis A in residents of that state, in residents of Alabama, and even in a visitor from Hawaii.[148] However, the champion food-borne epidemic, which affected 290,000 people in China, came from (not so silent) clams.[149]

A public swimming facility may have been contaminated by a cross-connecting sewage line.[150] The chlorine in the pool did not prevent HAV infection.

What about the role of environmental surfaces? Rajaratnam et al.[151] claimed that hepatitis A was transmitted by toilet seats (or at least by restroom facilities). At 20° C and 25% relative humidity, HAV remains viable (by in vitro assays) for many days (half-life, 8 days); an increased temperature or relative humidity reduces the half-life.[152] The calculated half-life on fingers was 2 hours, and the transfer of viruses to surfaces was directly related to the pressure applied by the finger.[153]

Various fluids and objects have been postulated to be passive carriers of HBV. We may have a new biological vector, the leech.[154] An outbreak of acute hepatitis B was allegedly caused by a contaminated culture medium used for in vitro fertilization.[155] The tears and aqueous humor of hepatitis B carriers were also often HBsAg positive[156]; the latter fluid is only a risk for a limited population (ophthalmologists, pathologists, and eye-pokers).

The interior surfaces of dental equipment can be contaminated with HBV-DNA.[157] Although the risk of this equipment was not directly assessed, it has been recognized since 1926,[158] when silent movies were still being produced and sold, that various medical devices transmit hepatitis.

Last year we asked whether organs from anti-HCV–positive donors transmitted hepatitis C.[14] We noted then that a large number of anti-HCV–negative recipients failed to seroconvert after receiving kidneys from anti-HCV–positive donors. More recently, Roth et al. documented anti-HCV in only one patient (chronic hepatitis also developed) out of 46 recipients of kidneys from positive donors.[159] Because all of the patients had little morbidity and no mortality from hepatitis, the authors stated that anti-HCV–positive donors should not be excluded. This conclusion was supported by Morales et al. who also saw that such recipients had, at worst, asymptomatic seroconversions.[160]

Unfortunately, the long-term fate of these patients is unknown. If end-stage liver disease appears many years later (a subject for the next chapter), the relative risk of that consequence must be balanced against the relative shortage of viable organs. Pereira et al. questioned the value of looking for anti-HCV seroconversions as evidence of HCV infection.[161] These workers found HCV-RNA in almost all recipients of organs from anti-HCV–positive donors, even in the absence of a seroconversion to any HCV antibody. The authors attributed the lack of antibody response to the immunosuppression. I am still concerned about the specificity of the HCV-RNA assay.

The same investigators who raised this issue[14] and did the HCV-RNA work just noted also evaluated patients who received more inert tissues (cornea, bones, or heart valves) from anti-HCV–positive donors.[162] In only one patient, who had other risk factors, did posttransplantation liver disease develop. The authors attributed this lack of risk to a lower transplanted tissue mass, no posttransplantation immunosuppression, and pretransplantation treatment of the tissue. It was interesting to me that the one case of hepatitis in this series was attributed to other risk factors but these authors put much less emphasis on these factors when discussing organ recipients in their previous work.[14]

Health Care Institutions and Workers

Two serologic surveys of the developmentally disabled failed to implicate HCV as an important issue in outpatients[163] and inpatients.[164] Hepatitis B was not a problem in patients with Down syndrome who are able to live at home.[165]

Remember the *Our Gang* comedies of the 1920s? Seventy years later a gang of investigators have been testing patients in renal failure for HCV markers.[166–185] These data are summarized in Table 5. Several conclusions can be made. EIA-2 identifies more patients than EIA-1 does.[172, 176, 177] Among hemodialysis patients, anti-HCV positivity rates are usually higher in patients from the Orient[172–177] than in those from Europe,[166–170] except perhaps in Italy.[171] Anti-HCV positivity was correlated with the duration of hemodialysis* and prior blood transfusions[168, 169, 171, 176]; these associations were identified in earlier studies.[14]

---

*References 166, 168, 169, 171, 173, 174, 176, 177.

TABLE 5.

Hepatitis C Antibodies in Patients With Renal Disease

| Patient Population | Reference | Location | Anti-HCV* Positivity by | | Associated Risk Factors* |
			EIA-1*	EIA-2*	
Hemodialysis	166	Germany	14/188 (7%)		Dur'n HD
	167	Belgium	3/57 (5%)		
	168	Spain	71/387 (18%)		Dur'n HD, Blood
	169	Greece	9/51 (18%)		Dur'n HD, Blood†
	170	Greece	6/66 (9%)		
	171	Italy	74/247 (30%)		Dur'n HD, Blood
	172	Taiwan	40/125 (32%)	59/125 (47%)	
	173	Taiwan	122/261 (47%)		Dur'n HD‡
	174	Japan	312/1,386 (23%)		Dur'n HD
	175	Japan	70/393 (18%)		
	176	Japan	20/184 (11%)	32/146 (22%)	Dur'n HD, Blood†
	177	Japan	100/489 (20%)§	204/489 (42%)§	Dur'n HD
	178	Hong Kong		11/51 (22%)	
	179	Saudi Arabia	21/52 (40%)		
	180	New Zealand		2/71 (3%)¶	
	170	Greece	8/43 (19%)		
Renal transplant	181	Spain	11/35 (31%)		
	182	Spain	28/67 (42%)		
	183	Austria	43/324 (13%)		Dur'n HD
	184	Italy	8/66 (12%)		
	185	Hong Kong	20/130 (15%)		

*Anti-HCV = antibody to hepatitis C virus; EIA-1 = first-generation enzyme immunoassay for anti-HCV; EIA-2 = second-generation enzyme immunoassay for anti-HCV; Dur'n HD = duration of hemodialysis; blood = blood transfusion.
†Arithmetic trend for transfused patients to be more likely to be anti-HCV positive.
‡No association was found for blood transfusion.
§Noncommercial assays employed.
¶Home hemodialysis patients.

In one study, the anti-HCV positivity rate in home hemodialysis patients was remarkably low.[180]

Three of the Oriental groups also sought HCV-RNA in their patients.[172, 176, 178] Although more of the anti-HCV–positive patients were HCV-RNA positive, each group did find this RNA in antibody-negative patients.

The prevalence of anti-HCV positivity in the dialysis patients was, as a first-order approximation, equivalent to that in transplant patients from the same geographic locations. This is of interest because of our previous discussion regarding the role of immunosuppression in masking anti-HCV responses (although the transplant and hemodialysis populations may not be strictly comparable).

All of these studies were conducted at one point in time; such prevalence data do not account for the development or loss of antibody in individual patients. In

Saudi Arabia, 11% of the seronegative patients became positive, but one patient (5% of the seropositives) became negative.[179] By prospectively following transplant patients in Hong Kong, Chan et al. estimated that there was an annual anti-HCV seroconversion rate of 5%.[186] Interestingly, three of four patients who were initially positive for HCV-RNA but negative for anti-HCV did become antibody positive during the follow-up; if seroconversion is an independent gold standard, this molecular biological assay was correct at least a majority of the time.

A common theme in early comedies is the dire things that befall patients who visit dentists, the title of Mack Sennett's first directorial comedy *(Lucky Tooth-ache)* notwithstanding. Two more health care workers (HCWs), both surgeons (not dentists), have been retrospectively identified as being the sources of HBV infections.[187, 188] The Centers for Disease Control has recommended that HBeAg-positive HBsAg carriers seek counsel before doing high-risk procedures but specifically declined to endorse mandatory hepatitis B screening of HCWs.[189]

In the prevaccination era HBsAg-negative HCWs with frequent exposures to blood seroconverted (to hepatitis B) at a rate of 1% per year.[190] If this risk lasts over a lifetime (30-year career), the probability of seroconversion is 0.26. These numbers were used to support universal vaccination.

Most of the seroconversions were manifested only by the development of antibody; the 1-year risk of HBsAg positivity developing was only 0.4% per year. If 10% of these individuals become carriers, the 30-year risk of a chronic HBV infection developing could be calculated to be 0.012. Assuming that the risk in the 1990s remains this high and that the vaccine prevents most or all of these people from becoming carriers, the investment for vaccination is still cost-effective.

Emergency personnel are at risk of viral hepatitis exposure. (Did you ever wonder whether the *Keystone Kops* got hepatitis? Since their movies were not in color, detecting jaundice would be difficult.) At Johns Hopkins, which services lower socioeconomic areas, 18% of the emergency department patients were anti-HCV positive by EIA-1 testing.[191] Reports of individual HCWs contracting hepatitis C from needlestick exposures continue to appear.[192-194] However, no more than 7 of 68 potential HCV needlestick exposees were infected by the virus (measured by a second-generation-equivalent anti-HCV assay), and in none did chronic hepatitis develop.

As each virus has earned its letter, it finds its way to HCWs. Hepatitis E virus infected at least one nurse assisting an icteric pregnant women in South Africa.[195] Acute hepatitis also developed in two other HCWs, but they were seronegative for anti-HEV.

COURSE AND PROGNOSIS

Easy Street (Charlie Chaplin, 1917) is not always the route that acute viral hepatitis pursues. Relapsing hepatitis A, where the relapse is usually considered to be a reappearance of the typical signs and symptoms (especially abnormal aminotransferase values), has been a topic here before[5–12]; in hepatitis A, these relapses have usually been progressively less severe.[11] Glikson et al. reported 14 patients with "relapsing hepatitis A"[196]; in 9 of them the relapse was at least as severe as the initial episode, including 1 patient with FHF. However, some of these 14 patients may not have had so much of a relapse as a progression of the disease into a cholestatic phase (characterized by the development of pruritus and more marked abnormalities in the alkaline phosphatase concentration).

John Bunny was America's first comedy star. Although rabbits are not susceptible to hepatitis viruses, other animal models have been used to look at host immunity in the development of chronic hepatitis after a hepadnavirus infection. Congenitally infected ducks always became chronic carriers, but ones challenged during "adolescence" rarely did so.[197] Woodchucks failed to clear the infection when they were given concomitant, but not subsequent, cyclosporin.[14, 198] Both of these studies suggest that the host immune state is important.

Alcoholics and nonalcoholics hospitalized with acute hepatitis B were compared.[199] Although the alcoholics may have taken longer to clear HBsAg, at the end of 6 months the only two carriers were both nonalcoholics. However, alcoholism may not be the best model of "immunosuppression," and retrospective data such as these cannot assure us that the two groups were otherwise comparable. Certainly, other data in humans would suggest that immunosuppressed individuals are at higher risk of becoming carriers after HBV infection.[9, 11, 14]

With most hepatitis viruses, we assume that immunity exists once an infection clears. In chimpanzees reexposed to HCV, disease again developed, albeit perhaps less severe.[200]

Buster Keaton was known as the *Great Stone Face* because he could freeze all emotional reaction. My colleagues and I used frozen sera to ascertain whether cases of NANB posttransfusion hepatitis (PTH) were due to HCV or not.[201] Among the patients with PTHC, chronic hepatitis developed in more men (16/18, 89%) than women (4/10, 40%), a phenomenon already appreciated for hepatitis B.

Furthermore, in agreement with several other groups,[14, 202] the 12 patients who did not have evidence of HCV exposure had less severe disease, and chronic hepatitis never developed.[201] Similarly, Dasarathy et al. did not see chronic hepatitis in any patient who failed to undergo anti-HCV seroconversion.[203] Although none of these data prove that there is another virus, it does raise the possibility that there is a hepatitis "F." (Only 3 of our 12 patients manifested evidence of CMV or Epstein-Barr virus exposure, and all 12 were HCV-RNA negative.)

A case of relapsing hepatitis was ascribed to CMV.[204] However, the IgM for CMV was probably a false positive related to high levels of IgM in the patient's serum.

Deshpande et al. treated 67 patients for tuberculosis at a time when they also had hepatitis.[205] The authors stated that the three-drug antituberculosis regimen (isoniazid, ethambutol, and streptomycin) had no adverse effect on the liver disease, but they only observed the patients for 15 days.

COMPLICATIONS

Just Gold, with Lillian Gish, was produced in 1913. It would be nice if hepatitis patients just got jaundice, but this is not the case.

Thrombocytopenia developed in one patient during the incubation of hepatitis B.[206] This "idiopathic thrombocytopenia purpura" resolved without therapy over a period of 4 days; it may have been due to a transient megakaryocyte dysfunction rather than an immune-mediated platelet destructive process.

Aplastic anemia has been associated with NANB hepatitis.[3, 6, 7, 9, 11–13] In two separate studies (of different groups of patients), Hibbs and Young (with different coinvestigators) could not implicate HCV.[207, 208]

Fred Evans was a comedian who played the character *Pimple*. Dollberg et al. saw two patients with urticaria early in the course of hepatitis A.[209] Kanzaki and Tsuda saw one severely icteric patient who had green and brown spots on his toes in a distribution resembling that of sweat pores[210]; the discoloration resolved after the jaundice did. The authors attributed the finding to the deposition of bilirubin in the horny layer of the skin by sweat.

Elevated amylase levels, with or without pancreatitis, has been reported in patients with acute hepatitis.[3, 4, 8, 10] In a young man with otherwise uncomplicated hepatitis A, acute pancreatitis developed.[211] Acute pancreatitis was found at autopsy in 14% of patients dying of FHF.[212]

Investigators still report abnormal gallbladder ultrasound findings, thickened walls in particular, in patients with acute hepatitis.[213, 214] I already got the message.[7, 9, 11, 13, 14] Black and Mann described a 6-year-old boy who required emergency surgery for gangrenous acalculous cholecystitis.[215]; almost serendipitously he was found to be positive for IgM–anti-HA, and anicteric (? asymptomatic) hepatitis subsequently developed. I am unconvinced that HAV had anything at all to do with the gallbladder disease.

Acute oliguric renal failure developed in a patient with mildly icteric hepatitis (attributed to HAV, although the IgM–anti-HA test was described as being both positive and negative).[216] He required dialysis, but he did recover.

Rheumatoid arthritis developed in a Japanese man after he had PTHC diagnosed.[217] We do not know whether the HCV triggered the rheumatologic process.

Two years ago we noted a case of "hepatitis A" in which the biopsy demonstrated ring granulomas.[13] That case was very atypical for HAV infection; the ALT concentration was near normal, the alkaline phosphatase level was more markedly elevated, and the patient's symptoms were high fever and arthralgias. Now Ruel et al. describe an alcoholic woman with a history of urticaria and fever who, on admission, had a more typical biochemical picture of hepatitis.[218] She was IgM–anti-HA positive (with rising titers), and her liver biopsy did show lobular ring granulomas. It is still unclear whether the preceding symptoms were a prodrome of the hepatitis A or actually a second disease; if the latter, the granulomas could have been residual evidence of that process.

FULMINANT HEPATITIS

In 1914, Lillian Gish played *The Green-Eyed Devil*. Patients with FHF and early encephalopathy may fit this description.

Precore mutants of HBV have been implicated in the etiology of FHFB.[13, 14] Since putative contacts have had the same mutations, it has been suggested that the mutant is responsible for the disease rather than being a consequence of it.[13, 14] Yotsumoto et al. compared HBV-DNA isolated from three Japanese patients with FHFB with that from their anti-HBe–positive hepatitis B carrier spouses.[219] Similar mutations were observed in both pairs.

Actually the data were not quite this clean. One of the patients with "fulminant hepatitis B" was only positive for anti-HBs (although HBV-DNA was purportedly isolated from his serum). One of the other patients was HBeAg positive in spite of being infected by a putative precore variant. Also, why don't the carriers of the precore mutant get FHF?[14]

Most patients with acquired immunodeficiency syndrome (AIDS) have relatively mild viral hepatitis. However, one AIDS patient was concomitantly infected with HBV and the hepatitis delta virus (HDV) and succumbed to FHF shortly thereafter.[220]

What agent(s) is(are) responsible for NANB FHF? Wright and coworkers found HBV-DNA by PCR in the livers of 6 of 12 such patients undergoing therapeutic transplantation.[221] The posttransplant sera from 4 of these 6 patients were positive for HBV-DNA, and at least 2 of these 4 became HBsAg positive. Sallie et al. could not find hepatic HBV-DNA in their patients.[222] Feray et al. only found HBV-DNA in 1 (out of 23) serum specimen of patients with NANB FHF.[223] Liang et al. could not find any HBV-DNA in such serum.[224]

Is HCV involved? Feray et al. did not find HCV-RNA in any of their 23 patients,[223] although, curiously, they did find this RNA in 8 of 17 patients with FHFB! Liang et al. found HCV-RNA in the sera of only 2 of 17 patients with NANB FHF.[224] A Japanese group found HCV-RNA in four of seven NAB cases, but they also found it in half of their eight patients with FHFB and even in one patient with FHFA.[225]

The HCV can probably cause FHF. Posttransfusion hepatitis C developed in two patients with acute leukemia who, after both being immunosuppressed undergoing bone marrow transplantation, died of FHF.[226]

Two groups sought evidence for HEV infection in NANB FHF. Neither could implicate the virus in patients seen in France[223] or Florida.[224]

Of course, not all NANB FHF is due to viruses. One patient had severe hepatitis that progressed to FHF; steroid therapy improved the situation, but the patient returned 2 months later with fever and more prominent alkaline phosphatase abnormalities. Ultimately, the diagnosis of Hodgkin's disease was made.[227]

Wilson's disease can also manifest itself as FHF, and a classic diagnostic tetrad (relatively low aminotransferase levels, relatively high bilirubin, hemolytic anemia, and increased urine and serum copper levels) has been described.[5, 8, 9, 11] In

1991, two diagnostic ratios (low alkaline phosphatase/bilirubin and high AST/ALT) were proposed.[13] Although the classic tetrad may have been useful for identifying Wilson's disease, these two ratios were not.[228]

What about treating FHF? Spanish workers retrospectively compared a consecutive series of patients treated with "selective intestinal decontamination" (poorly absorbed broad-spectrum oral antibiotics) with an earlier group not so treated.[229] The group receiving the antibiotics had fewer infections but no better survival.

Such retrospective data cannot *prove* that antibiotic therapy is of benefit since other differences also existed between the two groups. A prospective randomized controlled trial (PRCT) compared selective parenteral and enteral antibiotics with no such treatment in patients with mostly acetaminophen-induced FHF who were not thought to be infected.[230] A significant reduction in infections was seen in those receiving antibiotics (although it should be remembered that the parenteral antibiotics could have masked this end point by impairing the ability of cultures to demonstrate organisms). There was also an arithmetic trend for the recipients of the antibiotics to have improved survival (68% vs. 45%).

Lidofsky et al. described their uncontrolled experience with intracranial pressure monitoring in FHF.[231] Over 20% of the patients (5/23) had a clinically significant monitor-induced intracranial hemorrhage (which contributed to 2 deaths). Nevertheless, the authors thought that the monitor was of benefit in identifying patients with unresponsive intracranial hypertension (who would not be transplant candidates) and in managing patients before and during transplant surgery.

We previously reviewed an uncontrolled report of prostaglandin E in FHF.[13, 14] A PRCT of this agent could not demonstrate any treatment-associated improvements in survival or other clinical parameters.[232]

Charlie Chaplin's first film was *Making a Living*. What about making a liver? Extracorporeal cadaver livers (which had been rejected for transplantation) were used as temporary support in three patients with FHF.[233] One survived after receiving a standard transplantation; the extracorporeal livers functioned for up to 3 days.

We are beginning to see "liver machines." Two reports have described the development of encapsulated isolated hepatocytes that have been used on animals with experimental liver failure.[234, 235] Some isolated parameters have improved, but much work remains to be done.

POSTTRANSFUSION HEPATITIS

Hot Blood, a 1911 Danish film, did not describe the dangers people faced when they got transfused. That problem has become all too apparent in the subsequent eight decades.

Another miniepidemic of hepatitis A due to contaminated blood has occurred.[236] The original donation was obtained from a woman during that short period of time when she was viremic; before the talcum powder (it was a neonatal intensive care unit) settled, one baby, its mother, and nine nurses had been infected.

Let us now consider an epiphenomenon of the movie business, fan mail. Last year we briefly noted an outbreak of hepatitis A in some Italian hemophiliacs.[14] A subsequent barrage of letters was published by *Lancet*. Gerritzen et al. described a similar outbreak in Germany[237]; this group found HAV-RNA in a commercial clotting factor.[238] The manufacturers responded that previous seroepidemiologic studies could not support the hypothesis that clotting factors were a risk.[239] A letter in that same issue noted that a hepatitis A outbreak was associated with a particular product in Ireland.[240] A month later, a Belgium group added more cases.[241] Pasteurized products were not associated with HAV infections in a seroepidemiologic survey.[242] The same claim was made for preparations treated with solvents and detergents.[243] Nowicki and coworkers documented anti-HAV seroconversions in hemophiliac patients but noted that many of these may have been due to the passive receipt of globulin.[244] My perspective of all this is similar to my view of HBsAg-positive HCWs.[4, 8, 9] Most concentrates, like most of these HCWs, do not present a risk to patients, but occasional transmission probably does occur. Will the hepatitis A vaccine be of use in hemophiliacs?

Like the theme of this chapter, two patients with PTHC were alleged to have serologically silent infections with HBV.[245] Although both individuals failed to demonstrate any of the conventional HBV markers, both were positive for HBV-DNA by PCR, as was one of the donors in one of the cases. The authors speculated that the failure of both patients to manifest serologic evidence of hepatitis B was due either to a mutation in the HBV (a genetic variant unable to produce the usual antigens) or to a suppressive effect by the HCV. I would only add (again) the possibility of a false positive DNA assay. Wang et al. found no suppressive effect of HCV when chronic HBsAg carriers were superinfected.[246]

In Japan, PTH occurred in 10% to 20% of patients receiving blood between 1982 and 1987.[247] The risk increased with the volume transfused; it was unstated what, if any, screening of blood was done. This high rate was attributed to a high rate of HCV carriers in Japan.

In Italy, the incidence of PTH was 10%.[248] The rate declined from 1982 to 1990. Surrogate screening was employed for the entire period; the rate reduction may have been due to reduced usage with more emphasis on autologous donations.

In the United States, anti-HCV screening was associated with a reduced rate of "post-transfusion HCV infection," i.e., rate of anti-HCV seroconversions[249]; the study did not evaluate the rate of PTH as ascertained by ALT abnormalities. Anti-HCV screening has been associated with a reduced incidence of NANB PTH (as identified by ALT abnormalities).[250]

The Pawn Shop (Charlie Chaplin, 1916) reminds us that medicine is sometimes the business of trading benefits and risks. We have already discussed the problem of clotting factors and HAV; what about a more important infectious agent, hepatitis C?

Work done many years ago suggested that some blood components were less dangerous because of the physical properties of the virus; for example, in the process of Cohn fractionation, Dane particles did not separate out in the albumin/plasma protein fractions.[2, 3] Now Yei and coworkers have analyzed the various Cohn fractionations for HCV-RNA.[251] Coagulation factors were the components in which the HCV-RNA was mostly found. Some viral RNA was also found in the albumin and other protein components, but the heating to which these fractions are subjected may cause viral inactivation. Small amounts of the viral RNA were also present in the globulin component; there are reports of intravenous immunoglobulin transmitting disease.[9, 11, 12, 14]

Some type of heat sterilization has been used to reduce the risk of clotting factor–associated HCV transmission; wet-heat techniques may be better than dry-heat ones.[14] Hepatitis C virus markers were not found in hemophiliacs receiving only vapor-heated[252] or "super dry–heat treated"[253] concentrates. Although the way in which the clotting factor was treated was probably an important issue, the recipients of these treated factors received fewer units of clotting products overall.

Hepatitis C has occurred in hemophiliacs given only pasteurized product.[14, 254] Pollman and Jurgens, who have not observed any such incidents in 27 hemophiliacs, wondered whether these events were due to a non–clotting factor route of transmission.[255]

Solvent/detergent sterilization techniques have also been proposed as useful.[14] Three of five hemophiliacs treated solely by pasteurized or solvent/detergent-treated units had HCV markers.[256]

PROPHYLAXIS

Comedians treated females in different ways. Whereas Laurel and Hardy, W.C. Fields, and Buster Keaton tended to portray them derisively, Charlie Chaplin and Harold Lloyd put them on pedestals. There are two different approaches to hepatitis prophylaxis, passive techniques (immunoglobulins) and active ones (vaccination). Most of this section will concern itself with the hepatitis B and hepatitis A vaccines, but we will briefly consider two immunoglobulin reports.

Swedish investigators conducted a PRCT in 196 cardiac surgery patients to compare immune serum globulin with no prophylaxis in preventing NANB PTH.[257] The immune globulin was provided 1 to 2 hours before surgery and again 3 days after surgery (i.e., at or near the time of transfusion). The rate of NANB PTH was reduced from 10% (10/100 control patients) to 2% (2/96 treated patients). These data are consistent with previous reports that standard immune globulin is effective if given in close temporal proximity to the blood.[11] However, it should be noted that there was a large dropout rate in the trial (since 245 patients were initially randomized). Also, for unknown reasons, the study was completed in 1986 but not accepted for publication for 4 years.

Behren and Doherty saw two travelers who had received immune globulin 91 and 96 days before coming down with acute hepatitis A.[258] One of them died of fulminant hepatitis. The authors noted that the titers of anti-HA in the globulin preparations were relatively low; was it less effective, or at least did its protection wear off earlier?

Hepatitis B Vaccine

Harold Lloyd's trademark was his glasses. Since his movies were not in color, the rosy-pink hue of the lenses was not apparent. But one might wonder whether a number of advisory panels are not now looking through them. The Infectious Diseases and Immunization Committee of the Canadian Paediatric Society,[259] the Canadian National Advisory Committee on Immunization,[260] the United States Immunization Practices Advisory Committee (IPAC),[261] the Committee on Infectious Diseases of the American Academy of Pediatrics,[262] and the Italian Parliament[263] have all proposed that the hepatitis B vaccine be incorporated into the routine childhood vaccination series ("universal vaccination").

The rationale for this proposal relates in large part to the failure of most members of the high-risk populations to be vaccinated. However, I wonder whether there is not an underlying hope (? fantasy) that by performing early universal vaccination we will eliminate hepatitis B in the same way that smallpox was obliterated.

There are several major assumptions that this policy accepts without much if any direct proof. It is unknown whether early childhood vaccination will even afford long-term protection when these individuals enter the "at-risk" population as teenagers or adults. If boosters are needed, we will still be faced with the issues of compliance and inability to reach at-risk individuals. Universal vaccination assumes that society will be willing to pay for the vaccine; there has been no significant reduction in cost of the material. Unless we give more injections to infants, products combining the hepatitis B vaccine will have to be developed (assuming that the combination of vaccines will not result in any loss of efficacy of one or more of them).

The American Academy of Pediatrics and IPAC made even stronger recommendations.[261, 262] They proposed that universal HBsAg screening of all pregnant women continue (even though the implementation of universal vaccination would result in an even higher cost per case prevented [by screening] than the $180,000 I calculated several years ago.[12] The pediatric group called for universal adolescent vaccination "when resources permit".[262] It was suggested by IPAC that universal vaccination of teenagers be implemented in communities where behavioral risk factors are "common."[261] Both groups did acknowledge that protection is only known to last for up to 9 years; neither group considered who was to pay for all of this. While the implementation of this policy will get the vaccine to the groups who are less likely to need it (the middle and upper socioeconomic classes), its adoption will not improve the poor compliance of patients from the lower socioeconomic strata.

Cost analyses of universal vaccination strategies have appeared. Krohn and Detsky concluded that the critical factor will be the cost of the vaccine but that the duration of protection is also important.[264] They noted that the program would be economically attractive if the vaccine had a lower cost. However, unless protection lasts for decades, the burden of the disease would not be much diminished and the need for boosters would further decrease economic appeal.

Demicheli and Jefferson concluded that there was an unfavorable cost-benefit ratio for universal programs in Italy (where the disease is more prevalent), although vaccination of high-risk groups was probably efficient.[265] Two other analyses substantiated the benefit in high-risk patients.[266, 267]

Bloom et al. evaluated three approaches (universal vaccination, screen/vaccination, and no vaccination) in each of four populations (newborns, 10-year-olds, high-risk adults, all adults [aged 12 to 50]).[268] All of these strategies resulted in increased costs except vaccinating high-risk groups (our current policy). The least increase in cost was to screen pregnant females, vaccinate the neonates of carriers, and then provide universal vaccination for all 10-year-olds. Universal vaccination of neonates was ten times as expensive. (They did assume that protection only lasted 10 years.)

A Spanish cost-benefit analysis indicated that universal vaccination would only reduce direct costs if the attack rate (HBV infection) was 4.9% or greater per year.[269] By including the indirect costs, the "break-even" attack rate lowered to 0.9% per year. This will probably not be the case for *all* neonates.

In an interview Teele estimated that the cost of the vaccine alone, if all of the 4 million children born every year got all three doses, would be $250 to 500 million.[270] He estimated that there were 5,000 annual deaths (in all age groups) from hepatitis B. He then noted that dividing $250 to 300 (sic) million by 5,000 produces "a more cost-effective strategy." Avoiding an HBV-related death at a cost of $50,000 to $100,000 (since the higher numerator is $500 million, not $300 million) might be worthwhile. However, uncounted in his numerator are the other costs of prophylaxis (needles, syringes, nursing, anti-HBs monitoring, revaccination of the small number of nonresponders, etc.); the denominator assumes that all of the deaths would be prevented (the fantasy I noted earlier). The actual cost per life saved would be much higher; if protection wore off after 10 years, that cost could approach infinity (i.e., the denominator becomes zero).

Never Weaker, a Harold Lloyd comedy, might suggest that the vaccine effect remains forever. What long-term protection is afforded to neonates? After an average follow-up of 6 years, concomitant anti-HBc (presumably reflecting an asymptomatic, self-limited HBV infection) developed in 7 of 104 vaccinated infants of HBeAg-positive mothers.[271] Oon et al. found 1 similarly infected child out of 37 they followed for 4 years.[272] Hence, although such children (who are at much higher risk than those born into the general population) may become susceptible to HBV infection, the consequences of such an infection are clinically irrelevant. Unfortunately, we need much longer follow-up to know whether this level of protection persists.

Universal vaccination programs were undertaken many years ago in areas such as Africa or the South Pacific, where hepatitis B is also endemic but where childhood (not neonatal) infection is the issue. (Such "horizontal transmission," albeit in older people, is also the major problem in the United States and Canada.) Mahoney et al. did not find any HBsAg positivity in 95 children (aged 3 to 4 years) born during the vaccination period, although 2 may have been anti-HBC positive.[273] Chotard and coworkers did identify five previously vaccinated children who became HBsAg carriers, including one who had a satisfactory anti-HBs response and whose mother was HBsAg negative.[274] These four studies[271–274] suggest that the vaccine will not provide absolute protection from HBV infection in all children.

Farber, a practicing pediatrician, presented the human side of the dilemma regarding universal vaccination.[275] In his letter to the American Academy of Pediatrics, he stated his concern over the unproven long-term effect of the vaccine and his subsequent reluctance to put the recommendation into practice. He noted that he was left in an awkward position of "deciding not to go along" and asked the pointed question, "Was there really no member of the Committee who had sufficient reservations with the policy to offer a dissenting opinion?"

Dr. Caroline Hall, the chairperson of the committee (and also a member of IPAC) responded.[276] Her reply, longer than Dr. Farber's letter, reiterated data about vaccination schedules (Farber's other question) and lifetime risks, noted that regions with limited resources may not be able to implement the policy (but that it is "strongly recommended" where resources are not restricted), and observed that immunologic memory lasts at least 9 years. She wrote that the major message of the committee was "that universal immunization of children is essential to the eventual control of hepatitis B infection." (Again, is this part of the fantasy?) She did not respond to Dr. Farber's provocative question.

In *Streetcar Chivalry,* the men on a crowded streetcar pay no attention to a homely girl but rush to offer their seats to a pretty one. The plasma-derived vaccine was not accepted because of unfounded fears about AIDS transmission; the recombinant vaccine was more widely received, even though studies have suggested that it may be slightly less immunogenic.[10–14] One comparative trial of plasma-derived and genetically manufactured vaccines from the Pasteur Institute demonstrated that each product produced 100% seroconversions in children but that the anti-HBs titer was slightly higher in the recipients of the plasma product.[277]

Two PRCTs compared the Smith Kline (SK) recombinant vaccine (Engerix) to plasma-derived vaccines not available in the United States. When both were provided in a low-dose intradermal fashion, the recipients of the recombinant preparation had an arithmetically better response rate, and significantly higher titers of anti-HBs developed.[278] When employed as boosters to school children, both produced increased titers (arithmetically higher in the recipients of the recombinant product).[279]

Two recombinant vaccines are sold in the United States, the one noted above produced by S-K and one produced by Merck Sharp & Dohme (MSD). Comparative trials have not demonstrated any particular differences between them.[12, 280] This observation allows one to choose the cheaper product.

One way to reduce vaccine costs is to reduce dosages. This has usually produced a lower response rate and/or anti-HBs titer.[8-14, 281, 282] One PRCT compared 10- and 20-μg doses of the SK recombinant vaccine in neonates of HBeAg-positive carrier mothers.[283] Curiously the group receiving the lower dose had an arithmetically lower chronic carrier rate (1/56, 2%) than the one receiving the higher dose (4/54, 8%).

Had Fatty Arbuckle lived long enough, some disease related to his social excesses might have developed, such as diabetes, renal failure (from hypertension or diabetes), or even AIDS. He would then have had a less satisfactory response to the vaccine.[7-14, 284, 285] Dialysis patients may have more acceptable seroconversion rates if they are given renal doses (twice standard doses) of the vaccine four times.[14, 286]

One of the messages of *Streetcar Chivalry* is that beauty is only skin deep. Intradermal (even less deep) injections of very low doses have produced poorer response rates and anti-HBs titers.[11-14, 287-289] Commercial services are providing vaccinations to companies at rates comparable to the costs of intramuscular vaccine; the profit may come from the use of intradermal techniques, with less adequate responses.[290]

His Bitter Pill was a parody of the William S. Hart western. The vaccine's bitter pill is the poor responses some recipients have. There is an association between a poor response and histocompatibility leukocyte antigen (HLA) loci HLA-B8, SCO1, and DR3.[12, 291] Interleukin-2 did not enhance the antibody response of normal adults.[292]

We noted last year that there was no apparent interference between the hepatitis B vaccine and immunization for measles, mumps, or rubella.[14] We can add yellow fever,[293] bacille Calmette-Guérin (BCG),[294] polio,[294, 295] and diphtheria/tetanus[295] to the list.

Ben Turpin was known for his large Adam's apple and peculiar stare. Although otolaryngologic or neurologic complications of the vaccine were not recently reported, others were. Self-limited episodes of erythema multiforme developed in a nurse after each of the first two injections of a recombinant vaccine.[296] In another nurse with a past history of urticaria, urticaria again developed when she was given her first dose of a recombinant vaccine.[297] She subsequently had two similar reactions when given a thiomersol-free vaccine preparation, but not when given a placebo challenge; thiomersol, a preservation employed in standard vaccines, has been implicated in causing sensitivity reactions.[14] Skin tests against yeast antigens were negative.

Perhaps more because of coincidence than immunization, one man contracted acute glomerulonephritis after receiving the third dose of vaccine.[298]

A blood donor who had continually tested negative for the HIV antibody (using an EIA technique) turned positive after his second vaccine dose.[299] This result was thought to be a false positive one since Western blot and indirect immunofluorescence assays for HIV were negative. After a third dose of vaccine, the "HIV antibody" and anti-HBs titers rose in parallel; neither titer was boosted by an influenza/pneumococcus vaccine. If this is a true consequence of the vaccine, there is potential cause for much consternation as the vaccine is given to more people.

Unlike silent movies, our current entertainment media have the power to become stories unto themselves. For example, a Canadian nurse called a television program and alleged that she contracted chronic fatigue syndrome from the hepatitis B vaccine.[300] The program announced a toll free number, and at least 68 other similar claims were received. When 59 of these people were investigated, no conclusive epidemiologic association with the vaccine was established. However, one should never doubt the influence of the press. A medical student who read this reference[300] wrote a letter claiming he had been so affected by the vaccine.[301]

Which brings us to a word about sponsors. Two letters to the editor were published in response to articles about the infectious risks of HCWs.[302, 303] Both letters praised the articles ("otherwise excellent," "represent positive contributions to the issue of health care professional safety"), but noted that hepatitis B vaccination had been omitted. Although such an omission is appropriate to note, the authors of both letters were employees of a company that manufactures the vaccine. To the credit of the *Journal of the American Medical Association,* this fact was added by the editors.[303] Perhaps the *New England Journal of Medicine* should have done the same.[302]

Hepatitis A Vaccine

Pathe's newsreels were begun in 1910. If they were still being filmed, the hepatitis A vaccine might have received attention in the *News of the World,* where the disease is a particular problem.

Two vaccines have been developed, one by SK and one by MSD. Both are inactivated virus preparations.

The dose of the SK vaccine is expressed in arbitrary "ELISA units" (EU); the standard doses are 720 EU in adults and 360 EU in children. Field tests of this vaccine have produced nearly 100% seroconversion rates after the first two doses (given 1 month apart).[304–307] However, the anti-HA assay used to assess these responses was not the standard one but one developed by the manufacturer. Lower seroconversion rates were seen when the standard assay was used; only 67% were positive after the second dose, although there was 100% seroconversion after the third dose.[307] About half of the subjects had minor local or systemic side effects after the first injection, and a smaller number had subsequent problems.[305, 306]

The standard dosage of the MSD preparation is 25 units, which corresponds to 400 ng of viral antigen.[308] Two reports described greater than 90% seroconversion rates after the second dose, but again the anti-HA assay was a modification of the standard test.[308, 309]

Some PRCTs assessing the protective efficacy of these vaccines are being published.[310–312] The end point usually assessed is the occurrence of a clinical case; since hepatitis A does not produce chronic disease, this is what we want to prevent. In a brief report of the SK vaccine, 29 of the 30 cases of symptomatic HAV infection that were observed occurred in the placebo group[310]; about 40,000 Thai children were enrolled in this study.

Riedemann et al. gave 128 children the SK hepatitis A vaccine and 132 children the SK hepatitis B vaccine.[311] These investigators did look for subclinical disease. Seroconversions to IgM–anti-HA were seen in 1 of 128 and 3 of 132 children, respectively (differences not significant). Subclinical hepatitis A (asymptomatic ALT abnormalities) occurred in 2 of these 4 children (1 in each group). The number of children studied was too low to expect to see a significant therapeutic effect, and it is difficult to draw any conclusions.

The MSD vaccine was tested in 1,037 children living in an upstate New York community where hepatitis A is endemic.[312] The authors counted cases occurring after 7 weeks from the first injection to avoid including patients infected before the vaccine was administered. Although equal numbers of children were randomized to vaccine (519) or control (518), all 25 cases of clinical hepatitis A occurred in the placebo recipients ($P < .001$). Even if all of the cases of hepatitis were included, the differences still strongly favored the vaccine recipients. No cases occurred in the vaccinated group beyond 21 days after the first injection, which suggests that there was postexposure prophylaxis.

The SK vaccine is already licensed in parts of Europe.[313] Its cost is $24 per dose.[314] There is no cross-interference with the SK recombinant hepatitis B vaccine.[315]

Who should receive this vaccination? Certainly the long-term implications of hepatitis A are of much less concern that those of hepatitis B (or C, for that matter). Although there is some morbidity (and very occasional mortality) in the general population, an argument to use this expensive vaccine to eliminate the disease is even more unlikely to be economically defensible than that for universal hepatitis B immunization.

Jilg identified the groups at risk as being travelers (including military) to endemic areas, intravenous drug users, and day-care workers and others who have occupational risks.[316] I wondered about male homosexuals, residents of institutions for the developmentally disabled, and perhaps even hemophiliacs. Residents in the Third World could be considered, but a better overall solution would be to improve their public health facilities.

Margolis and Shapiro also addressed this issue.[317] They want to integrate the vaccine into childhood immunization schedules. They did state that we do not have proof of very long-term protection; they did not estimate what such a policy would cost. If history is a teacher, we will soon be hearing about plans to start such programs in the United States, where the need is the least (but where resources are perceived to be available).

A cost-effective analysis of hepatitis A prevention in travelers was published.[318] For an individual who spends 3 weeks a year for 10 years in a highly endemic area, the cheapest strategy was active immunization. However, the cost to prevent one case was almost $5,000. (This sounds like a good population for a PRCT.)

TREATMENT

The Cure, with Charlie Chaplin, was a short film. So is this section.

Three recent PRCTs have evaluated the role of interferon in acute NANB PTH[319–321]; the data are summarized in Table 6. (The trial by Omata et al. was mentioned last year.) The treated groups all appear to be more likely to have normal ALT values at the end of the follow-up. However, some problems exist.

In the first PRCT[319] it is not clearly stated how these patients were known to have "acute" disease (as opposed to a flare-up of chronic hepatitis), nor how long the acute process had been present before therapy. Furthermore, the interferon was given to each patient in increasing doses, with ALT normalization used as the end point.

In the second study[320] only 12 of 15 of the treated patients (vs. all 13 controls) had documented anti-HCV seroconversions (EIA-2). Although the interferon may have interfered with antibody development, it also may be that three patients had non-C disease (which, as we have seen, would be expected to resolve). If those three did have a self-limited process, the response rate in the remainder (33%) was not even arithmetically different from that of the controls (31%).

TABLE 6.

Interferon and Acute non-A, non-B Posttransfusion Hepatitis

| | Normalization of ALT* | | | | | |
| | 3 Months | | 12 Months | | Last Follow-up† | |
Reference	IF*	Control	IF	Control	IF	Control
319‡			7/11 (64%)	1/14 (7%)§	10/11 (91%)	3/11 (27%)§
320	11/15 (73%)	5/13 (38%)§	8/15 (53%)	4/13 (31%)		
321¶	22/26 (15%)	8/19 (42%)§	16/26 (62%)	6/19 (32%)	15/24 (63%)	7/18 (39%)

*ALT = alanine aminotransferase; IF = interferon.
†Last Follow-up: reference 319 = 3 years; reference 321 = 18 months.
‡Treated patients received β-interferon in doses that were increased until ALT became normal; patients with continuing abnormalities were retreated (the other two trials employed α-interferon, 3 million units three times weekly for 3 months).
§The frequency of normalization was significantly lower ($P < .05$) in the control group.
¶Data presented at Digestive Disease Week, San Francisco, May, 1992.

The last report[321] was an interval analysis of an ongoing study, and complete follow-up is not yet available on all participants.

If interferon will actually reduce the incidence of chronic hepatitis and, more importantly, the subsequent morbidity and mortality of cirrhosis or hepatomas, such treatment would be appropriate. Unfortunately, as we will again discuss in the next chapter, the transient normalization of a sign (the ALT) does not guarantee that present or future symptoms will improve. Such studies would require years (probably decades) to perform.

TRAILERS OF THINGS TO COME

This chapter has covered the developments related to acute hepatitis. I am still concerned that we need to be more cautious in interpreting many of the serologic (including molecular biological) assays for the various hepatitis viruses; optimally the development of gold standards with which we can compare these results will be forthcoming. It would be nice to have more information regarding exactly how easily HCV is transmitted among people in close contact so that we can be more definitive in our recommendations for alterations in behavior. Our desires to eliminate hepatitis viral infections from the face of the earth will need to be tempered by our limitations of resources, not only in the Third World but even (as our current health care crisis should be reminding us) in the United States.

It is time now for a brief (or long, if you wish) intermission. Then we will return with our feature films and a discussion of chronic hepatitis.

REFERENCES

1. Koretz RL: Acute and chronic hepatitis, in Gitnick GL (ed): *Current Gastroenterology and Hepatology*, Boston, Houghton Mifflin, 1979, pp 243–275.

2. Koretz RL: Hepatitis: problems and promises, in Gitnick GL (ed): *Current Hepatology*, vol 1. Boston, Houghton Mifflin, 1980, pp 1–39.

3. Koretz RL: Hepatitis: Retrospecti at prospecti, in Gitnick GL (ed): *Current Hepatology*, vol 2. New York, John Wiley & Sons, 1982, pp 1–54.

4. Koretz RL: Hepatitis: Same time, same station, in Gitnick GL (ed): *Current Hepatology*, vol 3. New York, John Wiley & Sons, 1983, pp 1–47.

5. Koretz RL: Hepatitis: Acute and chronic and Arthur Conan, in Gitnick GL (ed): *Current Hepatology*, vol 4. New York, John Wiley & Sons, 1984, pp 1–42.

6. Koretz RL: Hepatitis: Art and science, in Gitnick GL (ed): *Current Hepatology*, vol 5. St Louis, Mosby–Year Book, 1985, pp 1–47.

7. Koretz RL: Hepatitis: Serious papers, funny papers, in Gitnick GL (ed): *Current Hepatology*, vol 6. St Louis, Mosby–Year Book, 1986, pp 1–63.

8. Koretz RL: Hepatitis: The sports section, in Gitnick GL (ed): *Current Hepatology*, vol 6. St Louis, Mosby–Year Book, 1986, pp 1–34.

9. Koretz RL: Hepatitis: Words and music, in Gitnick GL (ed): *Current Hepatology*, vol 8. St Louis, Mosby–Year Book, 1988, pp 1–50.

10. Koretz RL: Hepatitis: Another fine mess, in Gitnick GL (ed): *Current Hepatology*, vol 9. St Louis, Mosby–Year Book, 1989, pp 1–54.

11. Koretz RL: Hepatitis: Facts and fables, in Gitnick GL (ed): *Current Hepatology*, vol 10. St Louis, Mosby–Year Book, 1990, pp 1–54.

12. Koretz RL: Hepatitis: Old pictures, new papers, in Gitnick GL (ed): *Current Hepatology*, vol 11. St Louis, Mosby–Year Book, 1991, pp 1–60.

13. Koretz RL: Acute hepatitis: Science and superstition, in Gitnick GL (ed): *Current Hepatology*, vol 12. St Louis, Mosby–Year Book, 1992, pp 1–51.

14. Koretz RL: Acute hepatitis: The short story, in Gitnick GL (ed): *Current Hepatology*, vol 13. St Louis, Mosby–Year Book, 1992, pp 1–42.

15. Johnson JR, et al: Hepatitis due to herpes simplex virus in marrow-transplant recipients. *Clin Infect Dis* 1992; 14:38–45.

16. Hayashi M, et al: Severe herpes simplex virus hepatitis following autologous bone marrow transplantation: Successful treatment with high dose intravenous acyclovir. *Jpn J Clin Oncol* 1991; 21:372–376.

17. Aboguddah A, et al: Herpes simplex hepatitis in a patient with psoriatic arthritis taking prednisone and methotrexate. Report and review of the literature. *J Rheumatol* 1991; 18:1406–1412.

18. Jacques SM, Qureshi FL: Herpes simplex virus hepatitis in pregnancy. *Hum Pathol* 1992; 23:183–187.

19. Miyazaki Y, et al: Disseminated infection of herpes simplex virus with fulminant hepatitis in a healthy adult, *APMIS* 1991; 99:1001–1007.

20. Brooks SEH, et al: Electron microscopy of herpes simplex hepatitis with hepatocyte pulmonary embolization in kwashiorkor. *Arch Pathol Lab Med* 1991; 115:1247–1249.

21. Takikawa T, et al: Liver dysfunction, anaemia, and granulocytopenia after exanthema subitum (letter). *Lancet* 1992; 340:1288–1289.

22. Makkonen M, et al: Cytomegalovirus hepatitis in late pregnancy. *Int J Gynaecol Obstet* 1992; 37:199–201.

23. Chang M-H, et al: Polymerase chain reaction to detect human cytomegalovirus in livers of infants with neonatal hepatitis. *Gastroenterology* 1992; 103:1022–1025.

24. Persing DH, Rakela J: Polymerase chain reaction for the detection of hepatitis viruses: Panacea or purgatory (editorial)? *Gastroenterology* 1992; 103:1098–1099.

25. Cames B, et al: Acute adenovirus hepatitis in liver transplant recipients. *J Pediatr* 1992; 120:33–37.

26. Gilger MA, et al: Extraintestinal rotavirus infections in children with immunodeficiency. *J Clin Gastroenterol* 1992; 15:251–255.

27. Devaney K, Goodman ZD, Ishak KG: Postinfantile giant-cell transformation in hepatitis. *Hepatology* 1992; 16:327–333.

28. De Vega T, et al: Acute hepatitis by *Listeria monocytogenes* in an HIV patient with chronic HBV hepatitis. *J Clin Gastroenterol* 1992; 15:251–255.

29. Samra Z, et al: Hepatitis in a family infected by *Chlamydia psittaci. J R Soc Med* 1991; 84:347–348.

30. Hervas JA, et al: Acute hepatitis as a presenting manifestation of Kala azar. *Pediatr Infect Dis J* 1991; 10:409–410.

31. Rex DK, et al: Post–cardiac surgery tamponade mimicking acute hepatitis. *J Clin Gastroenterol* 1992; 14:136–138.

32. Loeliger AE, et al: Eosinophilic fascitis presenting with a reactive hepatitis. *Clin Rheumatol* 1991; 10:440–444.

33. Mandell BF: Alanine aminotransferase: A nonspecific marker of this disease (letter). *Arch Intern Med* 1992; 152:212–213.

34. Morse RP, Rosman NP: Diagnosis of occult muscular dystrophy: Importance of the "chance" finding of elevated serum aminotransferase activities. *J Pediatr* 1992; 122:254.

35. Thieme T, et al: Clinical evaluation of oral fluid samples for diagnosis of viral hepatitis. *J Clin Microbiol* 1992; 30:1076–1079.

36. Bagg J, et al: The influence of dental status on the detection of IgG class anti-viral antibodies in human saliva. *Arch Oral Biol* 1991; 36:221–226.

37. Robertson BH, et al: Genetic relatedness of hepatitis A virus strains recovered from different geographic regions. *J Gen Virol* 1992; 73:1365–1377.

38. Lai C-L, et al: Significance of isolated anti-HBc seropositivity by ELISA. *J Med Virol* 1992; 36:180–183.

39. McIntyre A, et al: Isolated hepatitis B core antibody—can response to hepatitis B vaccine help elucidate the cause? *Aust N Z J Med* 1992; 22:19–22.

40. McMahon BJ, et al: Response to hepatitis B vaccine of persons positive for antibody to hepatitis B core antigen. *Gastroenterology* 1992; 103:590–594.

41. Iizuka H, et al: Correlation between anti-HBc titers and HBV DNA in blood units without detectable HBsAg. *Vox Sang* 1992; 63:107–111.

42. Medrano EJ, et al: Isolated anti-HBc and hepatitis B virus occult infection. *Vox Sang* 1991; 61:140.

43. Diamantis ID, et al: Polymerase chain reaction detects hepatitis B virus DNA in paraffin-embedded liver tissue from patients sero- and histo-negative for active hepatitis B. *Virchows Arch [A]* 1992; 420:11–15.

44. Smith HM, et al: Significance of serum IgM anti-HBc in chronic hepatitis B virus infection. *J Med Virol* 1992; 36:16–20.

45. Zoulim F, et al: New assays for quantitative determination of viral markers in management of chronic hepatitis B virus infection. *J Clin Microbiol* 1992; 30:1111–1119.

46. Blum HE, et al: Hepatitis B virus x protein is not central to the viral life cycle in vitro. *J Virol* 1992; 66:1223–1227.

47. Wirth S, et al: Detection of hepatitis B virus DNA by polymerase chain reaction in serum and liver of children with chronic hepatitis B negative for hepatitis B virus DNA by conventional hybridization tests. *Pediatr Infect Dis J* 1992; 11:209–212.

48. Wirth S, et al: Use of the polymerase chain reaction to demonstrate hepatitis B virus DNA in serum of children with chronic hepatitis B. *J Pediatr* 1992; 120:438–440.

49. Ohkoshi S: Detection of HBV DNA in non-A, non-B hepatic tissues using the polymerase chain reaction assay. *Gastroenterol Jpn* 1991; 26:728–733.

50. Dazza MC, et al: Polymerase chain reaction for detection of hepatitis B virus DNA in HBsAg seronegative patients with hepatocellular carcinoma from Mozambique. *Ann Trop Med Parasitol* 1991; 85:277–279.

51. Luo K-X, et al: Is non-responsiveness to hepatitis B vaccine due to latent hepatitis B virus infection (letter)? *J Infect Dis* 1992; 165:777–778.

52. Lyra L, Parana R, Cotrim H: Knowledge of the pre-core mutation variant of the hepatitis B virus (letter). *Am J Gastroenterol* 1991; 86:1851–1852.

53. Hatzakis A, et al: Antibody responses to hepatitis C virus by second-generation immunoassays in a cohort of patients with bleeding disorders. *Vox Sang* 1992; 93:204–209.

54. Yuki N, et al: Improved serodiagnosis of chronic hepatitis C in Japan by a second-generation enzyme-linked immunosorbent assay. *J Med Virol* 1992; 37:237–240.

55. Nakatsuji Y, et al: Detection of chronic hepatitis C virus infection by four diagnostic systems: First-generation and second-generation enzyme-linked immunosorbent assay, second-generation recombinant immunoblot assay and nest polymerase chain reaction analysis. *Hepatology* 1992; 16:300–305.

56. Bresters D, et al: Enhanced sensitivity of a second generation ELISA for antibody to hepatitis C virus. *Vox Sang* 1992; 62:213–217.

57. Puchammer-Stockl E, et al: Prevalence of hepatitis-C virus infection in children with chronic post-transfusion hepatitis. *J Med Virol* 1992; 37:298–302.

58. Larsen J, Skaug K, Maeland A: Second-generation anti-HCV tests predict infectivity. *Vox Sang* 1992; 63:39–42.

59. Kleinman S, et al: Increased detection of hepatitis C virus (HCV)-infected blood donors by a multiple-antigen HCV enzyme immunoassay. *Transfusion* 1992; 32:805–813.

60. Giuberti T, et al: Long-term followup of anti-hepatitis C virus antibodies in patients with acute non-A non-B hepatitis and different outcome of liver disease. *Liver* 1992; 12:94–99.

61. Kawano S-I, et al: Clinical evaluation of these anti-HCV ELISAs in patients with various liver disease. *Dig Dis Sci* 1992; 37:1268–1274.

62. Setoguchi Y, et al: Overlap and discrepancy between tests for anti-C100, anti-GOR and anti-CP9 in patients with chronic liver disease and inhabitants in Soga, Japan. *Gastroenterol Jpn* 1992; 27:502–507.

63. Sugitani M, et al: Sensitivity of serological assays to identify blood donors with hepatitis C viraemia. *Lancet* 1992; 339:1018–1019.

64. Hosoda K, et al: Non-A, non-B chronic hepatitis is chronic hepatitis C: A sensitive assay for detection of hepatitis C virus RNA in the liver. *Hepatology* 1992; 15:777–781.

65. Claeys H, et al: Association of hepatitis C virus carrier state with the occurrences of hepatitis C virus core antibodies. *J Med Virol* 1992; 36:259–264.

66. Prohaska W, et al: High rate of false positives in blood donor screening for antibodies to hepatitis C. *Klin Wochenschr* 1991; 69:294–296.

67. Martinot-Peignoux M, et al: Reactivity to c33c antigen as a marker of hepatitis virus multiplication (letter). *J Infect Dis* 1992; 165:595–596.

68. Da Silva Cardosa M, et al: Evaluating recombinant protein immunoblot assay and polymerase chain reaction for diagnosis of non-A, non-B hepatitis (letter). *J Infect Dis* 1992; 166:450–451.

69. De Beenhouwer H, et al: Confirmation of hepatitis C virus positive blood donors by immuno-blotting and polymerase chain reaction. *Vox Sang* 1992; 63:198–203.

70. Romeo JM, et al: Analysis of hepatitis C virus RNA prevalence and surrogate markers of infection among seropositive voluntary blood donors. *Hepatology* 1992; 12:188–195.

71. Yun Z-B, et al: Detection of hepatitis C virus (HCV) RNA by PCR related to HCV antibodies in serum and liver histology in Swedish blood donors. *J Med Virol* 1993; 39:57–61.

72. Garson JA, et al: Hepatitis C viraemia in United Kingdom blood donors. *Vox Sang* 1992; 62:218–223.

73. Serfaty L, et al: Risk factors for hepatitis C virus infection in hepatitis C virus antibody ELISA-positive blood donors according to RIBA-2 status: A case-controlled survey. *Hepatology* 1993; 17:183–187.

74. Czaja AJ, et al: Duration and specificity of antibodies to hepatitis C virus in chronic active hepatitis. *Gastroenterology* 1992; 102:1675–1679.

75. Bode JC, et al: High incidence of antibodies to hepatitis C virus in alcoholic cirrhosis: Fact or fiction? *Alcohol Alcohol* 1991; 26:111–114.

76. Laurent-Puig E, et al: Prevalence of anti–hepatitis C virus antibodies among patients with alcoholic liver disease, supplemented by 4-RIBA (letter). *Dig Dis Sci* 1992; 37:156–157.

77. Nicholson S, et al: Hepatitis C antibody testing: Problems associated with non-specific binding. *J Virol Methods* 1991; 33:311–317.

78. Lelie PN, et al: Patterns of serological markers in transfusion-transmitted hepatitis C virus infection using second-generation HCV assays. *J Med Virol* 1992; 37:203–209.

79. Vallari DS, et al: Serological markers of post-transfusion hepatitis C viral infection. *J Clin Microbiol* 1992; 30:552–556.

80. Dourakis S, et al: Serological response and detection of viraemia in acute hepatitis C virus infection. *J Hepatol* 1992; 14:370–376.

81. Wang J-T, et al: Improved serodiagnosis of post-transfusion hepatitis C virus infection by a second-generation immunoassay based on multiple recombinant antigens. *Vox Sang* 1992; 62:21–24.

82. Yoshikawa A, et al: Serodiagnosis of hepatitis C virus infection by ELISA for antibodies against the putative core protein (p 20^c) expressed in *Escherichia coli*. *J Immunol Methods* 1992; 148:143–150.

83. Beach J, et al: Temporal relationships of hepatitis C virus RNA and antibody responses following experimental infection of chimpanzees. *J Med Virol* 1992; 36:227–237.

84. Farci P, et al: The natural history of infection with hepatitis C virus (HCV) in chimpanzees; comparison of serologic responses measured with first- and second-generation assays and relationship to HCV viremia. *J Infect Dis* 1992; 165:1006–1111.

85. Chau KH, et al: IgM-antibody response to hepatitis C virus antigens in acute and chronic post-transfusion non-A, non-B hepatitis. *J Virol Methods* 1991; 35:343–352.

86. Clemens JM, et al: IgM antibody response in acute hepatitis C viral infection. *Blood* 1992; 79:169–172.

87. Brillanti S, et al: Significance of IgM antibody to hepatitis C virus in patients with chronic hepatitis C. *Hepatology* 1992; 15:998–1001.

88. Quiroga JA, et al: Immunoglobulin M antibody to hepatitis C virus during interferon therapy for chronic hepatitis C. *Gastroenterology* 1992; 103:1285–1289.

89. Kikuchi T, et al: Anti-hepatitis C virus immunoglobulin M antibody in patients with chronic hepatitis type C. *Hepatogastroenterology* 1992; 39:525–528.

90. Constantine NT, et al: Detection of antibodies to hepatitis C virus in urine (letter). *Lancet* 1992; 339:1607–1608.

91. Wei-ran C, Okamoto H, Qi-min T: Similarity and diversity in sequence of HCV genome among Chinese, Japanese and American strains. *Chin Med J* 1991; 104:825–829.

92. Liu K, et al: Genomic typing of hepatitis C virus present in China. *Gene*. 1992; 114:245–250.

93. Dremsdorf D, et al: Partial nucleotide sequence analysis of a French hepatitis C virus: Implications for HCV genetic variability in the E2/NS1 protein. *J Gen Virol* 1991; 72:2557–2561.

94. Li J, et al: Two French genotypes of hepatitis C virus: Homology of the predominant genotype with the prototype American strain. *Gene* 1991; 105:167–172.

95. Fujio K, Shimomura H, Tsuji T: Genetic variation of putative core gene in hepatitis C virus. *Acta Med Okayama* 1991; 45:241–248.

96. Chan S-W, et al: Analysis of a new hepatitis C virus type and its phylogenetic relationship to existing variant. *J Gen Virol* 1992; 73:1131–1141.

97. Hada H, et al: Sequence variation in the envelope protein of the hepatitis C virus; comparison with partial cDNA sequence of a new variant virus obtained by the polymerase chain reaction. *Acta Med Okayama* 1991; 45:347–355.

98. Okamoto H, et al: Nucleotide sequence of the genomic RNA of hepatitis C virus isolated from a human carrier: Comparison with reported isolates for conserved and divergent regions. *J Gen Virol* 1991; 72:2697–2704.

99. Kato N, et al: Distribution of pleural HCV types in Japan. *Biochem Biophys Res Commun* 1991; 181:279–285.

100. Martell M, et al: Hepatitis C virus (HCV) circulates as a population of different but closely related genomes: Quasispecies nature of HCV genome distribution. *J Virol* 1992; 66:3225–3229.

101. Oshima M, et al: cDNA clones of Japanese hepatitis C virus genomes derived from a single patient show sequence heterogeneity. *J Gen Virol* 1991; 72:2805–2809.

102. Zaaijer HL, et al: Reliability of polymerase chain reaction for detection of hepatitis C virus. *Lancet* 1993; 341:722–724.

103. Wang J-T, et al: Effects of anticoagulants and storage of blood samples on efficacy of the polymerase chain reaction assay for hepatitis C virus. *J Clin Microbiol* 1992; 30:750–753.

104. Busch MP, et al: Impact of specimen handling and storage on detection of hepatitis C virus DNA. *Transfusion* 1992; 32:420–425.

105. Rooney PJ, Coyle PV: The role of herd immunity in an epidemic cycle of hepatitis A. *J Infect* 1992; 24:327–331.

106. Skidmore SJ, et al: Hepatitis E virus: The cause of waterborne hepatitis outbreak. *J Med Virol* 1992; 37:58–60.

107. Favorov MO, et al: Serologic identification of hepatitis E virus infections in epidemic and endemic settings. *J Med Virol* 1992; 36:246–250.

108. Jameel S, et al: Enteric non-A, non-B hepatitis. *J Med Virol* 1992; 37:263–270.

109. Ticehurst J, et al: Association of hepatitis E virus with an outbreak of hepatitis in Pakistan. *J Med Virol* 1992; 36:84–92.

110. Lok ASF, et al: Seroepidemiological survey of hepatitis E in Hong Kong by recombinant-based enzyme immunoassays. *Lancet* 1992; 340:1205–1208.

111. Tsega E, et al: Acute sporadic viral hepatitis in Ethiopia: Causes, risk factors, and effects on pregnancy. *Clin Infect Dis* 1992; 14:961–965.

112. Hyams KC, et al: Acute sporadic hepatitis E in Sudanese children: Analysis based on a new Western blot assay. *J Infect Dis* 1992; 165:1001–1005.

113. Hyams KC, et al: Acute sporadic hepatitis E in children living in Cairo, Egypt. *J Med Virol* 1992; 37:274–277.

114. Zaaijer HL, et al: Hepatitis E in the Netherlands: Imported and endemic (letter). *Lancet* 1993; 341:826.

115. Chauhan A, et al: Hepatitis E virus transmission to a volunteer. *Lancet* 1993; 341:149–150.

116. Tor J, et al: Non-parenteral transmission of hepatitis C virus (letter). *Int J Stud AIDS* 1991; 2:449–450.

117. Kolko E, et al: Transmission of hepatitis C virus to sexual partners of seropositive patients with bleeding disorders: A rare event. *Scand J Infect Dis* 1991; 23:667–670.

118. Wang J-T, et al: Hepatitis C virus RNA in saliva of patients with post transfusion hepatitis and low efficiency of transmission among spouses. *J Med Virol* 1992; 36:28–31.

119. Deny P, et al: Low rate of hepatitis C virus (HCV) transmission within the family. *J Hepatol* 1992; 14:409–410.

120. Menendez SR, et al: Intrafamilial spread of hepatitis C virus. *Infection* 1991; 19:431–433.

121. Cilla G, et al: Possibility of heterosexual transmission of hepatitis C virus. *Eur J Clin Microbiol Infect Dis* 1991; 10:533–534.

122. Gordon SC, et al: Lack of evidence for the heterosexual transmission of hepatitis C. *Am J Gastroenterol* 1992; 87:1849–1851.

123. Akahane Y, et al: Transmission of HCV between spouses (letter). *Lancet* 1992; 339:1059–1060.

124. Kao J-H, et al: Intrafamilial transmission of hepatitis C virus: The important role of infections between spouses. *J Infect Dis* 1992; 166:900–903.

125. Peano GM, et al: Heterosexual transmission of hepatitis C virus in family groups without risk factors. *BMJ* 1992; 305:1473–1474.

126. Terada S, Kawanashi K, Katayama K: Minimal hepatitis C infectivity in semen (letter). *Ann Intern Med* 1992; 117:171–172.

127. Nishiguchi S, et al: Familial clustering of HCV (letter). *Lancet* 1992; 339:1486.

128. Osmond DH, et al: Risk factors for hepatitis C virus seropositivity in heterosexual couples. *JAMA* 1993; 269:361–365.

129. Weinstock HS, et al: Hepatitis C virus infection among patients attending a clinic for sexually transmitted diseases. *JAMA* 1993; 269:392–394.

130. Nakashima K, et al: Sexual transmission of hepatitis C virus among female prostitutes and patients with sexually transmitted diseases in Fukuoka, Kyushu, Japan. *Am J Epidemiol* 1992; 136:1132–1137.

131. Corona R, et al: Heterosexual and homosexual transmission of hepatitis C virus: Relation with hepatitis B virus and human immunodeficiency virus type 1. *Epidemiol Infect* 1991; 107:667–672.

132. Osmond DH, et al: Comparison of risk factors for hepatitis C and hepatitis B virus infection in homosexual men. *J Infect Dis* 193; 167:66–71.

133. Liou T-C, et al: Detection of HCV-RNA in saliva, urine, seminal fluid, and ascites. *J Med Virol* 1992; 37:197–202.

134. Nakano I, et al: Hepatitis C virus RNA in urine, saliva, and sweat (letter). *Am J Gastroenterol* 1992; 87:1522.

135. Ogasawara S, et al: Hepatitis C virus RNA in saliva and breast milk of hepatitis C carrier mothers (letter). *Lancet* 1993; 341:561.

136. Fried MW, et al: Absence of hepatitis C viral RNA from saliva and semen of patients with chronic hepatitis C. *Gastroenterology* 1992; 102:1306–1308.

137. Takamatsu K, et al: Hepatitis C virus propagates in salivary glands (letter). *J Infect Dis* 1992; 165:973–974.

138. Reinus JF, et al: Failure to detect vertical transmission of hepatitis C virus. *Ann Intern Med* 1992; 117:881–886.

139. Westjal R, et al: Mother-to-infant transmission of hepatitis C virus. *Ann Intern Med* 1992; 117:887–890.

140. Kuroki T, et al: Transmission of hepatitis C virus from mothers with chronic hepatitis C without human immunodeficiency virus (letter). *J Infect Dis* 1992; 166:1192–1193.

141. Inoue Y, et al: Silent mother-to-child transmission of hepatitis C virus through two generations determined by comparative nucleotide sequence analysis of the viral cDNA. *J Infect Dis* 1992; 166:1425–1428.

142. Graham JM, Blanco JD, Magee KP: Screening for hepatitis B among pregnant patients in a rural population. *South Med J* 1992; 85:594–596.

143. Kuller JA, et al: Efficacy of hepatitis B screening in a private obstetrical population. *J Perinatol* 1991; 11:164–167.

144. Hill LL, Hovell M, Benenson AS: Prevention of hepatitis B transmission in Indo-Chinese refugees wtih active and passive immunization. *Am J Prev Med* 1991; 7:29–32.

145. Audet A-M, Delage G, Remmis RS: Screening for HBsAg in pregnant women: A cost analysis of the universal screening policy in the province of Quebec. *Can J Public Health* 1991; 82:191–195.

146. Rosenblum LS, et al: A multifocal outbreak of hepatitis A traced to commercially distributed lettuce. *Am J Public Health* 1990; 1075–1080.

147. Niu MT, et al: Multistate outbreak of hepatitis A associated with frozen strawberries. *J Infect Dis* 1992; 166:518–524.

148. Desenclos JA, et al: A multistate outbreak of hepatitis A caused by the consumption of raw oysters. *Am J Public Health* 1991; 81:1268–1272.

149. Tang YW, et al: A serologically confirmed, case-control study, of a large outbreak of hepatitis A in China, associated with consumption of clams. *Epidemiol Infect* 1991; 107:651–657.

150. Mahoney FJ, et al: An outbreak of hepatitis A associated with swimming in a public pool. *J Infect Dis* 1992; 165:613–618.

151. Rajaratnam G, et al: An outbreak of hepatitis A: School toilets as a source of transmission. *J Public Health Med* 1992; 14:72–77.

152. Mbithi JN, Springthorpe VS, Sattar SA: Effect of relative humidity and air temperature on survival of hepatitis A virus on environmental surfaces. *Appl Environ Microbiol* 1991; 57:1394–1399.

153. Mbithi JN, et al: Survival of hepatitis A virus on human hands and its transfer on contact with animate and inanimate surfaces. *J Clin Microbiol* 1992; 30:757–763.

154. Narendranathan M: Leeches and hepatitis B (letter). *Lancet* 1992; 339:1362.

155. Van Os HC, et al: The influence of contamination of culture medium with hepatitis B virus on the outcome of in vitro fertilization pregnancies. *Am J Obstet Gynecol* 1991; 165:152–159.

156. Koksal I, Cetinkaya K, Aker F: Hepatitis B surface antigen in tears and aqueous humor. *Ophthalmologica* 1992; 204:19–22.

157. Lewis DL, et al: Cross-contamination potential with dental equipment. *Lancet* 1992; 340:1252–1254.

158. Schmid R: Transmission of hepatitis B by a finger-stick device (letter). *N Engl J Med* 1992; 370:476–477.

159. Roth D, et al: Detection of hepatitis C virus infection among cadaver organ donors: Evidence of low transmission of disease. *Ann Intern Med* 1992; 117:470–475.

160. Morales JM, Andres A, Campistol JM: Hepatitis C virus and organ transplantation (letter). *N Engl J Med* 1993; 328:511–512.

161. Pereira BJG, et al: Prevalence of hepatitis C virus RNA in organ donors positive for hepatitis C antibody and in the recipients of their organs. *N Engl J Med* 1992; 327:910–915.

162. Pereira BJG, et al: Low risk of liver disease after tissue transplantation from donors with HCV (letter). *Lancet* 1993; 341:903–904.

163. Levinson WM, et al: Hepatitis C virus seroprevalence in the developmentally disabled. *Arch Intern Med* 1992; 152:2309–2311.

164. Chaudhary RK, et al: Hepatitis B and C infection in an institution for the developmentally handicapped (letter). *N Engl J Med* 1992; 327:1953.

165. Pueschel SM, et al: The prevalence of hepatitis B surface antigen and antibody in home-reared individuals with Down syndrome. *Res Dev Disabil* 1991; 12:243–249.

166. Kallinowski B, et al: Prevalence of antibodies to hepatitis C virus in hemodialysis patients. *Nephron* 1991; 59:236–238.

167. Vanderschueren S, et al: Hepatitis C among risk groups for HIV and hepatitis B. *Int J Stud AIDS* 1991; 2:185–187.

168. San Miguel G, et al: Hepatitis C virus antibodies in patients on hemodialysis (letter). *Infect Cont Hospi Epidemiol* 1992; 13:254–256.

169. Elisaf M, et al: Antibodies against hepatitis C virus (anti-HCV) in hemodialysis patients: Association with hepatitis B serological markers. *Nephrol Dial Transplant* 1991; 6:476–479.

170. Alivanis P, et al: Hepatitis C virus antibodies in hemodialysed and in renal transplant patients: Correlation with chronic liver disease. *Transplant Proc* 1991; 23:2662–2663.

171. Mondelli MU, et al: Abnormal alanine aminotransferase activity reflects exposure to hepatitis C virus in haemodialysis patients. *Nephrol Dial Transplant* 1991; 6:480–483.

172. Sheu J-C, et al: Prevalence of anti-HCV and HCV viremia in hemodialysis patients in Taiwan. *J Med Virol* 1992; 37:108–112.

173. Lin H-H, et al: Prevalence of antibodies to hepatitis C virus in the hemodialysis unit. *Am J Nephrol* 1991; 11:192–194.

174. Machida A, et al: High incidence of hepatitis C virus antibodies in hemodialysis patients (letter). *Nephron* 1992; 60:117–118.

175. Tamura I, et al: Prevalence of four blood-borne viruses (HBV, HCV, HTLV-1, HIV-1) among haemodialysis patients in Japan. *J Med Virol* 1992; 36:271–273.

176. Sakamoto N, et al: Prevalence of hepatitis C virus infection among long-term hemodialysis patients. *J Med Virol* 1993; 39:11–15.

177. Fujiyama S, et al: Prevalence of hepatitis C virus antibodies in hemodialysis patients and dialysis staff. *Hepatogastroenterology* 1992; 39:161–165.

178. Chana TM, et al: Prevalence of hepatitis C virus infection in hemodialysis patients: A longitudinal study comparing the results of RNA and antibody assays. *Hepatology* 1993; 17:5–8.

179. Alfurayh O, et al: Hepatitis C virus infection in chronic haemodialysis patients, a clinicopathologic study. *Nephrol Dial Transplant* 1992; 7:327–332.

180. Hay NM, Lynn KL, Schousboe MI: The prevalence of antibody to hepatitis C virus in a dialysis population. *N Z Med J* 1992; 105:134.

181. Oliveras A, et al: Hepatitis C virus in renal transplantation. *Transplant Proc* 1991; 23:2636–2637.

182. Ponz E, et al: Hepatitis C virus infection among kidney transplant recipients. *Kidney Int* 1991; 40:748–751.

183. Klauser R, et al: Hepatitis C antibody in renal transplant patients. *Transplant Proc* 1992; 24:286–288.

184. Fabrizi F, et al: Hepatitis C virus infection in kidney graft recipients (letter). *Nephrol Dial Transplant* 1992; 7:274.

185. Chan TM, Lok ASF, Cheng IKP: Hepatitis C in renal transplant recipients. *Transplantation* 1991; 52:810–813.

186. Chan T-M, et al: A prospective study of hepatitis C virus infection among renal transplant recipients. *Gastroenterology* 1993; 104:862–868.

187. Anonymous: Surgeons who are hepatitis B carriers (letter). *BMJ* 1992; 303:184–185.

188. Prentice MB, et al: Infection with hepatitis B virus after open heart surgery. *BMJ* 1992; 304:761–764.

189. Centers for Disease Control: Recommendations for preventing transmission of human immunodeficiency virus and hepatitis B virus to patients during exposure-prone invasive procedures. *MMWR* 1991; 40(suppl RR-8):1–9.

190. Gibas A, et al: Prevalence and incidence of viral hepatitis in health workers in the prehepatitis B vaccination era. *Am J Epidemiol* 1992; 136:603–610.

191. Kelen GD, et al: Hepatitis B and hepatitis C in emergency department patients. *N Engl J Med* 1992; 326:1399–1404.

192. Tsude K, et al: Two cases of accidental transmission of hepatitis C to medical staff. *Hepatogastroenterology* 1992; 39:73–75.

193. Marranconi F, et al: HCV infection after accidental needlestick injury in health-care workers (letter). *Infection* 1992; 20:111.

194. Mitsu T, et al: Hepatitis C virus infection in medical personnel after needlestick accident. *Hepatology* 1992; 16:1109–1114.

195. Robson SC, et al: Hospital outbreak of hepatitis E (letter). *Lancet* 1992; 339:1424–1425.

196. Glikson M, et al: Relapsing hepatitis A. *Medicine (Baltimore)* 1992; 71:14–23.

197. Jilbert AR, et al: Rapid resolution of duck hepatitis B virus infection occurs after massive hepatocellular involvement. *J Virol* 1992; 66:1377–1388.

198. Cote PJ, et al: Immunosuppression with cyclosporine during the incubation period of experimental woodchuck hepatitis virus infection increases the frequency of chronic infection in adult woodchucks. *J Infect Dis* 1992; 166:628–631.

199. Laskus T, et al: Course and outcome of acute type B hepatitis in heavy alcohol abusers. *Digestion* 1991; 49:231–234.

200. Prince AM, et al: Immunity in hepatitis C infection. *J Infect Dis* 1992; 165:438–443.

201. Koretz RL, et al: Non-A, non-B posttransfusion hepatitis: Comparing C and non-C hepatitis. *Hepatology* 1993; 17:361–365.

202. Mattsson L, Grillner L, Weiland O: Seroconversion to hepatitis C virus antibodies in patients with acute posttransfusion non-A, non-B hepatitis in Sweden with a second generation test. *Scand J Infect Dis* 1992; 24:15–20.

203. Dasarathy S, et al: Prospective controlled study of post-transfusion hepatitis after cardiac surgery in a large referral hospital in India. *Liver* 1992; 12:116–120.

204. Galama JMD, et al: Relapsing hepatitis due to cytomegalovirus? *J Infect* 1991; 23: 175–178.

205. Deshpande DV, et al: Anti-tubercular treatment in patients with hepatitis. *J Assoc Physicians India* 1991; 39:599–601.

206. Korman SH: Thrombocytopenic purpura during the incubation of hepatitis B. *Acta Paediatr Scand* 1991; 80:975–976.

207. Hibbs JR, Issaragrisil S, Young NS: High prevalence of hepatitis C viremia among aplastic anemia patients and controls from Thailand. *Am J Trop Med Hyg* 1992; 46:564–570.

208. Hibbs JR, et al: Aplastic anemia and viral hepatitis. *JAMA* 1992; 267:2051–2054.

209. Dollberg S, Berkun Y, Gross-Kieselstein E. Urticaria in patients with hepatitis A virus infection (letter). *Pediatr Infect Dis J* 1991; 10:702–703.

210. Kanzaki T, Tsuda J: Bile pigment deposition at sweat pores of patients with liver disease. *J Am Acad Dermatol* 1992; 26:655–656.

211. Davis TV, Keeffe EB: Acute pancreatitis associated with acute hepatitis A. *Am J Gastroenterol* 1992; 87:1648–1650.

212. Ichihara S, Sato M, Kozuka S: Prevalence of pancreatitis in liver diseases of various etiologies: An analysis of 107,754 adult autopsies in Japan. *Digestion* 1992; 51:86–94.

213. Foulner D: Sonographic gallbladder wall thickening in children: Association with acute hepatitis A. *Australas Radiol* 1991; 35:333–335.

214. Sharma MP, Dasarathy S: Gallbladder abnormalities in acute viral hepatitis: A prospective ultrasound evaluation. *J Clin Gastroenterol* 1991; 13:697–700.

215. Black MM, Mann NP: Gangrenous cholecystitis due to hepatitis A infection. *J Trop Med Hyg* 1992; 95:73–74.

216. Geltner D, et al: Acute oliguric renal failure complicating type A nonfulminant viral hepatitis. *J Clin Gastroenterol* 1992; 14:160–162.

217. Sawada T, et al: Development of rheumatoid arthritis after hepatitis C virus infection (letter). *Arthritis Rheum* 1991; 34:1620–1621.

218. Ruel M, et al: Fibrin ring granulomas in hepatitis A. *Dig Dis Sci* 1992; 37:1915–1917.

219. Yotsumoto S, et al: Fulminant hepatitis related to transmission of hepatitis B variants with precore mutation between spouses. *Hepatology* 1992; 16:31–35.

220. Lichtenstein DR, Makadon HJ, Chopra S: Fulminant hepatitis B and delta virus coinfection in AIDS. *Am J Gastroenterol* 1992; 87:1643–1647.

221. Wright TL, et al: Hepatitis B virus and apparent fulminant non-A, non-B hepatitis. *Lancet* 1992; 339:952–955.

222. Sallie R, et al: Occult HBV in NANB fulminant hepatitis (letter). *Lancet* 1993; 341:123.

223. Feray C, et al: Hepatitis C virus RNA and hepatitis B virus DNA in serum and liver of patients with fulminant hepatitis. *Gastroenterology* 1993; 104:549–555.

224. Liang TJ, et al: Fulminant or subfulminant non-A, non-B viral hepatitis: The role of hepatitis C and E viruses. *Gastroenterology* 1993; 104:556–562.

225. Yanagi M, et al: Hepatitis C virus in fulminant hepatic failure (letter). *N Engl J Med* 1991; 324:1895–1896.

226. Kanamori H, et al: Case report: Fulminant hepatitis C viral infection after allogeneic bone marrow transplantation. *Am J Med Sci* 1992; 303:109–111.

227. Gunasekaran TS, et al: Hodgkin's disease presenting with fulminant liver disease. *J Pediatr Gastroenterol Nutr* 1992; 15:189–193.

228. Sallie R, et al: Failure of simple biochemical indexes to reliably differentiate fulminant Wilson's disease from other causes of fulminant liver failure. *Hepatology* 1992; 16:1206–1211.

229. Salmeron JM, et al: Selective intestinal decontamination in the prevention of bacterial infection in patients with acute liver failure. *J Hepatol* 1992; 14:280–285.

230. Rolando N, et al: Prospective controlled trial of selective parenteral and enteral antimicrobial regimens in fulminant liver failure. *Hepatology* 1993; 17:196–201.

231. Lidofsky SD, et al: Intracranial pressure monitoring and liver transplantatoin for fulminant hepatic failure. *Hepatology* 1992; 16:1–7.

232. Sheiner P, et al A randomized control trial of prostaglandin E$_2$ (PGE$_2$) in the treatment of fulminant hepatic failure (FHF) (abstract). *Hepatology* 1992; 16:88.

233. Fox IJ, et al: Successful application of extracorporeal liver perfusion for the treatment of fulminant hepatic failure: A technology whose time has come (abstract). *Hepatology* 1992; 16:88.

234. Sussman NL, et al: Reversal of fulminant hepatic failure using an extracorporeal liver assist device. *Hepatology* 1992; 16:60–65.

235. Rozga J, et al: Development of a bioartificial liver: Properties and function of a hollow-fiber module inoculated with liver cells. *Hepatology* 1993; 17:258–265.

236. Lee KK, et al: Transfusion-acquired hepatitis A outbreak from fresh frozen plasma in a neonatal intensive care unit. *Pediatr Infect Dis* 1992; 11:122–123.

237. Gerritzen A, et al: Acute hepatitis A in haemophiliacs (letter). *Lancet* 1992; 340:1231–1232.

238. Normann A, et al: Detection of hepatitis A virus RNA in commercially available factor VIII preparation (letter). *Lancet* 1992; 340:1232–1233.

239. Robinson SM, Schwinn H, Smith A: Clotting factors and hepatitis A (letter). *Lancet* 1992; 340:1465.

240. Temperley IJ, et al: Clotting factors and hepatitis A (letter). *Lancet* 1992; 340:1466.

241. Peerlinck K, Vermylen J: Acute hepatitis A in patients with haemophilia (letter). *Lancet* 1993; 341:179.

242. Kreuz W, et al: Absence of hepatitis A after treatment with pasteurized factor VIII concentrates in children with haemophilia A and von Willebrand disease (letter). *Lancet* 1993; 341:446.

243. Evensen SA, Rollag H: Solvent/detergent-treated clotting factors and hepatitis A virus seroconversion (letter). *Lancet* 1993; 341:971–972.

244. Nowicki MJ, et al: Passive antibody to hepatitis A virus in US haemophiliacs (letter). *Lancet* 1993; 341:562.

245. Baginski I, et al: Transmission of serologically silent hepatitis B virus along with hepatitis C virus in two cases of posttransfusion hepatitis. *Transfusion* 1992; 32:215–220.

246. Wang JT, et al: Posttransfusion hepatitis revisited by hepatitis C antibody assays and polymerase chain reaction. *Gastroenterology* 1992; 103:609–616.

247. Takano S, et al: Posttransfusion hepatitis in Japan. *Vox Sang* 1992; 62:156–164.

248. Meraviglia P, et al: Post transfusion hepatitis: Comparison between homologous and autologous blood transfusion. *Eur J Med* 1992; 1:75–79.

249. Donahue JG, et al: The declining risk of post-transfusion hepatitis C virus infection. *N Engl J Med* 1992; 327:369–373.

250. Mathiesen UL, et al: Anti-hepatitis C virus screening will reduce the incidence of post-transfusion hepatitis C also in low-risk areas. *Scand J Gastroenterol* 1992; 27:443–448.

251. Yei S, Yu MW, Tankersley DL: Partitioning of hepatitis C virus during Cohn-Oncley fractionation of plasma. *Transfusion* 1992; 32:824–828.

252. Blanchette VS, et al: Hepatitis C infection in children with hemophilia A and B. *Blood* 1991; 78:285–289.

253. Watson HG, et al: Use of several second generation serological assays to determine the true prevalence of hepatitis C virus infection in haemophiliacs treated with non–virus inactivated factor XIII and IX concentrates. *Br J Haemotol* 1992; 80:514–518.

254. Schulman S, et al: Transmission of hepatitis C with pasteurized factor VIII (letter). *Lancet* 1992; 340:305–306.

255. Pollman H, Jurgens H: Transmission of hepatitis in haemophiliacs (letter). *Lancet* 1992; 340:793.

256. Allain J-P, et al: Evidence for persistent hepatitis C virus (HCV) infection in hemophiliacs. *J Clin Invest* 1991; 88:1672–1679.

257. Al-Khaja N, et al: Gamma globulin prophylaxis to reduce post-transfusion non-A, non-B hepatitis after cardiac surgery with cardiopulmonary bypass. *Scand J Thorac Cardiovasc Surg* 1991; 25:7–12.

258. Behrens RH, Doherty JF: Severe hepatitis A despite passive immunisation (letter). *Lancet* 1993; 341:972.

259. Infectious Diseases and Immunization Committee, Canadian Paediatric Society: Hepatitis B in Canada: The case for universal vaccination. *Can Med Assoc J* 1992; 146:25–28.

260. Anonymous: Universal vaccination against hepatitis B. *Can Med Assoc J* 1992; 146:36.

261. Immunization Practices Advisory Committee: Hepatitis B virus: A comprehensive strategy for eliminating transmission in the United States through universal childhood vaccination. *MMWR* 1991; 40(suppl RR-13):1–25.

262. Committee on Infectious Diseases: Universal hepatitis B immunization. *Pediatrics* 1992; 89:795–800.

263. Da Villa G, et al: A pilot model of vaccination against hepatitis B virus suitable for mass vaccination campaigns in hyperendemic areas. *J Med Virol* 1992; 36:274–278.

264. Krahn MD, Detsky AS: Universal hepatitis B vaccination: The economics of prevention. *Can Med Assoc J* 1992; 146:19–21.

265. Demicheli V, Jefferson TO: Cost-benefit analysis of the introduction of mass vaccination against hepatitis B in Italy. *J Public Health Med* 1992; 14:367–375.

266. Hatziandreu EJ, et al: Cost-effectiveness of hepatitis-B vaccine in Greece. *Int J Technol Assess Health Care* 1991; 7:256–262.

267. Mauskopf JA, Bradley CJ, French MT: Benefit-cost analysis of hepatitis B vaccine programs for occupationally exposed workers. *J Occup Med* 1991; 33:691–698.

268. Bloom BS, et al: A reappraisal of hepatitis B virus vaccination strategies using cost-effectiveness analysis. *Ann Intern Med* 1993; 118:298–306.

269. Jonsson B, et al: Cost-benefit analysis of hepatitis-B vaccination. *Int J Technol Assess Health Care* 1991; 7:379–402.

270. Anonymous: Some concern over instituting hepatitis B vaccine into babies' routine vaccination schedules. *Infect Control Hosp Epidemiol* 1991; 12:745–746.

271. Stevens CE, et al: Prospects for control of hepatitis B virus infection: Implications of childhood vaccination and long-term protection. *Pediatrics* 1992; 90(suppl):170–173.

272. Oon CJ, Goh KT, Lim GK: Clearance of neonatal anti-HBs following hepatitis B vaccination: Relationship to anti-HBs level. *Ann Acad Med* 1991; 20:231–235.

273. Mahoney FJ, et al: Effect of a hepatitis B vaccination program on the prevalence of hepatitis B virus infection. *J Infect Dis* 1993; 167:203–207.

274. Chotard J, et al: The Gambia hepatitis intervention study: Follow-up of a cohort of children vaccinated against hepatitis B. *J Infect Dis* 1992; 166:764–768.

275. Farber JM: Hepatitis B immunization (letter). *Pediatrics* 1992; 89:981–982.

276. Hall CB: Hepatitis B immunization (reply). *Pediatrics* 1992; 89:982.

277. Coursaget P, et al: Comparative immunogenicity in children of mammalian cell–derived recombinant hepatitis B vaccine and plasma-derived hepatitis B vaccine. *Vaccine* 1992; 10:379–382.

278. Soyletir G, et al: Clinical evaluation of low dose intradermally administered hepatitis B vaccine: A comparison of plasma-derived and recombinant yeast–derived vaccines. *Vaccine* 1992; 10:301–304.

279. Chan C-Y, et al: Booster response to recombinant yeast–derived hepatitis B vaccine in vaccines whose anti-HBs responses were initially elicited by a plasma-derived vaccine. *Vaccine* 1991; 9:765–767.

280. Hammond GW, et al: Comparison of immunogenicity of two yeast-derived recombinant hepatitis B vaccines. *Vaccine* 1991; 9:97–100.

281. Goh KT, et al: Comparison of the immune response of four different dosages of a yeast-recombinant hepatitis B vaccine in Singapore children: A four-year follow-up study. *Bull World Health Org* 1992; 233:239.

282. Tsega E, et al: Immunogenicity reactogenicity and comparison of two doses of recombinant DNA yeast–derived hepatitis B vaccine in Ethiopian children. *Trop Geogr Med* 1991; 43:220–227.

283. Lee C-Y, et al: The protective efficacy of recombinant hepatitis B vaccine in newborn infants of hepatitis B e antigen–positive–hepatitis B surface antigen carrier mothers. *Pediatr Infect Dis J* 1991; 10:299–303.

284. Bouter KP, et al: Humoral immune response to a yeast-derived hepatitis B vaccine in patients with type 1 diabetes mellitus. *Diabetes Med* 1992; 9:66–69.

285. Zuin G, et al: Impaired response to hepatitis B vaccine in HIV infected children. *Vaccine* 1992; 10:857–860.

286. Guan R, et al: Hepatitis B vaccination in chronic renal failure patients undergoing haemodialysis: The immunogenicity of an increased dose of a recombinant DNA hepatitis B vaccine. *Ann Acad Med* 1990; 19:793–797.

287. Struve J, et al: Intramuscular versus intradermal administration of a recombinant hepatitis B vaccine: A comparison of response rates and analysis of factors influencing the antibody response. *Scand J Infect Dis* 1992; 24:423–429.

288. Hayashi J, et al: Cost effectiveness of intradermal vs. subcutaneous hepatitis B vaccination for the mentally handicapped. *J Infect* 1991; 23:39–45.

289. Coleman PJ, et al: Intradermal hepatitis B vaccination in a large hospital employee population. *Vaccine* 1991; 9:723–727.

290. Anonymous: Inadequate immune response among public safety workers receiving intradermal vaccination against hepatitis B—United States, 1990–1991. *MMWR* 1991; 40:569–572.

291. Kruskall MS, et al: The immune response to hepatitis B vaccine in humans: Inheritance patterns in families. *J Exp Med* 1992; 175:495–502.

292. Rose RM, et al: Failure of recombinant interleukin-2 to augment the primary humoral response to a recombinant hepatitis B vaccine in healthy adults (letter). *J Infect Dis* 1992; 165:775–777.

293. Coursaget P, et al: Simultaneous injection of hepatitis B and measles vaccines. *Trans R Soc Trop Med Hyg* 1991; 85:788.

294. Coursaget P, et al: Simultaneous injection of hepatitis B vaccine with BCG and killed poliovirus vaccine. *Vaccine* 1992; 10:319–321.

295. Giammanco G, et al: Immune response to simultaneous administration of a recombinant DNA hepatitis B vaccine and multiple compulsory vaccines in infancy. *Vaccine* 1991; 9:747–750.

296. Wakeel RA, White MI: Erythema multiforme associated with hepatitis B vaccine (letter). *Br J Dermatol* 1992; 126:94–95.

297. Hudson TJ, et al: Adverse reaction to the recombinant hepatitis B vaccine. *J Allergy Clin Immunol* 1991; 88:821–822.

298. Carmeli Y, Oren R: Hepatitis B vaccine side effect (letter). *Lancet* 1993; 341:250–251.

299. Lee DA, Eby WC, Molinaro GA: HIV false positivity after hepatitis B vaccine (letter). *Lancet* 1992; 339:1060.

300. Anonymous: Alleged link between hepatitis B vaccine and chronic fatigue syndrome. *Can Med Assoc J* 1992: 146:37–38.

301. House A: Alleged link between hepatitis B vaccine and chronic fatigue syndrome (letter). *Can Med Assoc J* 1992; 146:1145.

302. Krause DS: Hepatitis B in the emergency department (letter). *N Engl J Med* 1992; 327:1032.

303. Boscia JA: Surgery, AIDS, and hepatitis B (letter). *JAMA* 1991; 266:1361–1362.

304. Andre FE, et al: Clinical assessment of the safety and efficacy of an inactivated hepatitis A vaccine; rationale and summary findings. *Vaccine* 1992; 10(suppl 1):160–168.

305. Kallinowski B, et al: Immunogenicity, reactogenicity and consistency of a new, inactivated hepatitis A vaccine—a randomized multicentre study with three consecutive vaccine lots. *Vaccine* 1992; 10:500–501.

306. Tilzey AJ, et al: Clinical trial with inactivated hepatitis A vaccine and recommendations for its use. *BMJ* 1992; 304:1272–1276.

307. Lee S-D, et al: Immunogenicity of inactivated hepatitis A vaccine in children. *Gastroenterology* 1993; 104:1129–1132.

308. Ellerbeck EF, et al: Safety profile and immunogenicity of an inactivated vaccine derived from an attenuated strain of hepatitis A. *Vaccine* 1992; 10:668–672.

309. Nalin D, et al: Inactivated hepatitis A vaccine in childhood: Implications for disease control. *Vaccine* 1993; 11(suppl 1):15–17.

310. Innis BL, et al: Field efficacy trial of inactivated hepatitis A vaccine among children in Thailand (an extended abstract). *Vaccine* 1992; 10(suppl 1):159.

311. Riedemann S, et al: Placebo-controlled efficacy study of hepatitis A vaccine in Valdivia, Chile. *Vaccine* 1992; 10(suppl 1):152–155.

312. Werzberger A, et al: A controlled trial of a formalin-inactivated hepatitis A vaccine in healthy children. *N Engl J Med* 1992; 327:453–457.

313. Anonymous: Hepatitis A vaccines considered for licensing. *JAMA* 1992; 267:2007–2008.

314. Anonymous: Hepatitis A: A vaccine at last (editorial). *Lancet* 1992; 339:1198–1199.

315. Ambrosch F, et al: Simultaneous vaccination against hepatitis A and B: Results of a controlled study. *Vaccine* 1992; 10(suppl 1):142–145.

316. Jilg W: Adult use of hepatitis A vaccine in developed countries. *Vaccine* 1993; 11(suppl 1):6–8.

317. Margolis HS, Shapiro CN: Who should receive hepatitis A vaccine? Considerations for the development of an immunization strategy. *Vaccine* 1992; 10(suppl 1):85–87.

318. Tormans G, Van Damme P, Van Doorslaer E: Cost-effective analysis of hepatitis A prevention in travellers. *Vaccine* 1992; 10(suppl 1):88–92.

319. Omata M, et al: Resolution of acute hepatitis C after therapy with natural beta interferon. *Lancet* 1991; 338:914–915.

320. Viladomiu L, et al: Interferon-α in acute posttransfusion hepatitis C: A randomized, controlled trial. *Hepatology* 1992; 15:767–769.

321. Lampertico P, et al: A randomized multicenter controlled trial of recombinant interferon alpha 2b in patients with acute posttransfusion non-A, non-B hepatitis (PTH) (abstract). *Gastroenterology* 1992; 102:838.

CHAPTER 2

Chronic Hepatitis: The Long Silents

Ronald L. Koretz, M.D.

Associate Chief, Division of Gastroenterology, Olive View Medical Center, Sylmar, California; Professor of Medicine, University of California, Los Angeles, California

If acute hepatitis took two reels, chronic hepatitis (CH) will need more. As we wander through some full-length soundless movies, we will stop the projector to consider a number of topics; many of them will be extensions of old thoughts.[1-13] This year our lens will focus on liver-kidney microsomal antibody (anti-LKM), viral genetic mutations, the natural history of chronic hepatitis C (CHC), the relationship of cryoglobulin to the hepatitis C virus (HCV), and the ever-popular interferon (IF). So, if your popcorn is popped and your soda poured (without any noise, of course), let's begin. Silents, please.

ETIOLOGIC CONSIDERATIONS

Several well-characterized variants of autoimmune chronic active hepatitis (aCAH) are separable by different autoantibodies. In particular, anti-LKM identifies a disease that classically affects children and adolescents.[9-11] Anti-LKM is directed at a specific isoenzyme of the cytochrome P-450 family.[10-12] Do such patients have an abnormal gene that creates a structurally different cytochrome P-450? When the DNA of ten such patients was isolated, no remarkable differences from the normal cytochrome P-450 gene were demonstrated.[14]

A number of histocompatibility leukocyte antigen (HLA) associations have been linked to aCAH,[1, 7–9, 13] most recently HLA-DR4.[13, 15] A Japanese group investigated the frequencies of different genotypes of various suballeles of the DR4 gene to look for differences between patients with and without aCAH.[16] Although some differences were found, they were discounted because the association was less strong than for DR4 in general. Perhaps these genotype findings were also disregarded because this same group did not find them in an earlier published work.[16] (The disparate results in the two papers seem mostly related to different frequencies in the control groups.)

Lon Chaney was the *Man With a Thousand Faces*. Are there that many cytokines released in response to disease? Serum levels of various ones, including interleukins, are elevated in chronic hepatitis B (CHB).[10, 11, 13, 17, 18] This may be a nonspecific epiphenomenon since the levels are also elevated in other chronic hepatitides.[18]

Several investigators examined lymphocyte subpopulations in the livers of patients with CHC.[19–23] Hata et al. extracted lymphocytes from hepatic tissue and found that there were almost twice as many suppressor cells as helper cells.[19] The lobular inflammation was mostly composed of suppressor cells.[20–22] The portal tract had a higher proportion of helper cells,[21–23] especially in the follicles.[23] The pathophysiologic meaning of this is unclear, but it is refreshing to have agreement in the findings. Similar lobular findings have been described in CHB, although the portal tract data have not always agreed.[7]

Hepatitis B core antigen (HBcAg) may be an important target for the host immune system.[10] One chronic hepatitis B surface antigen (HBsAg) and hepatitis B e antigen (HBeAg) carrier did not have antibody to HBcAg (anti-HBc).[24] His serum was positive for hepatitis B virus (HBV) DNA that had no core or precore mutations. His serum alanine aminotransferase (ALT) concentration was normal, and his lymphocytes did not proliferate in vitro in response to HBcAg. The authors speculated that the patient had a selective immunologic defect preventing both HBcAg recognition and subsequent hepatitis.

Since patients with porphyria cutanea tarda usually had evidence of HCV infection, it was hypothesized that the chronic liver disease seen in this metabolic disorder is actually due to a virus.[25] In another metabolic condition, nonalcoholic steatohepatitis in diabetics, HCV was not implicated.[26]

Alstrom disease is a rare syndrome characterized by retinal degeneration, obesity, diabetes, sensorineural deafness, acanthosis nigricans, and in males, hypogenitalism. One such patient, an 11-year-old girl, had mildy abnormal aminotransferase levels, jaundice, and pruritus for 3 years.[27] Tests for hepatitis B, Wilson's disease, α-fetoprotein (AFP), and aCAH (antinuclear antibody [ANA] and smooth muscle antibody [SMA] only) were negative or normal. A liver biopsy revealed mild chronic active hepatitis (CAH), and she responded to immunosuppressive therapy. Was this part of the underlying syndrome, or did she have aCAH (perhaps the anti-LKM variant)?

DIAGNOSTIC CONSIDERATIONS

Positivity for anti-LKM and antibody to HCV (anti-HCV) are sometimes found in the same patient, usually an adult.[13] When anti-LKM–positive patients with anti-HCV are compared with those without anti-HCV, the former patients are older, more likely to be male, and have lower ALT values.[13, 28–30] They are more likely to have HCV-associated RNA (HCV-RNA)[29] and to respond to IF.[13] They are less likely to respond to immunosuppressives.[28] These patients probably have CHC with false positive anti-LKMs.

More specific antigen targets may differentiate patients with anti-LKM that is due to aCAH from that seen in CHC. Recently proposed tests are antibodies to an antigen from the cytochrome P-450 system[29] and to one from rat liver cytosol.[30]

It is claimed that anti-GOR, an antibody associated with CHC, is actually directed at a host-derived antigen. If true, this might explain how patients could have both autoimmune (anti-LKM) and HCV markers. Hosein et al. identified an HCV protein with significant amino acid homology with GOR, so the antigen may actually arise from the virus.[31]

Czaja et al. could not find anti-LKM in adult patients with aCAH (ANA and/or SMA positive), cryptogenic CAH, or viral CAH.[32] This observation reinforces our perspective that anti-LKM–positive aCAH is predominantly a disease of children.[8, 9, 12]

The Iron Horse was a John Ford western; *The Iron Mask* was Douglas Fairbanks' last silent swashbuckler. The iron liver could be confused with chronic viral hepatitis because the serum ferritin level is often, and the transferrin saturation sometimes, nonspecifically elevated in patients with CHB or CHC.[33] Coexistent hemochromatosis, defined by hepatic iron content, is usually absent, and the abnormal iron parameters are probably due to the release of iron and ferritin when hepatocytes are destroyed.

Are ultrasonographic and AFP screening useful for detecting early hepatocellular carcinoma (HCC)?[12] Italian and French groups were unimpressed that such diagnostic interventions were of any use when performed at least every 6 to 12 months.[34, 35]

Douglas Fairbanks' *Mark of Zorro* set the standard for tapping tense ascites. His sword fights were less successful attempts at liver biopsies.

Different investigators compared the histology of CHC with other forms of CH. Chronic hepatitis C was more likely to be associated with lymphoid follicles and fat than CHB[36, 37]; CHC may also have more prominent lobular but less severe portal tract inflammation[36] as well as bile duct damage and acidophilic bodies.[37] When aCAH was compared with CHC, the necroinflammatory response was more prominent and multinucleated giant hepatocytes were more commonly observed in the former[38]; however, it was unclear whether the two groups of patients were clinically comparable (i.e., had similar ALT abnormalities and/or clinical symptoms).

Freni et al. correlated the presence or absence of anti-HCV with histology in patients with presumed alcoholic liver disease.[39] Eleven patients who only had findings attributable to alcohol (fat, hepatocyte ballooning, megamitochondria, hyaline degeneration, and perivenular fibrosis) were anti-HCV negative, whereas the 16 who also had features of viral CAH (portal and/or periportal infiltrates, piecemeal and/or lobular necrosis) were anti-HCV positive. Although two other groups[40, 41] did not get such an absolute separation, the data from these three studies[39–41] substantiated previous reports[13] that anti-HCV–positive alcoholics are more likely to have histologic evidence of both alcoholic and viral disease.

The time may have come to discard the terms "chronic active" and "chronic persistent."[13, 42] Although these phrases were originally only intended to describe histologic findings, clinicians have adopted them as diseases and given them therapeutic relevance. From a clinical perspective, CH is better divided on an etiologic basis.

How safe are outpatient liver biopsies? At the Mayo Clinic, only 3% of patients undergoing such procedures even had to be hospitalized.[43] Only two (0.5%) required blood transfusions, and none had any more invasive therapy. Although only low-risk patients were offered the outpatient option, this appears to be a safe procedure in them.

In *The Magician*, Alice Tury is hypnotized by a madman who needs her heart for experimentation. In an eerily reminiscent report, Adams and Stenn hypnotized two patients in order to do liver biopsies.[44] One of the patients had severe anxiety, and the other was allergic to local anesthetics.

COURSE AND PROGNOSIS

In *Ben Hur*, 200,000 feet of film were exposed for the chariot race, but only 750 (<0.4%) appeared in the final film. Chronic hepatitis, especially if due to a viral cause, is present for years or decades, but we will read about it in a few minutes (<0.001%).

Hepatitis B (With or Without Delta)

Chronic HBsAg carriers who have normal ALT values generally have no or mild hepatitis.[2–4, 6, 8, 9] They also have good long-term prognoses, especially if the enzyme levels remain normal.[45]

In *The Big Parade*, John Gilbert loses his leg in a battle, a bad outcome. In the battle with CHB, losing HBsAg is presumably a better consequence. However, Mason et al. found HBV-DNA in the peripheral blood mononuclear cells of patients who had HBsAg clearance up to 4 years earlier following IF therapy.[46] Kuhns and her coworkers described patients who had HBV-DNA in their livers after HBsAg and HBV-DNA were no longer serologically demonstrable.[47] Since three of the four coworkers' names appeared on the paper by Mason et al., I wonder whether some of these patients weren't the same.

Adachi et al. followed seven patients with CHB after they cleared HBsAg (antibody to HBsAg [anti-HBs] even developing in six of them).[48] In at least five, HBV-DNA persisted in the serum. Of more concern, the progression of the liver disease may have continued; HCC developed in three of them 3 to 9 years later. The appearance of HCC years after HBsAg seroconversion has been described before.[11]

Acute hepatitis C developed in one patient with CHB, and then HBsAg spontaneously cleared.[49] Patients who had cleared HBsAg were anti-HCV positive more often than those who had not.[50] Unfortunately, among the group who lost HBsAg, those who were anti-HCV positive were more likely to have an abnormal ALT concentration; did they substitute one chronic viral infection for another? In Italy, patients with CHB who were also anti-HCV positive were more likely to have ongoing inflammation.[51] Although patients with CHB who are also infected by HCV may have reduced replication of HBV,[13] I am not sure that they are any better off.

In *Sunset Boulevard,* Gloria Swanson played a silent film star attempting a comeback. One of her famous lines was "We had faces then." Things change at all levels, even at the genetic one. Consider mutations in the core/precore region of the HBV genome.

Precore mutants contain a stop codon mutation in the precore region of the genome, and HBeAg is no longer synthesized. Such viruses continue to replicate even though their human hosts are positive for antibody to HBeAg (anti-HBe); they are said to be associated with more severe CH, although the evidence for this is circumstantial.[13] Indeed, in Israel carriers of precore mutants had a variety of histologic findings ranging from normal to CAH with cirrhosis.[52]

Carman et al. presented data purporting to show that patients infected with mutants had more severe disease.[53] Although an association may have existed, many exceptions occurred. Patients who were anti-HBe positive with abnormal ALT values had the wild-type, not mutant, virus. Some patients with the mutant infection had normal ALT levels.

If HBcAg is the target of the host immune response, the virus could protect itself by mutating the core region of the gene. Core mutations were found in patients with more severe histologic disease, although the correlation was not perfect.[54–56] Unfortunately such data do not allow us to distinguish between mutations that cause disease (the speculation) and disease that causes the mutations.

The Lodger was Alfred Hitchcock's first suspense film. It also describes what the delta virus does in an HBV-infected liver.

Hadler et al. prospectively identified 35 Yucpa Indian HBV carriers who became superinfected with delta.[57] Six of them died of fulminant hepatic failure (FHF) (5 in one family), and at least 13 others appeared to have an acceleration of their liver disease; 5 of those 13 died of hepatic insufficiency within 3 years. These authors also compared a population of concomitant HBV and delta carriers with a group only infected with hepatitis B and stated that the former individuals were more likely to have abnormal biochemical, clinical, and histologic findings. However, the wording of the paper makes it difficult to be sure that the two populations were comparable at baseline.

Delta superinfections of HBV carriers were clinically indistinguishable in anti-HCV–positive and anti-HCV–negative patients.[58] Hepatic delta antigen was less likely to be demonstrable in the anti-HCV–positive group, however.

Lee et al. obtained sera from individual delta carriers during three consecutive clinical flare-ups and looked for delta RNA mutations.[59] The calculated mutation rate of 0.003 substitutions per nucleotide per year was comparable to other RNA viruses. More severe flare-ups were associated with mutations. Although the flare-up could have been due to some mutational (and subsequent immunologic) change in the virus, flare-ups of disease may have produced the mutations; some of the mutations observed in the second isolate were not demonstrable in the third. It was also disconcerting that different clones from the same isolate had different nucleic acid sequences. Is this due to the presence of different genomic "strains" or to a problem with the assay?

Serials did exist in the silent film era. One French film maker released episodes irregularly, one at a time. Hepatitis viral reactivations also occur at unpredictable intervals.

One HBsAg chronic carrier received a bone marrow transplant from his sister, who was anti-HBc/anti-HBs positive.[60] Ten months later he had an icteric exacerbation, after which he cleared HBsAg and became anti-HBs positive. Was this a graft vs. host's virus reaction, and did the graft win?

Ackerman et al. observed 19 HBsAg/delta-positive carriers who had "reactivations" (defined by biochemical criteria).[61] Eleven were ascribed to delta (increase in delta virus RNA in the serum) and 3 to HBV (increased HBV-DNA). The remaining 5 were not attributable to delta, HBV, or HCV.

Hepatitis C

Gold Rush was a 1925 movie with Charlie Chaplin. Unlike the similarly colored mineral, jaundice (or any other evidence of liver failure) appears to be in no hurry to appear in patients with CHC.

Serial liver biopsies were obtained in 57 (out of 333) Japanese patients with CHC.[62] Over the years, histologic progression was seen in 35, which led the authors to conclude that "many patients with CHC show progression of their disease after a long and symptomless course." We do not know why these particular 57 had serial biopsies; although 35 of 57 (61%) is "many," 35 of 333 (11%) is a far less impressive number. Furthermore, there was no indication that any had clinical deterioration. Since these patients all had chronic disease when first seen, I concluded that CHC takes a very long time to become a clinical problem.

A long-term (approximately 8 years) follow-up of patients with community-acquired non-A, non-B (NANB) CH showed that most of them had HCV infection.[63] The focus of the paper was on the serologic outcomes; there was no mention of any overt liver disease. If this did not occur (rather than just not being mentioned), I would make the same conclusion again.

Seeff and many coauthors (including me) sought transfused patients in whom NANB hepatitis (posttransfusion hepatitis [PTH]) had or had not developed in the 1970s to see what happened to them 20 years later.[64] The overall mortality curves of the two groups were superimposable, although there were a few more hepatic deaths in the group with hepatitis.

This has been our experience at UCLA.[65] Fifteen years after contracting NANB PTH (mostly hepatitis C), the probability of survivors manifesting any evidence of liver failure was approximately 0.20.[65] During that time, the patients were twice as likely to die of some non–liver-related cause.

Chronic hepatitis C must take years and probably decades to become a clinically important problem in most patients. Before then, many of them (especially those who are transfused for other underlying conditions) will die of nonhepatic illnesses. As I have noted before,[11-13] we still need data from at least one long-term prospective randomized controlled trial (PRCT) showing that intervention prevents mortality or morbidity from end-stage liver disease.

Hepatitis B virus carriers with normal ALT values have good prognoses. What about such HCV carriers?

These people are identified because they are anti-HCV positive; many of them may not be infected with HCV (false positive anti-HCV assays). In one Italian study,[66] liver biopsies from nine anti-HCV/HCV-RNA–positive individuals demonstrated CH or cirrhosis in all, whereas those from seven anti-HCV–positive, HCV-RNA–negative people were all normal.

Positivity for HCV-RNA is not always such a good predictor. Another Italian group took biopsy samples from 19 patients with anti-HCV/HCV-RNA positivity and normal ALT values[67]; CH was found in 9, "slight changes" in 2, and normal histology in 8. However, these patients all had antibody to the human immunodeficiency virus (anti-HIV).

Four other Italian patients who also were anti-HCV/HCV-RNA positive with "persistently normal" ALT values had normal histology.[68] There was no indication that any of them was anti-HIV positive.

The early cowboy stars were real cowboys who came to Hollywood when their ranch jobs disappeared. After HCV infects the liver, does it move elsewhere? Hepatitis C virus–associated RNA has been found in peripheral blood mononuclear cells.[69]

Patients with NANB CH underwent biopsies, and the specimens from patients with HCV markers were compared with those from patients without.[70] The non-C patients were less likely to have CAH. They also had somewhat lower serum γ-globulin levels. However, some of the non-C patients may actually have had nonviral disease such as drug-induced hepatotoxicity.

Chronic Viral Hepatitis With Something Else

Eric von Stroheim had a cameo appearance in *Birth of a Nation* as a man falling off a roof. Do coexistent viral infections have more of a role to play in schistosomiasis?

Egyptian patients who had acute hepatitis B (defined by the presence of immunoglobulin M–specific anti-HBc) were evaluated for concomitant schistosomiasis.[71] The patients with both infections were more likely to have splenomegaly and to be identified as chronic carriers 1 year later. Among patients with schistosomiasis, those who were also anti-HCV positive were more likely to have ascites.[72] An association between hepatosplenic schistosomiasis and viral CH is slowly emerging,[7] although its pathophysiologic significance remains unclear.

Louise Brooks' private life was allegedly as sexually varied and indiscriminant as the roles she played. Fortunately for her, she lived before the acquired immunodeficiency syndrome (AIDS) became a problem.

Twu and colleagues have prospectively followed almost 5,000 homosexual males since the mid 1980s.[73] Those who had initial evidence of past or present HBV infection were more likely to become anti-HIV positive. Given the long observation period, this was probably not due to a lead-time bias (i.e., early seroconversions in latently infected). Furthermore, a risk persisted after the data were corrected for sexual behavior. Since association does not infer causation, it would be incorrect to presume that an HBV exposure caused HIV infection. Other unrecognized risk factors may have been operative that led first to HBV exposure and then to HIV infection.

In a French liver unit, anti-HIV/HBsAg–positive patients were more likely to die than were HBsAg-positive patients who were anti-HIV negative (5/25, 20% vs. 6/121, 5%; $P < .05$).[74] The cause of death in 4 of the 5 anti-HIV–positive patients was liver failure, whereas only 2 of the other 6 died of this. The investigators concluded that the HIV accelerated progression of the CHB. However, the other 4 deaths in the anti-HIV–negative group were due to HCC. Also, one must remember that the patients were not drawn from a random population of HBsAg/anti-HIV–positive individuals; rather, they were all being followed in a liver clinic where hepatic deaths are common. Among HIV-infected patients, overall survival was the same regardless of whether or not they were also HBsAg positive.[75]

Anti-HIV–positive patients coinfected with HBV may[9, 12, 13, 76] or may not[10, 13] have more evidence of viral replication. Even if they do, it may not be due to the HIV infection per se. Since HBV-DNA levels did not increase with time as cellular immunity declined, one could speculate that the phenomenon is due to more recent infections.[76]

COMPLICATIONS

One never knows how events shape history. Because Rin Tin Tin attacked movie crews, one director threatened to shoot the dog. Had this happened, Warners might have gone bankrupt before developing sound movies and the Great Depression would have further retarded this technology. It is also hard to predict what extrahepatic phenomena will occur in patients with CH.

Thirteen investigators tested 28 patients with polyarteritis nodosa for evidence of HBV infection.[77] Most were positive for HBsAg, 12 by standard assays and 9 others by a monoclonal antibody assay; this led to the conclusion that there was a "much higher rate of HBV infection in patients with polyarteritis nodosa than previously recognized." My concerns and those of the accompanying editorial[78] related to the specificity of the experimental assay. Hepatitis C could not be implicated in this disease.[79–81]

From 1913 to 1919, Mary Pickford may have been the most famous woman in the world. More recently, cryoglobulinemia appears to be the most popular (as measured by the number of papers) complication of HCV infections. Table 1 summarizes data from seven different groups regarding the incidence of anti-HCV or HCV-RNA positivity in patients with cryoglobulinemia.[82–88] Hepatitis C virus markers

TABLE 1.

Hepatitis C Markers in Cryoglobulinemia

Reference	Hepatitis C Marker (Assay)*	Number (%) Positive for Marker in	
		Serum	Cryoprecipitate
82	Anti-HCV (EIA-1)	5/15 (33%)†	
	HCV-RNA (PCR)	13/15 (87%)†	
83	Anti-HCV (EIA-1)	19/51 (37%)	21/51 (41%)
	(EIA-2)	50/51 (98%)	
	HCV-RNA (PCR)	13/16 (81%)	
84	Anti-HCV (EIA-1)	129/161 (80%)	
85	Anti-HCV (EIA-2)	38/42 (90%)	
	HCV-RNA (PCR)	36/42 (86%)	
86	Anti-HCV (EIA-1)	7/14 (50%)	
87	Anti-HCV (EIA-2)	13/26 (50%)	
88	Anti-HCV (EIA-2)	5/13 (38%)	
	HCV-RNA (PCR)	9/13 (69%)	

*Anti-HCV = antibody to hepatitis C virus; EIA-1/-2 = first/second-generation enzyme-linked immunoassay; HCV-RNA (PCR) = hepatitis C virus ribonucleic acid detected by polymerase chain reaction.
†Four patients with Waldenström's macroglobulinemia were excluded.

are commonly found in serum[82-89] and cryoprecipitate.[83, 90] Cryoglobulin may even disappear after IF therapy,[89, 91, 92] although one patient had the vasculitis worsen after treatment.[93]

It should be appreciated that cryoglobulinemia may be secondary to CHC.[12, 94] In such cases, it is difficult to label the disease "essential." At least some of the patients in most of the previously discussed works[83, 85-87, 89-93] did have CH.

Dr. Clodoveo Ferri and his many associates have produced a number of additions to this field. In 1991 they wrote a letter to the editor describing the observation of anti-HCV (first-generation assay) in the sera of patients with cryoglobulinemia[95] and then a five-page *Brief Report* in which a few more patients were added.[96] Another paper employed a second-generation anti-HCV assay,[97] as did the *Rapid Paper* used in Table 1.[85] When the 1991 work of Ferri et al. was reviewed in *Gastroenterology* in 1992, they were able to write a response and add some more patients to the total.[98]

Although each study did provide new data, I wonder how often any group needs to publish their findings. On average, more than seven authors wrote each of the cryoglobulin papers.[82-98] What is publication pressure doing to the sizes of libraries and the world's population of trees[12]?

Perhaps inappropriately, HBV was implicated in rheumatoid arthritis.[11] The high rate of anti-HCV positivity in this disease was probably due to a false positive assay,[99] as was a previously noted association[13] between HCV and Sjögren's syndrome.[100, 101]

Hashimoto's thyroiditis developed in two patients with CHC.[102] This is of note because thyroid disease has been a reported complication of IF treatment[11, 13] (see below).

Controversy exists regarding a possible association between lichen planus and CAH.[5-8] This skin condition developed in a man 9 years after having CHC diagnosed.[103] The seven authors of this one-page letter were not sure whether this was a coincidence or not. In a teenage girl anti-LKM–positive aCAH and lichen planus developed at about the same time.[104]

In *Sparrows*, Mary Pickford and a group of unwanted children were abused by the owner of a foster home. Chronic hepatitis B was kinder to Italian children; their nutritional status was normal.[105, 106]

Patients with aCAH have a variety of extrahepatic problems. When 105 such patients underwent "routine" sigmoidoscopy, 17 (16%) of them had ulcerative colitis[107]; most were symptomatic. In an infant with aCAH and an autoimmune hemolytic anemia, an interstitial pneumonitis developed several years after the baby was given immunosuppressive therapy[108]; we have previously noted an adult with aCAH, hemolytic anemia, and fibrosing alveolitis.[8] Were the lung problems part of the disease or a complication of the treatment? Mixed connective tissue disease has also been associated with aCAH,[7] as has thyroiditis[1]; one unfortunate woman got all three.[109]

In general, there is no early adverse effect from providing renal transplants to HBsAg-positive patients, although liver failure may develop years later.[7, 8, 10-13]

Recipients who are HBeAg and/or HBV-DNA positive at the time of transplantation may be at particular risk of having a subsequent fatal liver disease.[110]

Hepatocellular carcinoma has been considered to be a chronic sequela of either HBV or HCV infection.[1, 2, 8-13] Two studies sought HBV-DNA and HCV-RNA in the malignant and nonmalignant portions of the livers of patients with HCC who did not have circulating HBsAg (Table 2)[111, 112]: HBV-DNA was demonstrable in both the HCC and the nonmalignant tissue of patients with past HBV exposure, as well as in at least a few who had no serologic evidence of such an event; HCV-RNA was also found, but almost always only in those who were seropositive for anti-HCV.

TREATMENT CONSIDERATIONS

He Who Gets Slapped is one of the few surviving films that Swedish director Victor Sjostrom made in America. If "he" had chronic viral hepatitis today, instead of a slap, he would "get stuck" (IF injection).

One of the therapeutic end points for IF in CHB is the seroconversion of HBeAg to anti-HBe. Since these patients usually remain HBsAg positive, one might be concerned that precore mutants are evolving. Two groups sequenced portions of the HBV-DNA isolated from five responders.[113, 114] Precore mutations were found, including silent point changes, point changes causing substitutions, and start/stop codons as well as frameshift alterations.

TABLE 2.

Presence of Viral Genomes in Hepatic Tissues of Hepatitis B Surface Antigen–Negative Patients With Hepatocellular Carcinoma

	Reference 111			Reference 112		
Virus Sought*	Viral Antibody Status†	Tissue	Frequency Positive DNA/RNA	Viral Antibody Status†	Tissue	Frequency of Positive DNA/RNA
HBV	+	HCC*	2/3 (67%)	+	HCC	7/29 (24%)‡
	+	Non-HCC	2/3 (67%)	+	Non-HCC	7/29 (24%)‡
	−	HCC	3/5 (60%)§	−	HCC	0/2 (0%)
	−	Non-HCC	2/5 (40%)§	−	Non-HCC	0/2 (0%)
HCV	+	HCC	4/4 (100%)	+	HCC	12/21 (57%)‡
	+	Non-HCC	4/4 (100%)	+	Non-HCC	16/21 (76%)‡
	−	HCC	0/5 (0%)	−	HCC	1/10 (10%)
	−	Non-HCC	0/5 (0%)	−	Non-HCC	1/10 (10%)

*HBV = hepatitis B virus; HCV = hepatitis C virus; HCC = hepatocellular carcinoma.
†For HBV, +/− = with/without antibody to HBsAg or hepatitis B core antigen; for HCV, +/− = with/without antibody to HCV.
‡Not necessarily the same patients who were positive in the HCC and non-HCC groups.
§One specimen not available.

Hepatitis Be antigen– and/or HBV-DNA–positive HBsAg carriers are not considered to be good candidates for liver transplantation. Could these patients, who have manifestations of liver failure (from cirrhosis), be treated in order to achieve a "nonreplicative status"? Two groups provided IF, albeit often with lower than standard doses, to 19 patients.[115, 116] Six patients died within 6 months of treatment, some perhaps from IF-induced disease flare-ups. Most of the patients had relatively severe complications from the IF or a disease flare-up. A sustained loss of HBV-DNA was achieved in only 8 patients; they have apparently done well (without transplantation, in fact). The authors of both papers felt that such treatment was useful; I was more impressed by the associated morbidity and mortality. I also wondered whether such HBeAg-or HBV-DNA–negative patients have the same posttransplant prognosis as those whose replicative markers disappear as part of the natural history of their CHB.

Glycyrrhizin followed by human lymphoblastoid IF was given to 17 patients with CHB.[117] Ten ultimately lost HBeAg; only 3 seroconverted to anti-HBe. The authors stated that the glycyrrhizin (a licorice extract) may be an effective immuno-modulator. Although I have never been opposed to selling licorice in a movie theater, I will need more convincing data before recommending its sale to patients with CHB.

Several PRCTs have looked at aspects of IF therapy for CHB. Patients with and without abnormal ALT values were randomized to receive or not receive pretreatment with prednisone.[118] Steroid priming had no effect in patients with normal enzymes. In those with biochemical abnormalities, there may have been a small arithmetic trend for a better "partial response" (loss of replicative markers) in the prednisone recipients, 43% vs. 33%. However, the study design allowed some patients initially assigned to the untreated control group to cross over into a treatment group after 1 year. (Any patients destined to seroconvert in the second year would be added to the treatment arm of the study.) Given the overall small differences, there is still[12] no compelling reason to advocate corticosteroid "priming."

Patients with presumed precore mutant–related CHB (anti-HBe/HBV-DNA positive) were randomized to treatment with IF or control.[119, 120] In one trial[119] nothing appeared to change. In the other,[120] IF treatment was associated with more sustained loss of HBV-DNA and normalization of ALT.

Can the effect of IF be enhanced if one were to *(Tom) Mix* it with other agents? No real success has been seen in uncontrolled trials.[11] The outcome was no better when levamisole,[121] zidovudine (AZT),[122] or acyclovir[123] were tested in PRCTs.

What is new about IF for CHC? Several reports addressed aspects of the relationship between HCV-RNA and response (ALT normalization). Two groups observed a correlation, albeit not all or none, between low initial titers of RNA and response[124, 125]; a third group could not demonstrate this.[126] Among responders, the failure to lose, or the recurrence of, HCV-RNA usually identified patients whose biochemical disease relapsed.[126, 127] Hepatitis C viruses with different RNA genotypes may have different susceptibilities to IF.[128–130]

A small PRCT of IF was conducted in hemophiliacs with CHC.[131] ALT responses occurred in four of ten (one subsequent relapse) treated patients, but in none of the eight controls. These results are similar to what occurs in nonhemophiliacs[11–13]; this study has added one patient to each group since its publication as an abstract.[12]

The role of prednisolone priming in CHC was assessed.[132] There was no apparent effect of this therapy on the response rate. Although the authors concluded that the recipients of the steroids may have had fewer relapses, most of the patients either dropped out or were not followed for very long.

We still do not know whether IF will prevent end-stage liver disease or HCC. The established "benefit" is limited to changes in serologic or biochemical tests. Since the progression to symptomatic cirrhosis takes many years or even decades, it is unclear what we are really accomplishing. On the other hand, IF has side effects. Thyroid disease will develop in a small percentage of treated patients,[113] perhaps because of the development of thyrotropin receptor antibodies.[134] Thrombocytopenia may occur because of bone marrow suppression[135] or even from an IF-induced autoimmune thrombocytopenic purpura.[135, 136] A German group suggested that IF caused an exacerbation of preexistent lichen planus.[137] Hypertriglyceridemia developed in a diabetic patient on two occasions when IF was administered.[138]

Ben Hur was Metro-Goldwyn-Mayer's largest-grossing silent film, but it did not make a profit because of its expenses. Interferon will gross a great deal of money from its sales; I would like to feel more comfortable that patients will profit from its use.

Had King Vidor's *The Crowd* been produced this year, it could have included a number of other therapeutic agents that have been proposed. Two drugs used primarily to treat AIDS have again been tried in patients with viral CH. Dideoxyinosine did not benefit anti-HIV–negative[139] or anti-HIV–positive[140] patients with CHB. Eight of nine anti-HIV–positive patients with CHC who were given AZT had improved biochemical and histologic outcomes,[141] but AZT has not been useful in CHB.[11, 13]

Several years ago we read about an uncontrolled trial of an immunostimulant, *Propionibacterium granulosum* cell wall extracts.[7] A 5-year follow-up is now available.[142] Ten of the 14 patients with CHB became HBsAg negative, and the ALT concentration was normal in all of them. Another immunostimulant, AM3 (a macrophage enhancer), was given to 13 patients with CHB; 1 year later eight had lost HBV-DNA and seroconverted their HBeAg to anti-HBe.[143]

An extract of *Phyllanthus* reportedly successfully treated woodchucks and humans.[10] In a double-blind prospective randomized crossover trial in the Netherlands, this extract had no effect,[144] which confirmed observations that were subsequently made by the original and other investigators.[123] Another herb, shosaikoto, supposedly lowered abnormal ALT levels in patients with CAH[12]; it did not have any effect on HBeAg seroconversion rates.[145]

Ursodeoxycholic acid has reduced the levels of abnormal enzymes in a number of chronic liver diseases, including primary biliary cirrhosis,[11] primary sclerosing cholangitis,[11] and CH[11-13] (aCAH in particular[13]). In a PRCT of patients with mostly (at least 25 of the 26 participants) chronic viral hepatitis, it again improved serum enzyme values.[146] However, when use of the drug was stopped, the original abnormalities returned. Is improving a blood test result of any importance? If so, would we need to use this drug lifelong? Do you think that anyone will ever do that study?

MORE TRAILERS

As technology advanced, the silent film era ceased to exist. Ideally, as our research efforts similarly move forward, many of our current frustrations will also resolve.

Unfortunately, most of the long-term goals we have set in past years are still there. Some confusion still exists as to whether overlap between autoimmune and viral CH really exists or whether we have only been confused by our tests. We do not know whether genetic mutations in HBV and HCV are really important. Since the course of chronic viral hepatitis is so long, it would be nice to be able to differentiate the patients who are likely to get into trouble from their liver disease. Finally, as we enter an era of medical cost constraint, we need to be sure that our current therapies are effective in a clinically meaningful way and to find out whether there are still other modes of treatment out there.

REFERENCES

1. Koretz RL: Acute and chronic hepatitis, in Gitnick GL (ed): *Current Gastroenterology and Hepatology*. Boston, Houghton Mifflin Co, 1979, pp 243–275.

2. Koretz RL: Hepatitis: Problems and promises, in Gitnick GL (ed): *Current Hepatology*, vol 1. Boston, Houghton Mifflin Co, 1980, pp 1–39.

3. Koretz RL: Hepatitis: Retrospecti et prospecti, in Gitnick GL (ed): *Current Hepatology*, vol 2. New York, John Wiley & Sons, 1982, pp 1–54.

4. Koretz RL: Hepatitis: Same time, same station, in Gitnick GL (ed): *Current Hepatology*, vol 3. New York, John Wiley & Sons, 1983, pp 1–47.

5. Koretz RL: Hepatitis: Acute and chronic and Arthur Conan, in Gitnick GL (ed): *Current Hepatology*, vol 4. New York, John Wiley & Sons, 1984, pp 1–42.

6. Koretz RL: Hepatitis: Art and Science, in Gitnick GL (ed): *Current Hepatology*, vol 5. St Louis, Mosby–Year Book, 1985, pp 1–47.

7. Koretz RL: Hepatitis: Serious papers, funny papers, in Gitnick GL (ed): *Current Hepatology*, vol 6. St. Louis, Mosby–Year Book, 1986, pp 1–63.

8. Koretz RL: Hepatitis: Words and music, in Gitnick GL (ed): *Current Hepatology*, vol 8. St Louis, Mosby–Year Book, 1988, pp 1–50.

9. Koretz RL: Hepatitis: Another fine mess, in Gitnick GL (ed): *Current Hepatology*, vol 9. St Louis, Mosby–Year Book, 1989, pp 1–54.

10. Koretz RL: Hepatitis: Facts and fables, in Gitnick GL (ed): *Current Hepatology*, vol 10. St Louis, Mosby–Year Book, 1990, pp 1–54.

11. Koretz RL: Hepatitis: Old pictures, new papers, in Gitnick GL (ed): *Current Hepatology*, vol 11. St Louis, Mosby–Year Book, 1991, pp 1–60.

12. Koretz RL: Chronic hepatitis: Science and superstition, in Gitnick GL (ed): *Current Hepatology*, vol 12. St Louis, Mosby–Year Book, 1992, pp 53–74.

13. Koretz RL: Chronic hepatitis: The novel, in Gitnick GL (ed): *Current Hepatology*, vol 13. St Louis, Mosby–Year Book, 1993, pp 43–67.

14. Yamamoto AM, et al: Study of CYP 2D6 gene in children with autoimmune hepatitis and P450 IID6 autoantibodies. *Clin Exp Immunol* 1992; 87:251–255.

15. Ota M, et al: A possible association between basic amino acids of position 13 of DRB1 chains and autoimmune hepatitis. *Immunogenetics* 1992; 36:49–55.

16. Seki T, et al: HLA class II molecules and autoimmune hepatitis susceptibility in Japanese patients. *Gastroenterology* 1992; 103:1041–1047.

17. Kakamu S, et al: Serum interleukin 6 levels in patients with chronic hepatitis B. *Am J Gastroenterol* 1991; 86:1804–1808.

18. Tilg H, et al: Serum levels of cytokine in chronic liver diseases. *Gastroenterology* 1992; 103:264–274.

19. Hata K, et al: Phenotypic and functional characteristics of lymphocytes isolated from liver biopsy specimens from patients with active liver disease. *Hepatology* 1992; 15:816–823.

20. Onji M, et al: Intrahepatic lymphocyte subpopulations and HLA class I antigen expression by hepatocytes in chronic hepatitis C. *Hepatogastroenterology* 1992; 39:340–343.

21. Wejstal R, et al: Lymphocyte subsets and β_2-microglobulin expression in chronic hepatitis C/non-A, non-B. Effects of interferon-alpha treatment. *Clin Exp Immunol* 1992; 87:340–345.

22. Mosnier J-F, et al: The intraportal lymphoid nodule and its environment in chronic active hepatitis C: An immunohistochemical study. *Hepatology* 1993; 17:366–371.

23. Hino K, et al: Analysis of lymphoid follicles in liver of patients with chronic hepatitis C. *Liver* 1992; 12:387–391.

24. Lee J-H, et al: Chronic hepatitis B virus infection in an anti-HBc–nonreactive blood donor: Variant virus or defective immune response? *Hepatology* 1992; 16:24–30.

25. Fargion S, et al: Hepatitis C virus and porphyria cutanea tarda: Evidence of a strong association. *Hepatology* 1992; 16:1322–1326.

26. Rogers DW, et al: Hepatitis C virus does not cause nonalcoholic steatohepatitis. *Dig Dis Sci* 1992; 37:1644–1647.

27. Connolly MB, et al: Hepatic dysfunction in Alstrom disease. *Am J Med Genet* 1991; 40:421–424.

28. Lunel F, et al: Liver/kidney microsome antibody type 1 and hepatitis C virus infection. *Hepatology* 1992; 16:630–636.

29. Ma Y, et al: Case against subclassification of type II autoimmune chronic active hepatitis (letter). *Lancet* 1993; 341:60.

30. Abuaf N, et al: Characterization of the liver cytosol antigen type 1 reacting with autoantibodies in chronic active hepatitis. *Hepatology* 1992; 16:892–898.

31. Hosein B, Fang X, Wang CY: Anti-HCV, anti-GOR, and autoimmunity (letter). *Lancet* 1992; 339:871.

32. Czaja AJ, Manns M, Homburger HA: Frequency and significance of antibodies to liver/kidney microsome type 1 in adults with chronic active hepatitis. *Gastroenterology* 1992; 130:1290–1295.

33. DiBisceglie AM, et al: Measurements of iron status in patients with chronic hepatitis. *Gastroenterology* 1992; 102:2108–2113.

34. Colombo M, et al: Hepatocellular carcinoma in Italian parents with cirrhosis. *N Engl J Med* 1991; 325:675–680.

35. Durand F, et al: Hepatocellular carcinoma (letter). *N Engl J Med* 1993; 328:64.

36. Scheuer PJ, et al: The pathology of hepatitis C. *Hepatology* 1992; 15:567–571.

37. Lefkowitch JH, et al: Pathological diagnosis of chronic hepatitis C: A multicenter comparative study with chronic hepatitis B. *Gastroenterology* 1993; 104:595–603.

38. Bach N, Thung SN, Schaffner F: The histological features of chronic hepatitis C and autoimmune chronic hepatitis: A comparative analysis. *Hepatology* 1992; 15:572–577.

39. Freni MA, et al: HCV infection, hepatic HLA display and composition of the mononuclear cell inflammatory infiltrate in chronic alcoholic liver disease. *Eur J Clin Invest* 1991; 21: 586–591.

40. Nalpas B, et al: Hepatitis C viremia and anti-HCV antibodies in alcoholics. *J Hepatol* 1992; 14:381–384.

41. Halimi C, et al: Pathogenesis of liver cirrhosis in alcoholic patients: Histological evidence for hepatitis C virus responsibility. *Liver* 1991; 11:329–333.

42. Zetterman RK: Chronic hepatitis: Is it persistent, active, or just chronic (editorial)? *Am J Gastroenterol* 1993; 88:1–2.

43. Jones CH, Lindor KD: Outcome of patients hospitalized for complications after outpatient liver biopsy. *Ann Intern Med* 1993; 118:96–98.

44. Adams PC, Stenn PG: Liver biopsy under hypnosis. *J Clin Gastroenterol* 1992; 15:122–124.

45. De Franchis R, et al: The natural history of asymptomatic hepatitis B surface antigen carriers. *Ann Intern Med* 1993; 118:191–194.

46. Mason A, et al: Hepatitis B virus DNA in peripheral-blood mononuclear cells in chronic hepatitis B after HBsAg clearance. *Hepatology* 1992; 16:36–41.

47. Kuhns M, et al: Serum and liver hepatitis B virus DNA in chronic hepatitis B after sustained loss of surface antigen. *Gastroenterology* 1992; 103:1649–1656.

48. Adachi H, et al: Clearance of HBsAg in seven patients with chronic hepatitis B. *Hepatology* 1992; 16:1334–1337.

49. Liaw YF, et al: Acute hepatitis C virus seroconversion followed by spontaneous HBeAg seroconversion and HBsAg elimination. *Infection* 1991; 19:250–251.

50. Sheen I-S, et al: Role of hepatitis C virus infection in spontaneous hepatitis B surface antigen clearance during chronic hepatitis B virus infection. *J Infect Dis* 1992; 165:831–834.

51. Fiore G, et al: Hepatitis C virus infection in anti-HBe–positive HBsAg carriers with chronic liver diseases. *Digestion* 1991; 50:121–126.

52. Tur-Kaspa R, Klein A, Aharonson S: Hepatitis B virus precore mutants are identical in carriers from various ethnic origins and are associated with a range of liver disease severity. *Hepatology* 1992; 16:1338–1342.

53. Carman WF, et al: Precore sequence variation in Chinese isolates of hepatitis B virus. *J Infect Dis* 1992; 165:127–133.

54. Ehata T, et al: Variations in codons 84-101 in the core nucleotide sequence correlate with hepatocellular injury in chronic hepatitis B infection. *J Clin Invest* 1992; 89:332–338.

55. Chuang W-L, et al: Precore mutations and core clustering mutations in chronic hepatitis B virus infection. *Gastroenterology* 1993; 104:263–271.

56. Wakita T, et al: Detection of pre-C and core region mutants of hepatitis B virus in chronic hepatitis B virus carriers. *J Clin Invest* 1991; 88:1793–1801.

57. Hadler SC, et al: Epidemiology and long-term consequences of hepatitis delta virus infection in the Yucpa Indians of Venezuela. *Am J Epidemiol* 1992; 136:1507–1516.

58. Liaw Y-F, et al: Concurrent hepatitis C virus and hepatitis delta virus superinfection in patients with chronic hepatitis B virus infection. *J Med Virol* 1992; 37:294–297.

59. Lee C-M, et al: Evolution of hepatitis delta virus RNA during chronic infection. *Virology* 1992; 188:265–273.

60. Lok ASF, Kiang RHS, Chung H: Recovery from hepatitis B (letter). *Ann Intern Med* 1992; 116:957.

61. Ackerman Z, et al: Spontaneous exacerbation of disease activity in patients with chronic delta hepatitis infection: The role of hepatitis B, C, or D? *Hepatology* 1992; 16:625–629.

62. Takahashi M, et al: Natural course of chronic hepatitis C. *Am J Gastroenterol* 1993; 88:240–243.

63. Alter MJ, et al: The natural history of community-acquired hepatitis C in the United States. *N Engl J Med* 1992; 327:1899–1905.

64. Seeff L, et al: Long-term mortality after transfusion-associated non-A, non-B hepatitis. *N Engl J Med* 1992; 327:1906–1911.

65. Koretz RL, Abbey H, Gitnick G: Non-A, non-B (NANB) post-transfusion hepatitis (PTH)—the second decade (abstract). *Hepatology* 1992; 16:69.

66. Alberti A, et al: Hepatitis C viraemia and liver disease in symptom-free individuals with anti-HCV. *Lancet* 1992; 340:697–698.

67. Vento S, et al: Hepatitis C viraemia with normal liver histology in symptomless HIV-1 infection (letter). *Lancet* 1992; 340:1161.

68. Brillanti S, et al: Persistent hepatitis C viraemia without liver disease. *Lancet* 1993; 341:464–465.

69. Wang J-T, et al: Detection of replicative form of hepatitis C virus RNA in peripheral blood mononuclear cells. *J Infect Dis* 1992; 166:1167–1169.

70. Chemello L, et al: Patterns of antibodies to hepatitis C virus in patients with chronic non-A, non-B hepatitis and their relationship to viral replication and liver disease. *Hepatology* 1993; 17:179–182.

71. Ghaffar YA, et al: The impact of endemic schistosomiasis in acute viral hepatitis. *Am J Trop Med Hyg* 1991; 45:743–750.

72. Bassily S, et al: Hepatitis C virus infection and hepatosplenic schistosomiasis (letter). *Scand J Infect Dis* 1992; 24:687–688.

73. Twu SJ, et al: Relationship of hepatitis B virus infection to human immunodeficiency virus type 1 infection. *J Infect Dis* 1993; 167:299–304.

74. Hausset C, et al: Interactions between human immunodeficiency virus-1, hepatitis delta virus and hepatitis B virus infections in 260 chronic carriers of hepatitis B virus. *Hepatology* 1992; 15:578–583.

75. Scharschmidt BF, et al: Hepatitis B in patients with HIV infection: Relationship to AIDS and patient survival. *Ann Intern Med* 1992; 117:837–838.

76. Koblin BA: Effect of duration of hepatitis B virus infection on the association between human immunodeficiency virus type-1 and hepatitis B viral replication. *Hepatology* 1992; 15:590–592.

77. Marcellin P, et al: Latent hepatitis B virus (HBV) infection in systemic necrotizing vasculitis. *Clin Exp Rheumatol* 1991; 9:23–28.

78. Christian CL: Hepatitis B virus (HBV) and systemic vasculitis (editorial). *Clin Exp Rheumatol* 1991; 9:1–2.

79. Quint L, et al: Hepatitis-C virus in patients with polyarteritis nodosa. Prevalence in 38 patients. *Clin Exp Rheumatol* 1991; 9:253–257.

80. Bonacorsi S, Quint L: Association between hepatitis C virus and polyarteritis nodosa (letter). *Clin Exp rheumatol* 1992; 10:319–324.

81. Cacoub P, Lunel-Fabiani F, Du LTH: Polyarteritis nodosa and hepatitis C virus infection (letter). *Ann Intern Med* 1992; 116:605.

82. Agnello V, Chung RT, Kaplan LM: A role for hepatitis C virus infection in type II cryoglobulinemia. *N Engl J Med* 1992; 327:1490–1495.

83. Misiani R, et al: Hepatitis C virus infection in patients with essential mixed cryoglobulinemia. *Ann Intern Med* 1992; 117:573–577.

84. Galli M, et al: Hepatitis C virus and mixed cryoglobulinaemias (letter). *Lancet* 1992; 339:989.

85. Ferri C, et al: Association between hepatitis C virus and mixed cryoglobulinemia. *Clin Exp Rheumatol* 1991; 9:621–624.

86. Bambara LM, et al: Cryoglobulinemia and hepatitis C virus (HCV) infection (letter). *Clin Exp Rheumatol* 1991; 9:96–97.

87. Dammacco F, Sansonno D: Antibodies to hepatitis C virus in essential mixed cryoglobulinaemia. *Clin Exp Immunol* 1992; 87:352–356.

88. Werner C, Joller-Jemelka HI, Fontana A: Hepatitis C virus and cryoglobulinemia (letter). *N Engl J Med* 1993; 328:1122–1123.

89. De Bandt M, et al: Type II IgM monoclonal cryoglobulinemia and hepatitis C virus infection (letter). *Clin Exp Rheumatol* 1991; 9:659–660.

90. Marcellin P, et al: Cryoglobulinemia with vasculitis associated with hepatitis C virus infection. *Gastroenterology* 1993; 104:272:277.

91. Taillan B, et al: Type II cryoglobulinaemia associated with hepatitis C virus infection (letter). *Clin Exp Rheumatol* 1992; 10:320.

92. Johnson RJ, et al: Membranoproliferative glomerulonephritis associated with hepatitis C virus infection. *N Engl J Med* 1993; 328:465–470.

93. Zimmerman R, et al: Interferon alfa in leucocytoclastic vasculitis, mixed cryoglobulinaemia, and chronic hepatitis C (letter). *Lancet* 1993; 341:561–562.

94. Cocoub P, et al: Hepatitis C virus and cryoglobulinemia (letter). *N Engl J Med* 1993; 328:1121–1122.

95. Ferri C, et al: Hepatitis C virus antibodies in mixed cryoglobulinemia (letter). *Clin Exp Rheumatol* 1991; 9:95–96.

96. Ferri C, et al: Hepatitis C virus antibodies in mixed cryoglobulinemia. *Arthritis Rheum* 1991; 34:1606–1610.

97. Ferri C, et al: Antibodies against hepatitis C virus in mixed cryoglobulinemia patients. *Infection* 1991; 19:417–420.

98. Ferri C, et al: Hepatitis C virus and cryoglobulinemia: Unthawing the association (response). *Gastroenterology* 1992; 103:1110.

99. Borque L, et al: Rheumatoid arthritis and hepatitis C virus antibodies. *Clin Exp Rheumatol* 1991; 9:617–619.

100. Marson P, et al: Anti-hepatitis C virus serology in primary Sjögren's syndrome: No evidence of cross-reactivity between rheumatoid factor and specific viral proteins (letter). *Clin Exp Rheumatol* 1991; 9:661–662.

101. Aceti A, et al: HCV and Sjögren's syndrome (letter). *Lancet* 1992; 339:1425–1426.

102. Tran A, et al: Hepatitis C virus and Hashimoto's thyroiditis. *Eur J Med* 1992; 1:116–118.

103. Mokni M, et al: Lichen planus and hepatitis C (letter). *J Am Acad Dermatol* 1991; 24:792.

104. Cottoni F, et al: Lichen planus associated with anti–liver-kidney microsome–positive chronic active hepatitis and hyperthyroidism (letter). *Arch Dermatol* 1991; 127:1730–1731.

105. Vegnente A, et al: Nutritional status and growth in children with chronic hepatitis B. *J Pediatr Gastroenterol Nutr* 1992; 14:123–127.

106. Polito C, et al: Normal growth of children with HBsAg positive chronic active hepatitis (CAH). *Acta Paediatr Scand* 1991; 80:1231–1232.

107. Perdigoto R, Carpenter HA, Czaja AJ: Frequency and significance of chronic ulcerative colitis in severe corticosteroid-treated autoimmune hepatitis. *J Hepatol* 1992; 14:325–331.

108. Kayser K, et al: Alteration of the lung parenchyma associated with autoimmune hepatitis. *Virchows Arch [A]* 1991; 419:153–157.

109. Tomsic M, et al: Mixed connective tissue disease associated with autoimmune hepatitis and thyroiditis. *Ann Rheum Dis* 1992; 51:544–546.

110. Fairley CK, et al: The increased risk of fatal liver disease in renal transplant patients who are hepatitis Be antigen and/or HBV DNA positive. *Transplantation* 1991; 52:497–500.

111. Paterlini P, et al: Persistence of hepatitis B and hepatitis C viral genomes in primary liver cancers from HBsAg-negative patients: A study of a low-endemic area. *Hepatology* 1993; 17:20–29.

112. Sheu J-C, et al: Hepatitis C and B viruses in hepatitis B surface antigen–negative hepatocellular carcinoma. *Gastroenterology* 1992; 103:1322–1327.

113. Xu J, et al: Absence of hepatitis B virus precore mutants in patients with chronic hepatitis B responding to interferon-α. *Hepatology* 1992; 15:1002–1006.

114. Gunther S, et al: Frequent and rapid emergence of mutated pre-C sequences in HBV from e-antigen positive carriers who seroconvert to anti-HBe during interferon treatment. *Virology* 1992; 187:271–279.

115. Nevens F, et al: Treatment of decompensated viral hepatitis B–induced cirrhosis with low doses of interferon alpha. *Liver* 1993; 13:15–19.

116. Hoffnagle JH, et al: Interferon alfa for patients with clinically apparent cirrhosis due to chronic hepatitis B. *Gastroenterology* 1993; 104:1116–1121.

117. Hayashi J, et al: Glycyrrhizin withdrawal followed by human lymphoblastoid interferon in the treatment of chronic hepatitis B. *Gastroenterol Jpn* 1991; 26:742–746.

118. Lok ASF, et al: A controlled trial of interferon with or without prednisone priming for chronic hepatitis B. *Gastroenterology* 1992; 102:2091–2097.

119. Pastore G, et al: Anti-HBe–positive chronic hepatitis B with HBV-DNA in the serum response to a 6-month course of lymphoblastoid interferon. *J Hepatol* 1992; 14:221–225.

120. Fattovich G, et al: A randomized controlled trial of lymphoblastoid interferon-α in patients with chronic hepatitis B lacking HBeAg. *Hepatology* 1992; 15:584–589.

121. Fattovich G, et al: Therapy for chronic hepatitis B with lymphoblastoid interferon-α and levamisole. *Hepatology* 1992; 16:1115–1119.

122. Janssen HLA, et al: Interferon-α and zidovudine combination therapy for chronic hepatitis B: Results of a randomized, placebo-controlled trial. *Hepatology* 1993; 17:383–388.

123. Berk L, et al: Failure of acyclovir to enhance the antiviral effect of α lymphoblastoid interferon on HBe-seroconversion in chronic hepatitis B. *J Hepatol* 1992; 14:305–309.

124. Yamada G, et al: Quantitative HCV RNA and effect of interferon therapy in chronic hepatitis C (letter). *Dig Dis Sci* 1992; 37:1926–1927.

125. Hagiwara H, et al: Quantitative analysis of hepatitis C virus RNA in serum during interferon alfa therapy. *Gastroenterology* 1993; 104:877–883.

126. Shindo M, DiBisceglie AM, Hoofnagle JH: Long-term follow-up of patients with chronic hepatitis C treated with α-interferon. *Hepatology* 1992; 15:1013–1016.

127. Garson JA, et al: Hepatitis C viraemia rebound after "successful" interferon therapy in patients with chronic non-A, non-B hepatitis. *J Med Virol* 1992; 37:210–214.

128. Kanai K, Kako M, Okamoto H: HCV genotypes in chronic hepatitis C and response to interferon (letter). *Lancet* 1992; 339:1543.

129. Okada S-I, et al: The degree of variability in the amino terminal region of the E2/NS1 protein of hepatitis C virus correlates with responsiveness to interferon therapy in viremic patients. *Heptology* 1992; 16:619–624.

130. Yoshioka K, et al: Detection of hepatitis C virus by polymerase chain reaction and response to interferon-α therapy: Relationship to genotypes of hepatitis C virus. *Hepatology* 1992; 16:293–299.

131. Makris M, et al: A randomized controlled trial of recombinant interferon-α in chronic hepatitis C in hemophiliacs. *Blood* 1991; 78:1672–1677.

132. Liaw Y-F, et al: Effects of prednisolone pretreatment in interferon alfa therapy for patients with chronic non-A, non-B (C) hepatitis. *Liver* 1992; 13:46–50.

133. Lisker-Melman M, et al: Development of thyroid disease during therapy of chronic viral hepatitis with interferon alfa. *Gastroenterology* 1992; 102:2155–2160.

134. Fonseca V, Thomas M, Dusheiko G: Thyrotropin receptor antibodies following treatment with recombinant α-interferon in patients with hepatitis. *Acta Endocrinol (Copenh)* 1991; 125:491–493.

135. Hoofnagle JH: Thrombocytopenia during interferon alfa therapy. *JAMA* 1991; 266:849.

136. Lopez Morante AJ, et al: Immune thrombocytopenia after α-interferon therapy in a patient with chronic hepatitis C (letter). *Am J Gastroenterol* 1992; 87:809–810.

137. Protzker U, et al: Exacerbation of lichen planus during interferon alfa-2a therapy for chronic active hepatitis C. *Gastroenterology* 1993; 104:903–905.

138. Graessle D, Bonacini M, Chen S: Alpha-interferon and reversible hypertriglyceridemia (letter). *Ann Intern Med* 1993; 118:316–317.

139. Fried MW, et al: A pilot study of 2′,3′-dideoxyinosine for the treatment of chronic hepatitis B. *Hepatology* 1992; 16:861–864.

140. Caterall AP, et al: Dideoxyinosine for chronic hepatitis B infection. *J Med Virol* 1992; 37:307–309.

141. Vento S, et al: Zidovudine therapy associated with remission of chronic active hepatitis C in HIV-1 carriers. *AIDS* 1991; 5:776.

142. Gil J, et al: Immunotherapy of chronic active viral hepatitis B with *Propionibacterium granulosum* KP-45 (a 5-year follow-up report). *Hepatogastroenterology* 1992; 39:325–329.

143. Villarrubia VG, et al: Therapeutic response of chronic active hepatitis B (CAHB) to a new immunomodulator: AM3. Immunohematologic effects. *Immunopharmacol Immunotoxicol* 1992; 14:141–164.

144. Berk L, et al: Beneficial effects of *Phyllanthus amarus* for chronic hepatitis B, not confirmed (letter). *J Hepatol* 1991; 12:405–406.

145. Tajiri H, et al: Effect of sho-saiko-to (Xiao-chai-hu-tang) on HBeAg clearance in children with chronic hepatitis B virus infection and with sustained liver disease. *Am J Chin Med* 1991; 19:121–129.

146. Rolandi E, et al: Effects of ursodeoxycholic acid (UDCA) on serum liver damage indices in patients with chronic active hepatitis. *Eur J Clin Pharmacol* 1991; 40:473–476.

CHAPTER 3

Molecular Biology of the Hepatitis Viruses

George J. Dawson, Ph.D.
Research Fellow, Experimental Biology Research, Abbott Laboratories, North Chicago, Illinois

Larry T. Mimms, Ph.D.
Associate Research Fellow, Experimental Biology Research, Abbott Laboratories, North Chicago, Illinois

Richard R. Lesniewski, Ph.D.
Associate Research Fellow, Experimental Biology Research, Abbott Laboratories, North Chicago, Illinois

Aside from their potential to cause hepatitis, the five major hepatotropic viruses that infect humans (hepatitis A virus [HAV], hepatitis B virus [HBV], hepatitis C virus [HCV], hepatitis D virus [HDV], and hepatitis E virus [HEV]) have little in common. These five viruses are classified in separate viral families; none of them share common epitopes or extended regions of conserved homologous nucleotide sequences. Today, diagnostic tests, some in the research phase, are available to detect specific antibodies, antigens, or nucleic acids associated with exposure to these viruses. Many of the advances made in the discovery, classification, and diagnosis of these viruses and associated disease have relied on the techniques available through molecular biology. The following review is focused on providing an update on some of the recent advances made in our understanding of these viruses through the application of the methods and practices of molecular biology.

HEPATITIS A VIRUS

Introduction

As a result of considerable advances made in our understanding of HAV and of the immune response it elicits, the eradication of this virus could become a reality. Although infection with HAV may produce a clinically inapparent illness in children and in some adults, the majority of infected adults have clinical symptoms ranging in degree from mild or moderate (headache, fever, chills, nausea, vomiting, jaundice) to severe (encephalopathy, fulminant hepatitis). The control of HAV was the major topic at the International Symposium on Active Immunization Against Hepatitis A held in Vienna, Austria, in January 1992. The keynote speaker, Dr. Friedrich Deinhardt,* cited reasons for anticipating the eradication of HAV: cross-protection has been noted across many different HAV strains; there is no significant animal reservoir; and various HAV preparations have been successful as potential vaccine candidates.[1]

Selected highlights from both this symposium and some of the recent literature pertaining to the molecular biology of HAV and its relationship to the control of HAV are reviewed in this chapter.

General Virology

The HAV is a nonenveloped virus that is icosahedral in shape and has a diameter of 28 nm. The virion is extremely stable, resisting exposure to ether and to acid at pH 3, and is able to withstand temperatures as high as 80° C. The HAV genome is comprised of a linear, single-stranded, positive-sense RNA that is about 7.5 Kb[2-4] (Fig 1). The genome includes a 5' nontranslated region (743 nucleotides), a long open reading frame (6,681 nucleotides) encoding a large polyprotein of 2,227 amino acids, and a short 3' nontranslated region that is followed by a polyadenylic tract of 40 to 80 nucleotides.[3, 4] The 5' noncoding region of the HAV is highly conserved (nucleotide identity >95%) among different HAV strains and, as with HCV, nucleic acid probes from this region are used frequently for the detection of HAV RNA. There is a region within the 5' noncoding region that is required for internal ribosome binding and translation of the polyprotein. The 3' noncoding region is variable, with nucleotide homologies as low as 80% among different HAV strains.

The large polyprotein consists of three regions, P1, P2, and P3 (see Fig 1). The P1 region specifies four structural proteins (VP1-4) that comprise the viral capsid. The precursor structural protein VP0 likely is cleaved into separate viral proteins,

---

*Deceased April 30, 1992.

GENOMIC ORGANIZATION OF
HEPATITIS A VIRUS*

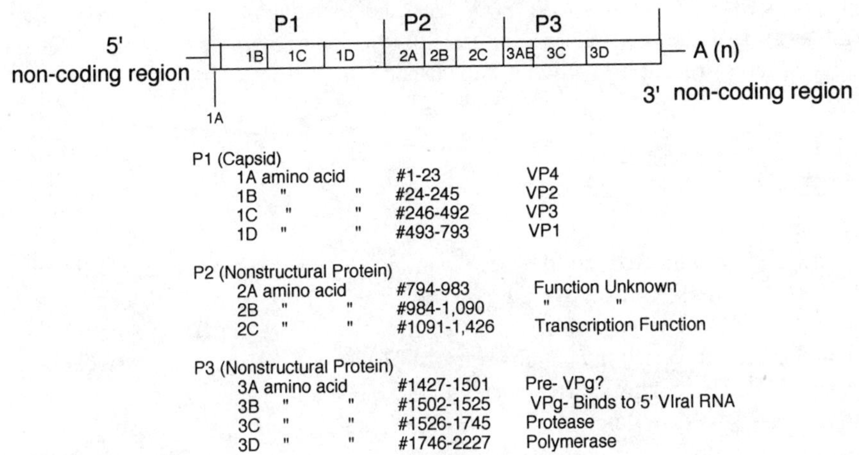

FIG 1.
Genomic organization of hepatitis A virus genome is depicted. The putative cleavage sites
for both structural and nonstructural proteins are indicated. (Adapted from Hollinger FB,
Ticehurst J: Hepatitis A virus, in Fields BN, Knipe DM (eds): *Fields Virology*, 2nd ed.
New York, Raven Press, 1990, pp 631–667.)

VP2 and VP4, as the viral proteins are processed. Three nonstructural proteins are
encoded by P2, including 2A (possibly a protease or autocatalytic site) and two
other proteins, 2B and 2C, whose functions are unknown. The P3 domain codes
for four nonstructural proteins, including protein 3A (function unknown, may be a
precursor to VPg), 3B, or VPg (which covalently binds to the 5' terminal region
of the viral RNA); 3C, a protease that probably cleaves most of the junctions between the mature viral proteins and the precursors); and 3D, an RNA-directed RNA
polymerase segment.[2–4] Although the overall genomic length and organization are
similar to the picornaviruses, the amino acid sequences of several of the mature
HAV viral proteins (VP4, VP1, 2A, 2B, and 3A) are unique.

The 11 HAV proteins are produced as a polyprotein that is processed cotransla-
tionally and posttranslationally. Until recently, the actual sizes, cleavage sites, and
mechanism by which cleavages occur have been based on models using other viruses of the picornavirus family. Recently, it has been shown that active proteinase 3C (a cysteine proteinase), expressed as a recombinant protein, catalyzes the
cleavages at the VP1/VP2 junction as well as catalyzing the VP0-VP3 cleavages.[5]
In a second study,[6] the parameters for the reactions catalyzed by the HAV 3C proteinase were studied. The efficiency of the 3C proteinase was determined in regard
to several parameters, including minimum substrate size, amino acid substitutions
at various positions along the substrate sequence, and the optimum pH for successful cleavage.[6]

It has been recommended that HAV be considered a new genus in the Picornaviridae family because of its unique properties, including a pronounced tropism for liver cells, the small size of VP4, and the few overall sequence similarities with viruses of the other genera comprising the Picornaviridae.[2, 7, 8] There is no antigenic cross-reactivity with any known hepatitis viruses.

Genetic Variability

Earlier work indicated that the HAV genome is conserved more highly than are other RNA viruses, with an overall base sequence identity between different strains being greater than 90%.[9] Two regions of the P1 gene of the HAV genome were studied for their variability among various HAV strains, including the carboxyl region of VP3 (a highly conserved region of VP3) and a more variable region at the putative VP1/2A junction.[10-13] In these studies, various HAV isolates were classified into different genotypes (defined as a group of viruses that have 85% or more of their base sequences conserved) based on nucleotide sequence differences at the putative site of the VP1/2A junction (Fig 2). Two genotypes (I and III) are split into two subgenotypes that differ by about 7.5% at the nucleotide level.[13] Geographic clustering of particular genotypes and subgenotypes has been noted; in one instance, over a 15-year period, there was less than 3% diversity in nucleotide sequences among multiple HAV isolates obtained from different infected individuals residing in the same geographic region.[11, 13] Among non–epidemiologic related strains, 82 of 104 were assigned as HAV genotype I (69 for subgenotype 1A and 13 for subgenotype IB) and 11 were assigned as genotype III.[13] There have been no reported differences in the pathogenicity of the various genotypes. Three genotypes (IV, V, and VI) have been recovered from Old World monkeys and are not believed to be associated with human disease.[13]

The HAV isolates exhibit amino acid differences to a lesser extent. These differences vary from about 3% (between subgenotypes) to as much as 18% among different genotypes.[13]

Virus Neutralization

X-ray crystallographic studies, which could elucidate the potential site(s) of neutralization of the virus, have not been performed on HAV in part because of difficulties in obtaining sufficient numbers of intact virions. Studies have been undertaken, however, to determine the position of the viral neutralization site(s) with the viral capsid.[14-16] In two of these studies, investigators have generated HAV escape mutants by exposing infectious HAV to monoclonal antibodies directed

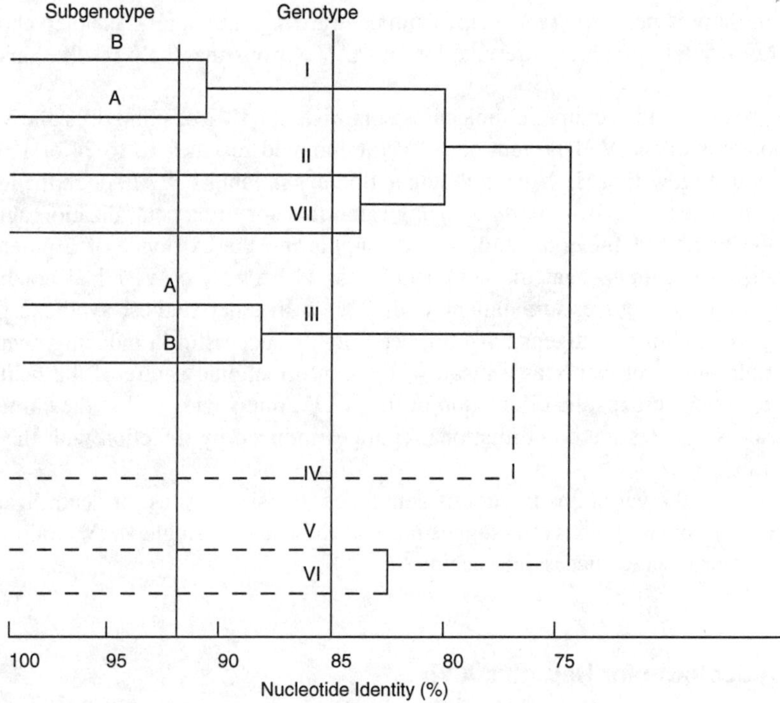

FIG 2.
The genetic relatedness of different strains of human *(solid line)* and uniquely nonhuman primate *(dashed line)* genotypes are depicted in this summary dendrogram. Most of the human strains that have been sequenced belong to genotypes I and III. (From Lemon SM, Jansen RW, Brown EA: *Vaccine* 1992; 10[suppl]:S40–44. Used by permission.)

against neutralization sites on the viral capsid.[14, 15] Escape mutant sequences were amplified by polymerase chain reaction (PCR) and sequencing was performed. In one of the studies, escape mutants had only single amino acid changes[14] either within VP3 (amino acid residue 70 or, to a much lesser extent, amino acid residue 74) or within VP1 (amino acid residues 102, 171, 176, or 221). Similar findings were reported in a second study using a modified method of selecting the escape mutants via monoclonal antibodies.[15] Escape mutants harboring one or more amino acid changes were noted frequently, again involving VP3 (amino acid residues 65 and 70) and VP1 (amino acid residues 104, 105, and 232). Taken together, these data suggest that the immunodominant epitope for virus neutralization is comprised of amino acid residues from different structural proteins, and that these two proteins must be aligned in such a way as to allow a single antibody molecule to bind to both proteins at the neutralization site. The current structural model of the hepatitis A virion does not permit alignment of these sites. Alternatively, it is possible that mutations in one protein may perturb the neutralization epitope on a second protein, thereby permitting its escape from neutralizing antibodies. As noted above, an x-ray crystallographic representation of HAV virions may help resolve this issue.

In a related study, chimeric molecules comprised of VP1 of poliovirus and various domains of the VP1 protein of HAV (amino acid residues 13 to 24 or 101 to 108) induced low-titer HAV neutralizing antibodies in rabbits.[16] Although the identification of residues 101 to 108 as being important for virus neutralization agrees with the results of previous studies, data supporting the existence of a potential neutralization domain near the amino terminus (13 to 24) of VP1 had not been noted in the previous escape mutant studies.[14, 15] In other studies, synthetic peptides or recombinant antigens have not been highly successful in inducing neutralizing antibodies, probably as a result of the conformational nature of the neutralizing epitope. Perhaps the orientation of the HAV amino acids within the chimeric molecule simulates the conformational epitopes induced by infection with the native virus.

In spite of the variations in various genotypes, the site or sites for neutralization of the virus remain conserved, suggesting that the use of a single HAV strain may suffice to produce a successful vaccine.

Why Vaccinate for Hepatitis A Virus?

In underdeveloped countries, HAV infections occur early in life, usually during childhood, typically producing as asymptomatic illness and lifelong immunity. The benefits of implementing a vaccine program in underdeveloped nations are not clear. First, the current vaccine is expensive. Second, after a mild or asymptomatic HAV infection, most of the population has lifelong immunity; it is unclear whether the vaccine will induce similar immunity. Yet, as developing countries improve sanitation and the standard of living, there is likely to be a decline in early childhood infection with HAV, which will result in an increase in the number of symptomatic infections occurring among adults.[17]

In developed countries, children usually escape HAV infection. The high-risk group for HAV infection include military personnel, people who travel to HAV-endemic areas for business or recreation, intravenous drug users, individuals who consume raw shellfish, and personnel at day-care centers. HAV infections in adults usually produce symptoms and in some cases require hospitalization. There is significant morbidity associated with HAV infection. Based on the number of cases reported to the Centers for Disease Control (CDC) and the Sentinel County Study, it is estimated that there are 35,000 nonhospitalized cases and 13,000 hospitalized cases of HAV in the United States each year, resulting in 54 deaths.[18] In this country alone, the annual cost of caring for individuals with acute HAV infection exceeds $200 million.[19]

Vaccine Studies

The demonstration that a formalin-inactivated preparation of HAV protected marmosets from challenge with live HAV was an important milestone in establishing the feasibility of producing an effective HAV vaccine.[20] A second milestone was the adaptation of HAV to cell culture in 1979 by Provost,[21] and by others,[22, 23] which provided the means to control virus yield and to monitor variability more closely. A third milestone was the demonstration that various preparations of HAV, including whole virions, subunit vaccines (recombinant proteins, synthetic peptides), and attenuated viruses have proven to be immunogenic and capable of inducing neutralizing antibodies to HAV.[23, 24] Although several approaches for the development of HAV vaccines have shown some promise, the vaccines most likely to be available in the near future make use of a classic approach for vaccine design (i.e., the use of an inactivated preparation of purified HAV virions).[24-28] A typical antibody profile observed in these studies indicates that antibodies are produced in most individuals in the first weeks after vaccination; antibody titers increase after additional doses of the vaccine (Table 1).[27, 28] This type of profile was demonstrated in several different studies.[28] In one study,[29] three different lots of vaccine produced similar immune responses to HAV, indicating the consistency of the vaccine production process. Previous studies had demonstrated that the inactivated vaccine induced neutralizing antibodies, and that antibody titers induced by the vac-

TABLE 1.

Seroconversion Rates and Geometric Mean Titers After the Administration of Hepatitis A Virus Vaccine*

		Seroconversion		Geometric Mean Titer	
Group†	Time of Sample (Mo.)	No. Positive/Total	Percentage	mIU/mL	Range
1 and 2	0	0/104	0		
	1	96/99	97	241	20–1,162
	2	102/102	100	300	25–3,230
1	3	50/50	100	916	214–5,597
		49/49	100	694	62–3,806
	7	48/48	100	543	77–2,777
	12	51/51	100	433	47–2,547
	24	29/29	100	361	45–2,093
2	3	48/49	98	286	33–1,273
	6	47/49	96	291	35–1,216
	7	49/49	100	2589	206–13,506
	12	49/49	100	1315	143–9,990
	24	24/24	100	593	53–2,678

*From Tilzey AJ, Palmer SJ, Barrow S: *Vaccine* 1992; 10(suppl 1):S121–123. Used by permission.
†Individuals were inoculated with 1.0 mL of vaccine containing 720 enzyme-linked immunosorbent assay units of inactivated hepatitis A virus. Group 1 was vaccinated at 0, 1, and 2 months, and group 2 was vaccinated at 0, 1, and 6 months.

cines were higher than those produced by the passive administration of immunoglobulins directed against HAV.

The use of an inactivated vaccine from a second source was effective in preventing HAV infection among children in an area where there had been recurrent outbreaks of HAV.[26] During the first few days after vaccination, there were acute cases of HAV infection in both the vaccinated group (7 cases) and the placebo group (4 cases). There were no cases of HAV infection among the vaccinated group from day 21 through day 137 after vaccination; 34 cases of HAV infection were reported in the placebo group during this same period. These data demonstrate the utility of the vaccine in preventing HAV infection in a natural setting.

Persistence of Hepatitis A Virus

There have been several reports of biphasic, relapsing HAV infections.[30–34] HAV infection resolves in most individuals within 3 to 5 weeks. It is estimated, however, that between 1.5% and 18.5% of individuals infected with HAV experience a second acute hepatitis infection after a remission phase lasting 4 to 15 weeks.[32] In a recent study, some 14 cases of protracted or relapsing hepatitis were reviewed; in 3 of 8 cases, HAV RNA was detected during the relapse phase of infection, in one case persisting for months after the initial infection.[32] In a separate study, HAV virus, HAV RNA, and HAV antigens were detected during the relapse phase of infection (days 30 to 90 after the initial illness), but not during the follow-up period at 6 and 12 months after infection.[33]

Recently, an outbreak of HAV occurred in a neonatal intensive care unit when an asymptomatic HAV carrier (who later had hepatitis) donated blood to an infant in whom acute HAV infection subsequently developed.[34] In the following weeks, the HAV infection spread to a total of 13 infants, 22 nurses, and 8 other staff members. In two cases, both HAV antigen and HAV RNA (via PCR) were detected for 4 to 5 months after the initial illness.[34] It was unclear as to whether the duration of infectivity was unusually long because these were infants whose immune systems still were developing, or whether viral persistence could be attributed to the particular virus strain initiating the outbreak.

The mechanism by which relapses of HAV infection occur has been discussed in a recent review.[32] The persistence potentially could be a function of the virus strain (e.g., a particular genotype or escape mutant) or, alternatively, the result of a host-related factor wherein an effective immune response has failed to develop in the host. Many of the individuals having relapse infections had been treated with steroids during the initial stage of infection.[32]

Further studies of this phenomenon should provide a clearer picture of protracted and relapsing HAV infections in the epidemiology of HAV. Is it possible that the evolution of HAV could be accelerated by such viral persistence? One could speculate as to whether persistent infections may provide a mechanism by which more diverse genotypes and serotypes may emerge in the future, serotypes that potentially could evade the immune response directed against a vaccine.

Summary

Application of the techniques of molecular biology to HAV supports earlier concepts of HAV infection in man. First, the fact that there is likely to be a single serotype of HAV that produces hepatitis in man is supported by the nucleotide sequencing studies indicating in general that the HAV genome is highly conserved. Second, the observation that inactivated virions are better inducers of neutralizing antibodies than are smaller epitopes is supported by the molecular biology studies identifying the major epitope as being highly conformational, with different proteins contributing to the neutralization epitope. Recent progress in HAV research continues to provide hope that the control of HAV and its possible eradication are within the bounds of our current knowledge and technology.

HEPATITIS B VIRUS

Introduction

HBV infection leads to a wide range of disease states from mild subclinical infection to chronic active and fulminant hepatitis. The complex interplay between host and virus is just beginning to be understood at the molecular level. In this review, recent findings concerning genetic variation in HBV and host immune response and induced selection, the HBV envelope and discovery of a hepatocyte receptor, and new methods for the diagnosis of HBV infection are discussed.

Hepatitis B Virus Genome and Gene Products

The hepatitis B genome is a circular, partially double-stranded DNA of about 3,200 base pairs that codes for seven viral proteins[35] (Table 2). As shown in Figure 3, the polymerase gene completely overlaps the viral envelope genes PreS1, PreS2, and S, and partially overlaps the X and core genes. The envelope of the hepatitis B virion consists of three proteins and their glycosylated derivatives. These proteins, termed small (S), middle (M), and large (L) hepatitis B surface (HBs) proteins, contain the S gene sequence.[36] The MHBs also contains the PreS2 sequence (55 amino acids) and the L protein contains the PreS1 sequence (108 or 119 amino acids), depending on subtype) plus the PreS2 sequence. In the blood of

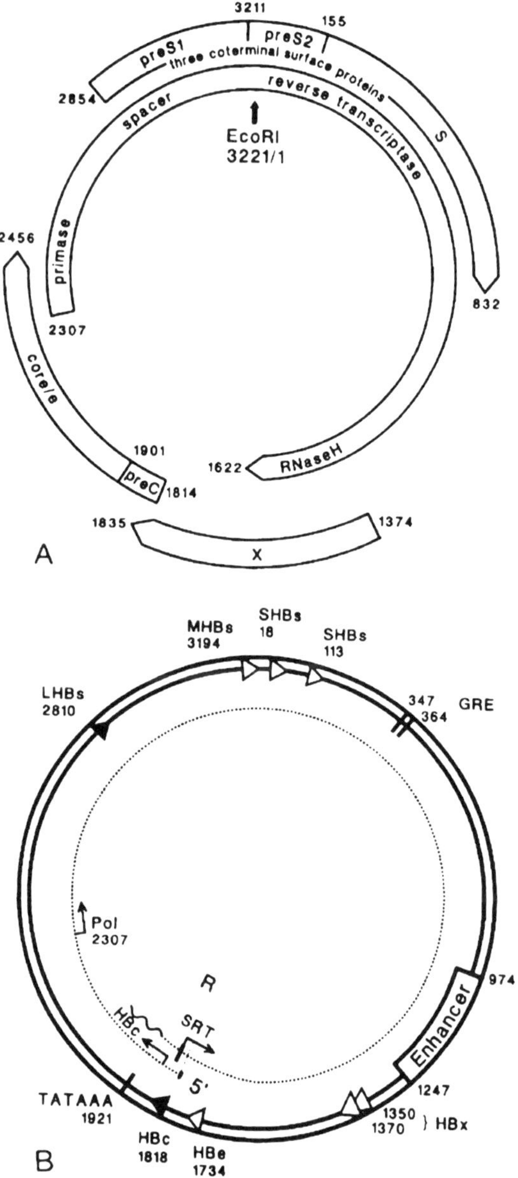

FIG 3.

Organization of the HBV genome. **A,** open reading frames (ORFs) are shown. ORFs start with the first AUG and end at the first stop codon. The largest ORF corresponds to the P, or pol, gene. **B,** start and stop sites of messenger RNAs encoding the HBV proteins. Only the major messenger RNAs consistently found in liver or transfected cells are shown. The *open triangles* indicate the messenger RNA start sites occurring in all HBV-expressing cells; the *closed triangles* refer to those that occur only in hepatic cells if no foreign promoter is in-

TABLE 2.

Hepatitis B Virus Genes and Proteins*

Gene	Nucleotide Location	Protein	Amino Acids	Apparent Molecular Weight (kd)
S	155–832	SHBs (HBsAg)	226	24, 27
PreS2+S	3211–832	MHBs	281	33, 36
PreS1+PreS2+S	2854–832	LHBs	400	39, 42
PreCore+C	1814–2456	HBeAg	157–170†	16–20
C	1901–2456	HBcAg	185	22
X	1374–1835	HBxAg	154	16
P	2307–1622	DNA polymerase	845	95

*Adapted from Gerlich WH, Hermann KH: Functions of hepatitis B virus protein and virus assembly, in Hollinger FB, Lemon S, Margolis H (eds): *Viral Hepatitis and Liver Disease*. Baltimore, Williams & Wilkins, 1991, pp 121–134.
†Multiple proteolytic cleavage sites at the C terminus.

HBV-infected individuals, only a very small portion of the total HBs antigen exists as complete virions or Dane particles. Two other morphologic forms, 22-nm spherical particles and filaments 22 nm in diameter and of variable length, lack capsid or DNA and are produced in huge excess over HBV virions. Virions are enriched in the PreS1 containing protein, LHBs, compared to incomplete 22-nm particles, which consist primarily of S gene product.

The core gene encodes the nucleocapsid protein (183 or 185 amino acids depending on subtype), HBcAg. Immediately upstream of the core gene is the precore region, which consists of 87 nucleotides encoding 29 amino acids in phase with the core gene.[36] The translation from the precore region, therefore, leads to the production of a protein that shares the HBcAg sequence. The first 19 amino acids of the precore region serve as a signal for membrane translocation and eventual secretion of the precore gene product termed HBeAg. Cotranslational cleavage of the N terminal signal and subsequent proteolytic cleavage at the C terminal end produces the mature HBeAg, which contains ten amino acids from the precore gene and the N-terminal three fourths of the HBcAg. The function of HBeAg is enigmatic, but it may help the virus to escape immune surveillance by inducing immune tolerance. The P gene product is a 95-kd protein containing four functional domains: a primase or terminal protein, a spacer, DNA polymerase/reverse transcriptase, and a ribonuclease H.[37] Finally, the X gene encodes a protein of

troduced. The common stop of all messenger RNA is behind the TATAAA box at 1921. Pregenomic RNA that encodes HBcAg and Pol is shown as a *dotted line. R* = terminal redundancy; *SRT* = signal sequence for reverse transcription; *GRE* = glucocorticoid responsive element. (From Gerlich WH, Hermann KH: Functions of hepatitis B virus protein and virus assembly, in Hollinger FB, Lemon S, Margolis H (eds): *Viral Hepatitis and Liver Disease*. Baltimore, Williams & Wilkins, 1991, pp 121–134. Used by permission.)

154 amino acids that functions as a transcriptional activator of the HBV genome and a variety of heterologous viral and cellular transcription control regions.[38] Because the entire viral DNA sequence codes for one or more translated proteins, all cis-acting elements that regulate gene expression also overlap functional genes. These regulatory sequences include four promoters, two enhancers, an encapsidation signal, and two direct repeats[39] (Table 3).

Hepatitis B Virus Mutability

Because of the genomic compactness and the extensive functional overlaps, one would expect significant constraints on DNA sequence divergence to maintain a genome capable of efficient replication and transmission. The HBV, however, shows greater mutability than previously appreciated.[40, 41] Similar to the human immunodeficiency virus, HBV uses reverse transcription as an essential step in the replication cycle. Reverse transcription has poor proofreading ability, leading to a high rate of nucleotide misincorporation. Calculations suggest the rate of HBV mutation at 2×10^{-4} base substitutions per site per year, which is 4 orders of magnitude higher than other DNA viruses.[42] Variability in the virus first was discovered through classic subtyping studies of HBsAg.[43] By applying modern molecular biology procedures, such as amplification of the viral DNA by PCR and rapid DNA sequencing techniques, the molecular basis of these subtype differences was identified.[44]

TABLE 3.

Hepatitis B Viral Regulatory Sequences and Overlapping Genes*

Regulatory	Element	Nucleotide Location†	Overlapping Gene
Promoters			
	S	3130–3220	PreS2/P (spacer)
	PreS1	2679–2824	P (terminal protein)
	C	1705–1805	X
	X	1250–1350	P (ribonuclease H)
Enhancers			
	I	1182–1216	P (reverse transcriptase/ ribonuclease H)
	II	1637–1764	X
Direct repeat			
	1	1826–1836	X/Precore
	2	1592–1602	X/P (ribonuclease H)
G R E		347–364	S/P (reverse transcriptase)
Encapsidation signal		1853–1937	Precore/C
Poly A		1914–1962	C

*Adapted from Yen TSB: *Seminars in Virology,* in press.
†Exact end points for many of the regulatory sequences have not been defined precisely.

Mutations may not be located randomly on the genome; at least one "hot spot" for mutation at the carboxy terminus of the precore gene has been identified in viremic patients lacking HBeAg.[42] Although multiple variants may arise in a virus population, the abundance of the variant depends on its ability to survive defense mechanisms of the host, to replicate efficiently, and to maintain infectivity. Recent reports have documented the emergence of other mutations in the precore, core, and envelope protein genes, PreS and S, which presumably give these mutants a selective advantage over wild type in evading the immune system.

Host Response to Hepatitis B Virus Infection

Evidence has accumulated that viral clearance and liver cell injury in HBV infection are mediated by a cytotoxic T lymphocyte (CTL) response to one or more HBV-encoded antigens expressed at the hepatocyte surface.[45] Only in a rare type of chronic HBV infection termed "fibrosing cholestatic hepatitis" are the unusually high levels of HBsAg observed thought to be directly cytotoxic.[46, 47] As reviewed recently,[45] a strong T cell response to HBcAg and HBeAg, but not to envelope antigens, was found in acute hepatitis B. Guilhot and colleagues[48] demonstrated that HBV transfectants stably expressing HBcAg serve as excellent targets for the detection of HLA class I–restricted CTLs, and Missale and coworkers[49] showed the existence of a class II CTL response to synthetic peptides of the HBcAg in patients with acute HBV infection. A study of vaccine recipients by Penna and associates[50] also suggests that HBV envelope–specific, HLA class II–restricted CD4+CTLs potentially can participate in the immune clearance of HBV-infected cells. Persistence of viral replication correlated with a blunted T cell response to HBcAg. Although T cell response to viral antigen may be abrogated in chronic HBV, CTL response may persist in chronic carriers. One study[51] demonstrated that at least two different class I–restricted CTLs exist in patients with chronic hepatitis B, one recognizing the envelope antigens and the other recognizing the core antigen. Barnaba and colleagues[52] demonstrated the presence of CTLs that were specific for the HBV envelope in intrahepatic lymphoid cells of patients with chronic active hepatitis. In a transgenic mouse system, Ando and coworkers[53] showed that CD8+, major histocompatibility complex class I cells specific for the S gene can recognize and destroy HBsAg transgenic hepatocytes in vitro and in vivo. Even though these cytopathic cells may exist as a very small proportion of the lymphatic infiltrate, they may cause disease by eliciting a nonspecific inflammatory response by secreting γ-interferon. In this regard, HBsAg-positive transgenic mouse hepatocytes were extremely sensitive to destruction by γ-interferon in vivo.[54]

There also is evidence of an ongoing humoral immune response in both symptomatic and asymptomatic carriers of hepatitis B. High levels of antibody to HBcAg (anti-HBc) are observed in almost all HBV carriers. Twenty percent of random HBsAg-positive specimens have detectable HBeAg and antibody to HBeAg (anti-HBe),[55] and 10% to 20% have detectable, but low-level antibody to HBsAg (anti-HBs). A recent report[56] using very sensitive detection methods claims that virtually all patients with HBV infection and liver disease, and about 50% of those with chronic hepatitis B without liver disease have demonstrable humoral immune responses specific for HBeAg, anti-envelope. Much of the anti-envelope response, however, may exist because of the different fine specificities of HBsAg and anti-HBs. These data support the thesis that there is ongoing immune surveillance of precore, core, and envelope gene products in chronic HBV carriers that could provide selective pressure for the emergence of HBV variants.

Precore/Core Mutants

In populations in which HBV is endemic in the Mediterranean and Far East, precore mutants have been observed in a large number of chronic carriers of HBV who are anti-HBe–positive and have high levels of HBV DNA.[40, 41, 57] The most common mutation observed in several studies was a G-to-A point mutation (A1896) in the penultimate codon (nucleotide 1896) of the precore region, creating a termination codon. This mutation in the precore region prevents the synthesis and secretion of the HBeAg. These variants appear to emerge spontaneously during seroconversion from HBeAg to anti-HBe in natural infection[58] or, in some cases, during interferon treatment.[59] Although the precore mutant A1896 has been observed in several cases of fulminant hepatitis and may be more pathogenic than is the wild type, it often is observed in patients with quiescent disease, suggesting that host factors or other mutations in the viral genome may have an effect on pathogenesis.[59–63]

It is important to note that precore mutants have been observed predominantly in endemic populations. Most anti-HBe–positive carriers in the United States and Western Europe do not have high viremia or fulminant hepatitis, and the A1896 mutant may not be the usual predicator of seroconversion in these populations. Although A1896 emergence has been reported in some patients responding to interferon treatment, precore mutants were not detected in responders or nonresponders in England.[64] Lo and associates[65] and Hasegawa and colleagues[66] reported that the precore mutant also was absent in cases of fulminant hepatitis in England and the United States, respectively. Manzin and coworkers[67] tested for the presence of A1896 in the HBV integrated into the human genome from tumorous tissue in patients with hepatocellular carcinoma. No A1896 mutations were found; however, seven of nine patients had missense mutations leading to the substitution of alternative amino acids for the distal cysteine (position −7) in the precore region. This cysteine has been shown to be important in determining the aggregation state and antigenicity of the HBeAg.[68] Interestingly, four of six nontumor regions had nonintegrated HBV genomes containing the A1896 mutants. These data suggested that an early HBV DNA integration event in some cells before the emergence of the A1896 mutant or negative selection against the A1896 mutant in tumor cells could account for its absence in these cells.

It also is notable that the A1896 mutation exists inside the hairpin structure of the core messenger RNA, which is involved in encapsidation and translation. Although this mutation apparently has little effect on encapsidation in an in vitro system,[69] it may interfere with translation. A second mutation, G-A 1899, often accompanies the A1896 mutation.[70] One hypothesis is that this second substitution may increase translation of the core and thereby provide a selective advantage to compensate for the deleterious effects of the A1896 mutant.

Another variant mutually exclusive of A1896 was found in HBeAg-negative Chinese patients.[60] This mutant had a substitution of one nucleotide (T1856) leading to the replacement of a proline residue with a serine at codon 15, which was as prevalent as the A1896 stop codon mutant. HBeAg-positive patients with the T1856 mutation had a worse prognosis after seroconversion to anti-HBe than did patients bearing the A1896 mutant. The effect of T1856 on HBeAg production is not clear; however, Carman and associates[60] hypothesize that transport or processing of the precore/core may be reduced, resulting in decreased secretion. Alternatively, the altered secondary structure may inhibit binding and secretion of signal peptide to the endoplasmic reticulum. Another mutant with a substitution at the precore initiation codon (1815) has been discovered[70, 71] that also would lead to the loss of HBeAg secretion and may aid in viral persistence. Chuang and coworkers[62] showed that clusters of missense mutations occur in core regions 48–60, 84–101, and 147–155 in Taiwanese patients with chronic HBV infection and severe liver disease. The regions of missense clustering mutations in the core may represent T cell recognition epitopes. These researchers found that A1896 was present in asymptomatic patients as well as those with chronic active hepatitis. In contrast, the core clustering mutants were associated closely with chronic active hepatitis. Taken together, these data indicate that the A1896 mutation decreases or eliminates the production of HBeAg, perhaps enhancing viral persistence, but does not necessarily lead to more severe hepatic disease. Additional mutations that promote improved replication or transmission may be selected positively, similar to A1899. The occurrence of these mutations, however, may expose (because of increased core production) the cells harboring these virus mutants to increased immune surveillance, leading to increased selective pressure on other genes, for example, the core. Because only the precore/core genes were sequenced in this study,[62] it is not known whether the core mutations are more pathogenic or whether they simply are indicative of the emergence of pathogenic variants with increased numbers of mutations occurring throughout the genome. Whether recurrent acute exacerbations of liver disease associated with the HBV chronic carrier state are related to the emergence of escape mutants or HBV variants, or simply are host related is under investigation. Possible deletion mutants in HBcAg also have been suggested.[72]

Envelope Mutants

The HBV envelope regions encompassing PreS1, PreS2, and the region 100–160 of S are exposed on the surface of the viral particles and would be expected to be targets of immune surveillance.[36] Some S mutants described to date have affected significantly the antigenicity of the "a" epitope(s), which is the common or group-specific determinant(s) of SHBs.[40] The "a" determinants are complex, conformational, and dependent on disulfide bonding among highly conserved cysteine residues. The "a" immunoreactivity can be mimicked partially by cyclic synthetic peptides. Although the "a" epitope(s) traditionally had been defined by reactivity to polyclonal antisera, the use of monoclonal antibodies has shown that the "a" region consists of at least five nonoverlapping epitopes.[73] Genetic variation in the "a" determinant leading to immune escape has been described in vaccinees in Italy and Japan, and in patients receiving liver transplants who are taking monoclonal anti-a antibody therapy.[74–78] The most common mutant thus far is a single nucleotide substitution leading to the replacement of a glycine with an arginine (Gly-Arg 145). This mutation destroys some, but not all, "a" epitopes.[79]

Other mutations in the "a" region lead to the loss of subtypic or type-specific determinants, *y/d* and *w/r*. Because these determinants overlap with "a" determinants and some subtypic variation leads to differential affinity of anti-"a" monoclonal antibody, it can become a semantic argument as to whether some HBV genomes bearing an S gene amino acid change(s) are "a" mutants. Some mutations lead to the loss of subtype reactivity, such as ASP-Gln(144) or Gly-Ala(145), which destroy *d* activity (they also likely affect some anti-a monoclonal antibody binding), or Lys-Asn(160), which destroys *w* or *r* reactivity.[80] High levels of subtypic antibody (anti-d or y) often develop in naturally infected and vaccinated individuals. In fact, some individuals have only an anti-subtypic antibody response. A child infected in a hemodialysis unit by multiple HBV carriers had an S point mutation substituting Pro-Gln 120 that led to complete loss of reactivity to subtyping polyclonal antibody and also to partial loss of "a" reactivity.[44] Another case involved a Thr/Ile-Asn 126 in an infant treated with hepatitis B immune globulin and vaccine,[75] and in yet another case, Lys-Glu 141 was demonstrated in a breakthrough infection in a child vaccinated with HB who had a high anti-HBs titer.[81] Finally, a patient who was HBsAg-negative but HBeAg- and HBV DNA–reactive had three point mutations in the "a" region: Thr-Ser 126, Thr-Asn 131, and Met-Thr 133.[82] This individual also had deletions in the PreS2 domain.

Several recent studies have documented the emergence of gross deletions and point mutations in the PreS1/PreS2 region, suggesting that the production of these envelope gene products also is under immune selection in chronically infected individuals.[83–86] Fernholtz and colleagues[83] showed that HBV with mutated PreS sequences is unable to express PreS2 antigen and occurs as a dominant or exclusive virus population in a highly viremic carrier. Gerken and associates[84] studied an HBsAg-positive, anti-HBe–positive patient whose chronic hepatitis B progressed rapidly to hepatocellular cancer and to death within 5 years. Nine of 12 clones isolated from this patient showed a 183–base pair deletion spanning the 3′ end of the PreS1 gene and the 5′ end of the PreS2 gene. This viral deletion eliminated B and T cell recognition sequences in PreS2, but did not affect the PreS1 hepatocyte receptor site.

Tran and coworkers[85] observed the emergence of rearrangements in the PreS/S and precore/core regions in several samples from chronic carriers of HBV who had been subjected to two rounds of interferon therapy 2 years apart. During the first 2 years, only wild type virus was seen. Later, the emergence of precore A1896 was observed, followed by additional point mutations and deletions in PreS1, PreS2, and S. These mutations were shown to exist on the same viral DNA molecule. Interestingly, this patient remained HBeAg-positive. In a final study, Santantonio and associates[86] tested 22 unselected carriers from Southern Italy. Six of them had deletions in the PreS region, mainly at the amino terminus of PreS2, plus another mutation in the PreS2 initiation codon, and, therefore, could not express M protein antigen. The emergence of PreS mutants occurred over the natural course of infection for 1 patient and after interferon treatment for 2 others.

Mutations in Nonstructural Genes

Most authors have focused on only the precore or PreS/S regions, but mutations may be accumulating throughout the genome over the decades of chronic viremia. The entire HBV genome was sequenced from the liver of a patient who was HBsAg-negative and anti-HBs–positive, but had a history of viral hepatitis.[87] Numerous point mutations were found throughout the genome; however, transfection experiments showed that a single missense mutation, a substitution of a proline for a threonine at the amino terminus of the P gene, resulted in the inability to package pregenomic messenger RNA into particles. This point mutation could be complemented by the wild type virus.

Repp and colleagues[88] found that 15% of the HBV genomes in the sera of a hepatitis B carrier had an 89–base pair deletion in the enhancer II region, truncating the X protein by 26 amino acids at the COOH terminal end. Whether this mutation offers some selective advantage is uncertain. A third example of a potential regulatory mutation was an insertion mutant producing an elongated X protein.[89] This protein was shown to retain transacting activity.

HBV mutants that cannot replicate because of deletions in the env, C, or P genes have been reported in plasma from HBV carriers. All coexist with HBV forms that are replication competent. Okamoto and associates[90] demonstrated that mutant genomes with gross deletions in the PreS/S, C, and P genes derived from the plasma of asymptomatic carriers may be complemented in hepatoma cells using transient expression systems. Complementation was measured as the ability to secrete viral particles with mutant genomes into the culture media. Interestingly, all mutants had an intact encapsidation signal. Complementation with predecessor wild type viruses, other mutants, and even with HBV DNA sequences integrated into host chromosomes was demonstrated in this in vitro system. These authors suggest that HBV mutants acting as defective interfering particles may attenuate wild type virus replication and thereby help to maintain persistence of infection.

Cryptic or Occult Hepatitis B Virus Infection

Infections in patients who have detectable HBV DNA in the serum or liver but no detectable serum HBsAg have been termed cryptic or occult. Not surprisingly, with the advent of PCR, numerous studies have documented new cases of cryptic HBV infection. PCR procedures can detect 1 to 10 viruses compared to 2,500 to 25,000 viruses (0.1 to 1.0 pg/mL of viral DNA per test) for standard HBV hybridization assays. The most sensitive HBsAg tests detected about 20 pg of HBsAg, or about 2 million particles. Because HBsAg particles may outnumber DNA-containing virions by factors as high as 1 million, the HBsAg test is a good measure of HBV infection. In most cases, the presence of low-level HBV DNA in individuals with cryptic infection appears to have no clinical relevance. Clinically significant cryptic infections, however, have been reviewed recently by Wands and coworkers.[91] In some patients, the HBsAg is present at vanishingly small quantities in sera, but in others, it may be undetectable because of masking by anti-HBs. Current commercial monoclonal antibody–based enzyme immunoassays have improved significantly the detectability of HBsAg in immune complex compared to the standard radioimmunoassay, and it is unfortunate that many researchers continue to use only the latter technique for classifying cryptic infection. Wright and colleagues[92] have PCR evidence for the presence of HBV DNA in 7 of 17 patients with apparent non-A non-B hepatitis, and suggest that latent HBV may be a common cause of posttransplant fulminant hepatitis. HCV PCR and anti-HCV testing gave no evidence for HCV infection. Other centers have been unable to find evidence for HBV latency in their patients with fulminant hepatitis.[93] There are several recent reports of DNA PCR–positive, anti-HBc–reactive, and anti-HBs–reactive or anti-HBc-only–reactive individuals among Taiwanese volunteer blood donors,[94] random Senegalese populations,[95] British patients with chronic liver disease,[96] patients with primary liver cancer,[97] and unselected hemophiliacs.[98] The actual etiologic role of HBV in these cases is unknown because HCV coinfection was not examined. These data suggest that some proportion of patients with high-titer anti-HBc in the presence or absence of low-titer anti-HBs may be cryptic HBV carriers. Five recent reports have documented the persistence of PCR-detectable DNA after the clearance of HBV in resolving cases of acute HBV infection,[99] in experimentally infected chimpanzees,[100] and in HBV carriers who responded to therapy with apparent recovery.[101, 102] Although DNA usually disappears weeks to months after therapy, some patients continue to have positive test results for HBV DNA in the liver and serum. The long-term consequences of this persistent low-level DNA are unknown.

PreS Serology and the Hepatitis B Virus Hepatocyte Receptor

During the acute and chronic phases of disease, PreS1, PreS2, and S antigens are codetected in serum and their serum concentrations tend to rise and fall in concert.[103, 104] Most carriers have detectable PreS antigens as well as S antigens, regardless of their HBe/anti-HBe status.[105] Loss of PreS-encoded antigens in acute HBV infection correlates with the resolution of infection and clearance of the virus.[103] In resolving infection, anti-PreS1 and anti-PreS2 often, but not always, appear earlier than does anti-HBs. Because anti-PreS antibody may be detected during acute-phase viremia, as well as in some chronic carriers, the presence of anti-PreS2 or anti-PreS1 antibodies has limited utility as a favorable prognostic sign.[106, 107] PreS1 and PreS2 antigens have been shown to be highly immunogenic in mice, and their presence together with the S antigen may potentiate the immune response to S.[108] Recent studies with a third-generation hepatitis B vaccine have shown that inoculation of a vaccine containing PreS1, PreS2, and S leads to higher anti-HBs titers and can overcome the lack of response to HBsAg vaccine that is observed in some individuals.[109]

HBV binding to hepatocytes is mediated by the PreS1 domain (amino acids 21–47),[110–114] but the identity of the HBV PreS1 receptor on the hepatocyte plasma membrane remained a mystery until recently. The HBV PreS1 receptors were detected not only on human liver and hepatoma cells, but also on B lymphocytes, and on monocytes and T cell lines activated by *Escherichia coli* lipopolysaccharides and concanavalin A, respectively.[115] Recent work in two laboratories has identified interleukin-6 (IL-6) as a cell attachment site for PreS1.[115–118] Interestingly, the PreS (21-42) does not bind the IL-6 receptor.[116] Nor is the IL-6 receptor required even directly for PreS (21-47) binding to the membrane. Chinese hamster ovary cells and ovarian insect cells (which presumably lack the IL-6 receptor) expressed receptors for the PreS (21-47) region only after transfection with human IL-6 complementary DNA. These findings confirm that IL-6 is expressed on the surface of these cells independent of the IL-6 receptor and that IL-6 is sufficient to endow cells with PreS (21-47) binding activity. The nature of the interaction between IL-6 and the cell surface is not well understood. IL-6 is a soluble protein lacking a transmembrane anchor. Treatment of transfected cells with phosphatidylinositol-specific phospholipase C releases IL-6 from the cell surface, with a subsequent decrease in PreS1 (21-47) binding activity. The terminus of IL-6 lacks the sequence requirements for the attachment of phosphatidylinositol glycans, however, suggesting that IL-6 is not tethered directly to the membrane via a lipid chain. Whether an association between cell surface–bound IL-6 and HBV env proteins is neccssary and sufficient for the entry of HBV into cells also is unknown.

Because the IL-6 binding site for HBV is distinct from that for the IL-6 receptor, it is possible that antiviral compounds could be developed that mimick and block the binding site for HBV on IL-6 but do not display undesirable biologic effects of the intact IL-6 molecule. Preliminary studies by Yang and colleagues[119] also have shown binding of the S gene product to cells, which may be mediated by apolipoprotein H. Much remains to be learned about the binding and entry of HBV into cells.

New Diagnostic Techniques

Significant advances also have been made in the diagnostic laboratory with the implementation of automated immunodiagnostic testing. Fully automated hepatitis immunoassays have been developed for the nonisotopic detection of HBsAg, anti-HBc IgG and IgM, anti-HBs, anti-HBe, and HBeAg on the IMx instrument.[55, 120–124] All steps of the assay except dispensing the speciman into the reaction are performed by the instrument. These assays are based on microparticle enzyme immunoassay (MEIA) technology. MEIA uses latex microparticles as a solid phase and separation of bound from unbound material is accomplished by capture of the microparticles in a glass fiber matrix. Alkaline phosphatase conjugated antibodies or antigens act as signal generators, catalyzing the conversion of methyl umbelliferyl phosphate (MUP) to its dephosphorylated fluorescent product. The instrument measures the fluorescence rate, which is a function of the concentration of analyte tested. The sensitivity and specificity of these assays has been reported to be equivalent to or better than that of traditional enzyme immunoassays or radioimmunoassays. The major advantages of the system over polystyrene 1/4 bead or microtiter tests are speed in obtaining results (<45 minutes); full automation, including specimen dilution, and improved precision.[121] Microparticles offer the advantage of ease of manipulation by a robotic pipette system. They are dispersed in solution, significantly reducing the "mean free path" for productive collisions between analyte in solution and capture solid phase, thereby significantly shortening the time of reaction. Another automated system uses microparticles as a capture phase along with chemiluminescent molecules attached directly to the detecting antibody.[125, 126] The detecting antibody is bound covalently to acrydinium orange, which emits photons of light when a "trigger" solution (containing peroxide in an alkaline buffer) is added. Emitted light is measured using an optical detector containing a photomultiplier tube. Other automated systems use paramagnetic microparticles as a solid phase and an alkaline phosphatase conjugate for detection with either fluorescent (MUP)[127] or chemiluminescent substrates.[128] The magnetic microparticles have the advantage that they may be manipulated in a magnetic field to allow thorough washing and removal of unbound reactants.

The improved precision of these robotic systems coupled with the expanded dynamic ranges afforded by fluorescent and chemiluminescent systems may stimulate the development of quantitative HBV tests, as already has occurred in the measurement of anti-HBs.[123] Quantitative values are determined automatically in the instrument by comparison to a stored, but adjusted, standard curve. Quantitative tests for HBeAg may be useful in monitoring patient response to HBV therapy.[129] Some investigators have used the levels of IgM anti-HBc as measured by the IMx as an indication of active liver disease in chronic carriers.[130] New, nonisotopic methods for HBV DNA quantitation of sera have been developed[131, 132] and may prove useful in both predicting and measuring response to therapy.

The PCR has become a valuable research tool; however, its routine use still is not within reach of most clinical laboratories. Even with automation and the development of procedures to reduce contamination and carryover between specimens, the clinical utility of such a sensitive test for HBV DNA awaits further investigation.

Summary

Ongoing immune surveillance in chronic HBV infection provides selective pressure for the emergence of HBV variants. Escape mutants in precore, core, PreS, and S genes may arise during the natural course of chronic infection or during vaccine or hyperglobulin therapy, and may correlate with increased severity of disease. Much work remains in defining the interplay between HBV, host immunologic responses, and the pathogenesis of HBV infection. New molecular biologic and diagnostic techniques provide important tools to aid in this understanding.

HEPATITIS C VIRUS

Introduction

A discussion of HCV molecular biology necessitates some knowledge of the virus genome sequence and organization, structural and nonstructural gene products, and the physical characteristics of the viral particle itself. It is a testament to the power of modern molecular techniques that such a discussion can occur regarding HCV, which never has been purified, conclusively visualized, or reproducibly cultured in the laboratory. Our knowledge of the virus is the consequence of having cloned molecularly and identified this agent from a pool of infectious chimpanzee plasma using immunoscreening techniques.[133] Since the successful cloning of HCV, we rapidly have accumulated knowledge of its sequence diversity, genomic organization, and encoded gene products, and of the immune response to this pathogen. We also have learned the tremendous potential for the application of these very powerful cloning and screening techniques to the discovery of new viral agents.

Physical Properties

Only limited data are available regarding the physical properties of HCV. Most of the early characterization of the virus was done by Bradley and coworkers.[134, 135] The size of the virus was determined by sequential filtration through polycarbonate filters of decreasing pore size[135, 136] and testing of the filtrates for infectivity in chimpanzees. Infectious virus appears to be between 30 and 60 nm in diameter, in agreement with the sizes of known flaviviruses and pestiviruses. The virus is thought to have a lipid envelope because treatment with chloroform destroys HCV infectivity.[137] Recent studies of the buoyant density of HCV[138, 139] further support a lipid-associated virus particle. Two bands of viral nucleic acid can be detected by PCR after density gradient centrifugation in sucrose or cesium. A distinct band of virus is observed at 1.18 to 1.21 g/cm^3, in agreement with the density of known flaviviruses (1.19 to 1.20 g/cm^3), and probably represents the density of the intact virus. A second band of HCV RNA is observed at the top of the gradient (<1.03 g/cm^3) and appears to be associated with the lipid fraction of the plasma. Even when infectious plasma is mixed with cesium chloride and self-forming gradients are generated, two separate bands of HCV RNA are detected, indicating that the band of low-density RNA is not an artifact observed on preformed gradients.[139] Whether this lighter material represents intact virus, defective virus, or simply lipid-associated replication complexes is unknown. The nucleocapsid of HCV, which can be liberated from the virion/lipid coat by detergent treatment, has an apparent density of 1.25 g/cm^3 in sucrose.[138]

The Viral Genome

HCV is an RNA virus. The genome consists of a positive-strand RNA molecule about 9.4 Kb in size.[140] A large open reading frame was identified that encodes a polyprotein of 3,011 amino acids. Genomic organization of the virus is similar to that of both flaviviruses and pestiviruses,[140, 141] with structural components encoded at the 5' end and nonstructural proteins encoded at the 3' end of the genome. In addition, the genome contains both a 5' noncoding region (also known as 5' untranslated region [5'-UTR]) and a 3' noncoding region.

Overall, the 5'-UTR is highly conserved among the HCV isolates sequenced to date.[142–144] That is not to imply that the entire 5'-UTR is conserved; in fact, recent work has shown that the overall conservation is a result of highly invariant stretches of sequence (nucleotides −263 to −246, −199 to −178, and −65 to −3) interspersed among smaller, more variable regions within the 5'-UTR.[145] High sequence conservation at the 5' and 3' ends of viral genomes generally reflects the important role these regions play as recognition sequences for genome replication (3') and ribosomal entry sites[146] for translation (5'). Recent experiments by Yoo and associates[147] demonstrated that the 5'UTR of HCV contains multiple *cis*-acting elements, some of which repress and others of which enhance translation of the genome. These regulatory functions were active only in constructs containing partially truncated 5'-UTR regions. Similar truncated species have been found circulating during natural infection, suggesting that these subgenomic species may play a role in translational control of virus expression. Although small open reading frames exist within the 5'-UTR, the encoded gene products and specific associated functions have not been identified. One important consequence of the sequence conservation within the 5'-UTR has been our ability to detect multiple genotypes of the virus using conserved PCR primers designed based on this region.[143, 144]

Unlike the 5'-UTR, the 3' noncoding region is poorly conserved among the different HCV genotypes, but is highly conserved within a given genotype.[142, 144] Hence, whereas the 5'-UTR may contain virus-specific sequences, the 3' noncoding region appears to contain group-specific sequences. Computer analysis of this region from all genotypes studied, independent of specific sequence, suggests the presence of stem and loop structures indicative of recognition sites used by viral RNA–dependent RNA polymerases.[148] The remaining portion of the HCV genome is organized into three structural and four or five nonstructural gene products. Assignment of individual functions encoded by the HCV genome was accomplished using a variety of molecular methodologies. First, the actual gene sequence was compared with those of known viruses to determine regions of homology. Very little sequence homology exists between HCV and other viruses, with the exception of limited regions within the 5'-UTR[142, 148] where similarity to the 5' noncoding region of a pestivirus, bovine viral diarrhea virus, was observed. A second, and more useful, analysis was done by translating the large open reading frame of the virus and searching for amino acid sequence similarities with other viruses. The hydrophobicity profiles and overall organizational layout of the polyprotein also were examined. Using these methods, additional information was obtained suggesting an association of HCV not only with pestiviruses and flaviviruses,[133, 140, 149–151] but also with a group of plant viruses known as potyviruses. It currently is thought that HCV is related distantly to both flaviviruses and pestiviruses, and perhaps even is related evolutionarily to certain plant viruses.

Two additional approaches were used to characterize the HCV gene products: *in vitro* translation/processing analysis of a partial viral genome and cloning of the whole viral genome into vaccinia virus followed by expression in mammalian cells. The first technique makes use of rabbit reticulocyte lysates that translate portions of viral RNA sequence to protein and canine pancreatic microsomal membranes, which process the translated polyprotein into its component proteins. Four colinear amino terminal proteins (p22-gp35-gp70-p19) were identified by this technique.[152]

Two groups[153, 154] have assembled the HCV genome and cloned it into vaccinia virus vectors. Using a cotransfection system with T7 RNA polymerase, these investigators characterized the resulting expressed HCV proteins. As in the case of the *in vitro* translation experiments, a 22-kd putative core protein was identified as the 5'-terminal gene product.[153] A second protein thought to be a 35-kd envelope protein also was identified at the 5′ end. A 65-kd protein was discovered, which was in good agreement with the expected size of the NS3 gene product, but only a 52-kd NS5 protein was observed where the predicted NS5 gene product would have a molecular weight greater than 110 kd. This suggests that the NS5 protein may be processed further. The results of these combined approaches to defining the HCV genome have been used to construct the genome map depicted in Figure 4.

Hepatitis C Virus Gene Products

The composite evidence of nucleotide and amino acid homology suggests that HCV is related more closely to pestiviruses than to flaviviruses.[140, 149, 155] The remaining discussion of HCV proteins is based on the interpretation of the HCV gene products as they relate to pestivirus genomes such as bovine viral diarrhea virus.

Amino acids 1–190 encode the nucleocapsid or core protein of HCV. This protein is not glycosylated and contains a large number of basic amino acid residues that are thought to bind the viral nucleic acid. A similar protein is encoded by the pestiviruses. The analogous protein in flaviviruses is smaller (~120 amino acids), and the remaining sequence up to amino acid 190 encodes a separate matrix protein.

Two envelope proteins are encoded between amino acid 191 and amino acid 729. The first of these, E1 (amino acid 191-383), is a glycoprotein of about 33 kd (~21 kd unglycosylated) analogous to the envelope glycoprotein gp33 of bovine viral diarrhea virus. The second envelope protein (E2/NS1, amino acid 384-729) also is glycosylated and has an apparent molecular weight of 72 kd (~38 kd unglycosylated). The E2/NS1 nomenclature results from earlier consideration of this gene product as analogous to the first nonstructural region (NS1) in flaviviruses and the later designation of this region as a second envelope protein (E2) analogous to a bovine viral diarrhea virus envelope protein, gp55. A key feature of this glycoprotein is a hypervariable region located at the 5′ end of E2/NS1 (amino acid 369-407)[156] that demonstrates extensive heterogeneity among HCV isolates sequenced around the world.

The remaining sequence of the HCV genome encodes nonstructural (NS) proteins. NS2 ((amino acid 730-1006) is an extremely hydrophobic domain encoding a 30-kd protein that has no known function at this time. The NS3 protein (amino acid 1007-1615, 65 to 70 kd) is the viral protease that contains consensus sequences of trypsinlike serine proteases.[157, 158] Similar NS3 proteases exist in both flaviviruses[159] and pestiviruses. Protease activity of NS3 actually has been demonstrated[154, 158] on the HCV polyprotein, suggesting its role in processing the viral polyprotein posttranslationally during infection. The HCV protease appears to be involved only in specific cleavages of nonstructural proteins. Grakoui and colleagues[154] demonstrated that the cleavage of several HCV proteins from the polyprotein was abolished by replacing amino acid 1165, serine, with alanine,

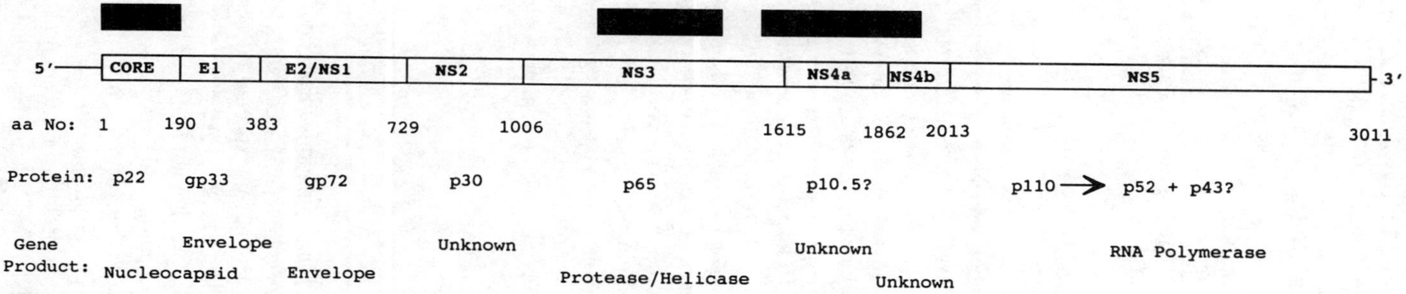

FIG 4.

Proposed organization of hepatitis C virus. Putative amino acid boundaries taken from Okayama et al.[160] Proteins shown are those identified by Manabe et al.[154] and Grakoui et al.[155] *Shaded bars* above genome show the approximate location of HCV antigens used in second generation HCV antibody EIAs.

concluding that the NS3 gene product was indeed a serine protease able to recognize and cleave nonstructural elements of the HCV polyprotein. Cleavage of individual structural proteins upstream from NS3 was unaffected by this amino acid substitution, suggesting a host cell protease role in cleavage of the structural proteins, as is supported by the *in vitro* processing of core/E1/E2 in the absence of NS3 by canine microsomal fractions.[152] A nucleotide triphosphate binding sequence, [Gly-X-Gly-Lys-(X) 39-105-Asp-Glu], conserved among flaviviruses and pestiviruses, also is observed in HCV NS3.[157] This motif is found commonly in helicase enzymes, which help to unwind the RNA genome so that replication can occur.

A defined function for the NS4 gene product(s) is unknown at this time. It appears that the NS4 region actually may encode two separate products, $NS4_a$ and $NS4_b$,[153, 154] analogous to the situation in flaviviruses.[141] Okayama and associates[160] propose that the putative $NS4_a$ and $NS4_b$ gene products span amino acids 1616-1862 and 1863-2013, respectively. It is notable that, although the NS4 sequence is very hydrophobic and probably is membrane associated, it was the first antigenic region of the virus to be discovered, and detection of antibodies to this region continues to be used as an index of exposure to HCV.

The gene product encoded by the virus NS5 region (amino acid 2014-3011) has an apparent molecular weight of 110 kd. Further processing to smaller components has been observed in the vaccinia system of Manabe and coworkers[153]; however, the size of the native NS5 gene product during natural infection is unknown. This region is thought to contain the RNA-dependent RNA polymerase activity of the virus and has been shown to have a known consensus sequence (GDD) in a location comparable to the RNA replicase proteins of flaviviruses and pestiviruses.[157, 161, 162] Overall sequence homology between HCV NS5 and flavivirus or pestivirus NS5 regions, however, is not statistically significant. This gene product of HCV actually may be related more closely to replicase proteins of certain plant viruses.[149]

Genomic Heterogeneity

HCV is a ubiquitous virus found in populations throughout the world. A number of these global isolates have been sequenced. Extensive heterogeneity is observed among HCV isolates, a result that is not unexpected because most RNA viruses demonstrate significant genomic heterogeneity. As of this writing, at least five related, but distinct, major genotypes are thought to exist.[144, 163, 164] Multiple genotypes can coexist within a given population and minor subtypes may be present also. Although isolates of a given genotype demonstrate a high degree of amino acid conservation for the HCV gene products, isolates from any two of the different major genotypes will show significant heterogeneity in the amino acid sequences of most gene products, including E1, E2/NS1, NS2, NS4, NS5, and 3' noncoding regions. The 5'UTR, core, and NS3 regions are more highly conserved among the major genotypes. An example of sequence conservation within genotypes and heterogeneity between genotypes is shown in Table 4.[163] The implications of HCV genomic heterogeneity are significant for vaccine and diagnostic test development, and also may be of concern to physicians treating HCV-infected patients with antiviral drugs, especially if the different viral genotypes manifest themselves as phenotypes with different virulence and susceptibility to treatment, as previously suggested.[165]

HCV sequences also are heterogeneous within the infected individual. Although a predominant genotype usually will represent about half the viral species circulating, the remaining half is composed of a wide variety of heterogeneous species with predominantly first and second base mutations.[166, 167] More extensive mutations occur within the E2/NS1 region that give rise to amino acid changes as well. Hence, HCV is thought to exist as a "quasispecies" in the circulation of infected patients. This, too, raises concerns for the success of future vaccines. In addition, the wide variety of viral genomes that coexist may be responsible for the high rate of chronic infection that is associated with HCV. The existence of quasispecies can provide the virus with a high degree of adaptability when host immune responses to the virus occur. As neutralizing or cytotoxic T cell responses develop to the major phenotype of the virus, selective replication advantage may be provided to a minor variant, allowing further replication and viral persistence in the host.

Another selective advantage for HCV may result from the high mutation rate that is observed within defined domains of the virus envelope proteins. Two distinct hypervariable regions have been described.[168, 169] The 5' end of the second envelope protein (E2/NS1) is hypervariable with respect to both nucleotide and amino acid sequence. This heterogeneity is observed among all isolates, independent of major genotype. The mutation rate within E2/NS1 is high and comparable to that observed for the hypervariable V3 loop of the envelope protein, gp120, from the human immunodeficiency virus.[141, 156, 170] A selective advantage for HCV will exist if virus-neutralizing epitopes are encoded within this highly mutable region. Recent work[156, 171] using E2/NS1 synthetic peptides demonstrated the presence of multiple epitopes within this region and provided evidence that the genotypic variation observed within E2/NS1 results in antigenically distinct variants of

TABLE 4.

Homology of Nucleotide and Amino Acid Sequences of Two Hepatitis C Virus (HCV) Isolates Compared to Type I Isolate HCV-H From the United States*

Isolate	Percent Homology With HCV-H									
	5'-UTR	Core	E1	E2/NS1	NS2	NS3	NS4A	NS4B	NS5	3'NC
HCV-1†	99.7‡	98.9	94.1	92.9	95.1	97.2	95.5	96.7	96.7	83.3‡
HCV-J§	98.2‡	98.9	78.8	79.3	80.0	92.2	87.0	84.8	83.2	73.6‡

*Adapted from Inchauspe G, Zebedee S, Lee S, et al: *Proc Natl Acad Sci U S A* 1991; 88:10292–10296. Used by permission.
†Type I United States isolate.
‡Refers to homology at the nucleotide level; all other numbers refer to amino acid sequence homology.
§Type II Japan isolate.

HCV. These data support the hypothesis that neutralizing epitopes could be located within this region. Genetic drift of the virus resulting in multiple amino acid substitutions within the E2/NS1 hypervariable region was observed to occur in a chronically infected chimpanzee that was observed over an 8.5-year period.[172] During this time, 12 of 25 amino acid positions in the hypervariable region had undergone substitution. Because of hypermutation in this region, the overall mutation rate of E2/NS1 is calculated at 2.7×10^{-3} base substitutions per year, nearly double the mutation rate for the viral genome as a whole (1.44×10^{-3}).

Protective Immunity to Hepatitis C Virus

In light of the observed mutation rate of HCV and hypervariability within the envelope domains, it is not surprising that protective immunity to HCV has not been demonstrated. Farci and colleagues[173] have shown that chimpanzees convalescent from HCV infection (as defined by normalized alanine aminotransferase values and undetectable levels of RNA by PCR) are not protected from subsequent infection when they are inoculated with either a homologous or a heterologous infectious serum. Some animals were challenged and reinfected as many as four times, with new viremia developing each time. Virus was rescued from each acute infection and sequenced. In each case, the rescued virus had an identical sequence to that of the inoculating strain, indicating that a new infection had been established.

Lack of a cell culture system producing sufficient quantities of native HCV is the largest obstacle to a successful attempt at identifying neutralizing antibodies. Investigators at Chiron,[174] however, have described at least one vaccine attempt using recombinant proteins. Vaccinia viruses containing HCV E1 and E2/NS1 inserts were inoculated into chimpanzees. In some cases, the animals' immune systems were primed further with recombinant envelope proteins expressed in yeast. Even after the development of anti-envelope responses, these animals were not protected from subsequent HCV infection because they all had elevation of the alanine aminotransferase level and detectable RNA in the sera after challenge. Some delay or moderation of disease may have occurred; however, the number of animals was too small to determine whether either of these observations was statistically significant.

Hepatitis C Virus Detection

The only method (excluding biologic assays in chimpanzees) for detecting hepatitis C viremia in acute or chronically infected patients is the PCR assay. No test for HCV viral proteins or components (such as that for HbsAg) are known. Because of viral heterogeneity, the selection of appropriate PCR primers is crucial. Fortunately, the 5'-UTR is well conserved among all HCV isolates reported so far, and primers designed from this region[141, 142] permit the detection of all known viral isolates. Viral nucleic acid can be detected during the early acute phase of infection, even before alanine aminotransferase levels rise. The virus remains detectable in the circulation of chronically infected individuals as well. Many papers on PCR have been published describing the viremia that occurs in the chimpanzee model and during the natural history of the infection in man.[175–180] Sensitivity of PCR below ten copies of viral RNA has been described.[177] The detection of HCV RNA is our best approximation of infectivity second to inoculation into experimental animals. Most anti-HCV–positive individuals (71% to 100%) are HCV PCR–positive.[178] Cases of antibody-negative, PCR-positive cases have been described during early acute phase infection, however, highlighting the utility of PCR for HCV detection in these cases.

Recombinant HCV antigens, expressed in yeast and *E. coli*, have been used to produce enzyme immunoassays to detect antibodies to HCV. These tests have both research and commercial utility. Most blood banks worldwide screen blood carefully for HCV antibodies using a second-generation enzyme immunoassay. The second-generation test uses three antigenic targets from the HCV genome. The three antigens are encoded by the core, NS3, and NS4 regions of the virus. Use of this assay has reduced significantly the risk of posttransfusion hepatitis[181, 182] and enabled the detection of HCV exposure in many groups of high-risk patients, such as intravenous drug users, hemophiliacs, transfusion recipients, and patients with clinically diagnosed chronic non-A, non-B–related liver disease.[183, 184] Antibodies to HCV are present in most patients with chronic non-A, non-B hepatitis (70% to 100%), as well as in high numbers of intravenous drug users (50% to 90%) and hemophiliacs (64% to 83%).[183]

New markers of HCV infection are under development. IgM antibodies to the nucleocapsid (core) of HCV have been described[185–187] and may have some utility in staging disease. Antigens representing the NS5 region occur at frequencies similar to those for the other nonstructural (NS3/NS4) antigens.

Expression of the envelope proteins of HCV has presented a more significant challenge. Both the E1 and E2/NS1 proteins are glycosylated heavily and contain hydrophobic membrane-anchoring regions. Generally, more complex expression systems such as baculovirus vectors in insect cells or SV40 vectors in mammalian cells are required to obtain appropriate glycosylation and secretion of these molecules. One of the authors' (RRL) laboratories recently has succeeded in expressing and secreting sufficient HCV E2/NS1 protein to permit its purification for use in enzyme immunoassays. Our preliminary data demonstrate that antibodies to this protein are found more frequently than are other markers in PCR-positive patients with non-A, non-B hepatitis and often occur earliest after virus exposure. The data suggest that further improvements in the sensitivity of screening or diagnostic assays may be possible.

Summary

Our knowledge of HCV has increased dramatically since its reported cloning in 1989. This virus exists globally, is heterogeneous, and appears to be related distantly to flaviviruses and pestiviruses. Both structural and nonstructural components are encoded by a single-stranded RNA genome of positive polarity. The expression of cloned sequences enabled the manufacture of assays capable of detecting HCV-infected patients and identifying HCV-infected blood donors. Although much progress has been made, we have a long way to go before we understand completely the genetic complexities and replication strategies of this virus that allow it to cause acute and often chronic persistent liver disease.

HEPATITIS D VIRUS

Introduction

HDV is a defective virus in that it requires HBV as a helper for its full range of infectivity. In infected individuals, HDV coinfection with HBV results in acute or fulminant hepatitis, but the risk of progression to chronicity is similar to that of HBV infection alone. HDV also may superinfect a chronic HBV carrier, resulting in severe chronic hepatitis and a more aggressive form of disease.[188] In this review, we discuss recent findings concerning HDV structure, requirements for HBV helper function, HDV mutability, and the role of the two forms of hepatitis D antigen (HDAg) in control of the viral life cycle.

Hepatitis D Virus Genome and Structure

HDV is a 36-nm virus containing a single-strand, circular RNA genome of 1.7 Kb[188] (Fig 5). This is the smallest genome of any known animal virus and most closely resembles plant viroids or satellites. The HDV genome forms an unbranched, rodlike structure with 70% of the genome internally base paired. In vitro studies have shown that both genomic and antigenomic RNA are capable of self-cleavage and self-ligation reaction.[189, 190] Current models for the replication of HDV involve these reactions in a double rolling circle mechanism similar to that proposed for viroids. HDV replication occurs in the nucleus of the infected cells. Unlike viroids, the HDV genome codes for at least one protein, HDAg, from its antigenomic strand. The genome is bound to HDAg, which in turn is enveloped by HBsAg. Only recently have HDV RNA/HDAg corelike structures

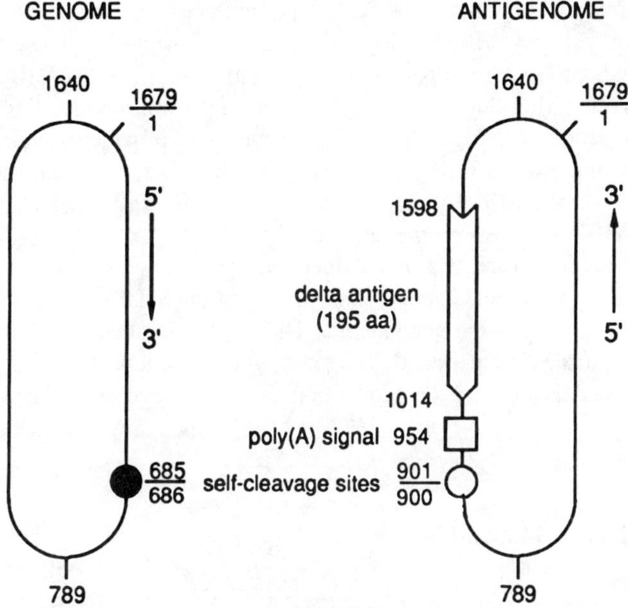

FIG 5.
Organization of the hepatitis D virus genome and antigenome. The opening reading frame for the delta antigen is indicated on the antigenome. Self cleavage sites in the genome and antigenomic are also indicated. (From Taylor JM, Chao M, Hseih SY, et al: Structure and replication of hepatitis delta virus, in Hollinger FB, Lemon SM, Margolis HS (eds): *Viral Hepatitis and Liver Disease*. Baltimore, Williams & Wilkins, 1991, pp 460–463. Used by permission.)

been identified.[191] These contain about 40 HDAg molecules per HDV RNA molecule. HDV virions contain almost exclusively genomic RNA[192]; however, HDV ribonuclear particles also have been isolated from the cell nucleus that contain both genomic and antigenomic RNA.[191]

Requirements for Hepatitis B Virus Helper Function

Although HDV requires an HBV coat for infectivity in a natural setting, Sureau and coworkers[193] demonstrated that a typical HDV infection could be initiated by direct inoculation of recombinant HDV complementary DNA into the liver of an HBV-infected chimpanzee. Interestingly, progeny viruses were indistinguishable from native HDV. Tissue culture studies have shown that, although it requires HBV (or woodchuck hepatitis virus) for infectivity, HDV does not require HBV for genomic replication.[194–197] HBV/HDV-cotransfected cells, but not HDV-transfected cells alone, could produce infectious HDV particles in vitro. These particles displayed all the HBV envelope epitopes on their surface[198] and antibodies against the HBV envelope proteins could neutralize HDV infectivity. Studies in patients undergoing liver transplantation indicate that HDV infection can be observed earlier than can HBV infection in the transplanted liver, although histologic evidence of hepatocyte damage occurs only in patients with coincident HBV reinfection and proliferation.[199, 200] Furthermore, in one study, HDV infection was transmitted to the donor liver despite the apparent absence of replicating HBV in either the native diseased organ or the transplanted liver.[201, 202] Liver disease was not evident in these patients, even though HDV RNA and HDAg were detectable in these livers throughout follow-up, suggesting that HDV alone is not very pathogenic. These reports taken together show that HDV can replicate independently of the HBV infection, but that significant hepatocyte transmission and the production of hepatic disease requires help from HBV.

Hepatitis D Virus Mutability

Similar to HCV and HBV, HDV has significant sequence variability and mutability.[203, 204] RNA sequences from various geographic areas of the world differ by 11% to 17%. Four HDV genomic regions are highly conserved: two corresponding to the catalytic sequences on the genomic and antigenomic sense RNAs and two within the HDAg coding region of the antigenomic HDV RNA. The mutation rate of HDV from the HDAg coding region was estimated at 0.6 × 10 E-3 per site per year[203] and between 0.3 and 3.0 × 10 E-2 when the entire genome is considered,[204] suggesting some greater constraints on mutation within the HDAg coding region. In one study,[204] HDV sequences were obtained at three time points in one patient over the course of two years. Periods of increased mutational rate tended to correlate with more dramatic changes in symptoms. Unfortunately, multiple independent PCRs were not performed at each point, so the relative abundance of mutated forms could not be evaluated; therefore, the estimated mutation rates may be suspect as a result of sampling errors. Little is known about the extent to which HDV is under immune selective pressure to escape host defenses or about the effects of individual point mutations on replicating ability. Whether HDV antigens are presented on the surface of infected cells, whether there is a significant cellular immune response to HDV infection, and whether the increased disease severity in HDV coinfection is the result of the direct pathogenesis of HDV or is mediated by cellular immunity also is not known. Because there is a strong humoral immune response to HDAg,[188] some surveillance on the B and T cell level would be likely. Minimal, but tantalizing, evidence exists that acute exacerbations and flares in chronic HDV disease may represent the reactivation of HDV replication resulting from the emergence of immune escape mutants.[204]

Functional Regions of the Genome

The functional regions of the genome have been mapped partially. Regions 659-772 in the genomic sense and 847-966 in the antigenomic sense are required for autocatalytic, cleavage activity. This self-cleavage activity has been localized further to an antigenomic stretch of only 90 nucleotides.[205] Although the sequence requirements and conditions of this ribozymal activity have been studied extensively in vitro,[206–209] little is known about how this autocatalytic activity works in HDV's own replication in vivo. HDAg consists of two forms coded by the region 1598-1014 or 1598-957: S, which is 24 kd (195 amino acids), and L, which is 27 kd (214 amino acids), respectively. The two forms are identical in sequence, but the L form contains an additional 19 amino acids at the C terminus. The production of the L form occurs through an important RNA editing phenomenon during the normal HDV life cycle. In this RNA editing, the stop codon for S, UAG, is changed to UGG, allowing production of the L form. Two reports indicate that the editing involves a highly specific U to C conversion in genomic RNA.[210, 211] This sequence change occurs independently of viral replication, does not require HDAg, and can be catalyzed in vitro by adding purified HDV RNA to a nuclear extract of cells from a variety of species.[211] This U-to-C conversion requires an amination reaction and a double-stranded HDV RNA conformation at the modification site. Preliminary evidence suggests that the amino donor for this reaction may be glutamine.[212]

Structure of Hepatitis D Antigen: Role of L and S Forms

The HDAg is highly basic at the amino terminal two thirds of the molecule. It contains a nuclear localization signal within the N terminal one third (amino acids 69-88) that directs HDAg to the nucleus of infected cells.[213] RNA binding domains are localized to the middle one third (two arginine-rich regions at 97-107 and 136-146) of the protein.[214] Both L and S HDAg forms bind specifically to HDV RNA, and at least six subregions on the HDV rodlike genome have HDAg binding capacity.[192] No difference in binding affinity was observed between the two forms in an in vitro assay.[215] A leucine-zipper–like sequence (amino acids 30-51) is required for dimerization or oligomerization of HDAg.[214, 216] The L form exhibits a much higher degree of phosphorylation than does the S form,[215] but the significance of this posttranslational modification is unclear. The L form also is isoprenylated near the C terminal end; however, the S form lacks the isoprenylation motif.[217] Because the L form, but not the S form, is required for HDV virion assembly,[215, 217, 218] this isoprenylation or C terminal extension on the L form may play some role in enabling interactions with HBsAg. The S form can be packaged into virions only if the L form is present.

Data indicate that the S form transactivates HDV replication, but the L form suppresses replication in a transdominant mode.[214, 218] The mechanism of S HDAg promotion of HDV replication is unclear. Hypotheses include aiding transport of HDV RNA to the nucleus, stabilizing HDV RNA or interacting with RNA polymerase II, or transcriptional factors leading to improved efficiency of the replication process. Xia and Lai[214] suggest that the S HDAg participates in HDV replication as an oligomeric form, and that the L form binds to S oligomers, forming a complex that is not able to transactivate. Interestingly, the presence of 12% L form in a pool of S form can inhibit HDV RNA replication by 90%. Therefore, the presence of one L form for every eight S forms in a complex may be sufficient to disrupt S function.

What is the significance of the fact that a fraction of HDV genomes encoding the S form are changed specifically to encode the L form? Ryu and associates[219] suggest that this RNA modification is an essential step in the life cycle of the virus. The appearance of the L form turns off genomic replication by binding to the S complexes and also serves as an essential facilitator of viral assembly. Therefore, the virus shifts from a replicating mode to a virus production mode. No direct evidence exists that the relative amount of L and S is an important survival factor in natural infections, however, or that the S HDAg producing HDV RNA is packaged preferentially in virions compared to the L producing RNA.

Hepatitis D Virus Downregulation of Hepatitis B Virus

It is well documented that HDV superinfection of HBV carriers often leads to dramatic, transient reductions in HBV replication and serum HBsAg concentrations in these patients.[188] How does HDV cause this suppression? This phenomenon has been studied recently in tissue culture systems.[196] Expression of both the 3.5- and 2.1-Kb RNAs of HBV was decreased dramatically by the presence of HDV in a cotransfected human hepatoma cell line, HuH-7.[220] The amount of HBV virions released was also reduced. This reduction appeared to result solely from the action of the HDAg, because cotransfection with HBV and an HDAg expression vector led to reductions comparable to those induced by cotransfection with the entire HDV genome. These authors suggest that suppression is mediated by HDAg binding to HBV RNA or to transcriptional regulatory factors.

Summary

Although HDV is a small virus, it possesses unique and interesting properties that are only beginning to be unraveled. Many questions have been addressed, but many remain unanswered concerning the control of HDV replication and viral assembly.

HEPATITIS E VIRUS

After serologic tests to detect antibodies or antigens associated with recent HAV or HBV infection came into widespread use, it became clear that there was an enterically transmitted non-A, non-B hepatitis (ET-NANBH) virus producing both epidemic and sporadic cases of viral hepatitis, mainly in developing nations.[221–223] Infection with ET-NANBH virus often results in acute hepatitis with symptoms similar to those of HAV infection. Most infections attributed to ET-NANBH virus are resolved completely within 3 to 4 weeks; there have been no reports of chronic infection. There is, however, a high incidence of fulminant hepatitis among infected pregnant women, often resulting in mortality rates of 10% to 20%.[221–223] The etiologic agent of ET-NANBH virus, now named HEV, has been molecularly cloned and is classified tentatively as being similar to caliciviruses in genomic organization.[224]

A brief summary of some of the recent research is presented, emphasizing the role of molecular biology in both the discovery and the characterization of HEV.

General Virology

Viral-like particles 27 to 30 nm in diameter first were visualized by electron microscopic examination of filtered stool extracts obtained from an individual who was infected voluntarily with HEV.[225] The authors also reported on the transmission of HEV to nonhuman primates inoculated intravenously with filtered fecal extracts from the infected volunteer. Over the next several years, additional studies[222, 226, 227] expanded the knowledge base to the point that HEV was believed to be related closely to members of the calicivirus family.[227] The key observations leading to this conclusion were based on the biophysical properties of the ET-NANBH virus agent. Specifically, the computed sedimentation coefficient of ET-NANBH virus was 183S and the buoyant density was 1.29 g/cm^3, similar to the caliciviruses and different from the picornaviruses.

Two different cloning strategies were implemented by the scientists at GeneLabs, Inc. in successfully cloning HEV.[224, 228, 229] First, using a differential hybridization screening protocol, one clone (ET1.1) was identified in the complementary DNA library generated from the bile of a cynomolgus macaque experimentally infected with filtered stool extracts from an individual from Burma with acute ET-NANBH.[224, 228] The ET1.1 sequences were proven to be exogenous to the human and primate genomes, and were shown to be associated with infection by the agent of NANBH virus. ET1.1 sequences hybridized specifically to RNA from the liver of an infected macaque, but not to RNA from uninfected liver.[224] In addition, ET1.1 sequences hybridized specifically to stool specimens obtained from ET-NANBH outbreaks, after the nonspecific amplification[230] of complementary DNA constructed from partially purified stool extracts. These data further established the relationship between ET1.1 and ET-NANBH virus.[224] The second cloning strategy used an immunoscreening protocol to identify putative ET-NANBH virus sequences; two clones (designated M 3-2 and M 4-2) were identified in the complementary DNA library constructed directly from human fecal material obtained from an outbreak of HEV in Mexico (M).[229] These clones were verified as being linked to ET-NANBH virus both by serologic studies and by PCR. After the publication of these two manuscripts, the term "HEV" came into popular use to refer to cases of ET-NANBH.

Once HEV-specific clones had been confirmed, contiguous sets of overlapping complementary DNA clones representing the entire genome of the Burmese (B) HEV strain and the M strain were generated.[231, 232] The HEV genome was found to be comprised of three discontinuous open reading frames[231–233] (Fig 6). The first open reading frame (ORF 1) is preceded by 27 nucleotides from a 5′ noncoding region. ORF 1 begins with nucleotide position 28 and extends through position 5107. Several conserved motifs have been identified within ORF 1,[231–235] including a putative methyltransferase (amino acid 56-240), a putative papainlike proteinase (amino acid 433-592), an RNA helicase domain (amino acid 960-1204), and a putative RNA-dependent RNA polymerase (amino acid 1207-1693).[235] The relative positions of these domains within the HEV nonstructural region are different than their positions in other viral genomes within the picornavirus family, but

GENOMIC ORGANIZATION OF
HEPATITIS E VIRUS

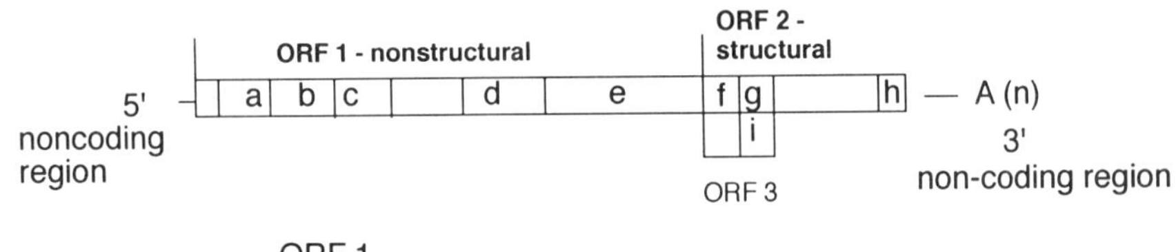

ORF 1
a putative methlytransferase
b putative papain-like domain
c hypervariable region
d RNA helicase domain
e RNA-dependent RNA polymerase domain

ORF 2
f 5' signal sequence
g basic amino acid residues
h epitope B 3-2/M3-2

ORF 3
i epitope B 4-2

FIG 6.
Genomic organization of hepatitis E virus genome is depicted. Several domains within ORF 1 have similarities to domains found in other RNA viruses.

resemble the domain organization of rubella virus (RubV), a flavivirus, and beet necrotic yellow vein virus (BNYVV), a plant furovirus.[235]

The second open reading frame (nucleotide 5147-7327) likely encodes for structural protein(s) (the putative capsid protein) and is translated in a plus 1 reading frame. At the 5' end of ORF 2 are consensus signal peptide sequences, followed by a region rich in basic amino acids, suggesting its association with viral RNA. There are about 150 to 200 adenosine residues at the 3' tail of ORF 2.[231]

A third, small open reading frame, ORF 3, read in the plus-2 frame, was identified by immunoscreening.[229] ORF 3 is situated at the 3' end of ORF 1 beginning with base pair 5106 and extending 369 base pairs through the 5' end of ORF 2. The function of this small protein is unknown.

Except for the regions within ORF-1 that contain conserved motifs, there is little homology with other known viruses.[224, 231, 233, 235] Scientists at GeneLabs, Inc. have proposed that HEV may represent a prototype for a new class of RNA virus, or, alternatively the prototype for a separate genus within the calicivirus family.[231] Phylogenetic analysis of the polymerases and helicases has indicated that HEV is related more closely to RubV and BNYVV.[235] The authors go on to suggest that HEV, BNYVV, and RubV have evolved from a common ancestor and should be grouped separately within the alphalike supergroup of positive-strand viruses.

Genetic Diversity

In studies characterizing the first two strains of HEV, it became apparent that there was a significant nucleotide sequence diversity between the M and B strains.[233] The ET1.1 regions from M and B strains of HEV were compared to a third strain of HEV obtained from an outbreak in Tashkent (in the former Soviet Union).[234] Results indicated that the B strain shared 93% nucleic acid identity with the Tashkent strain, but only 78% with the M strain; the Tashkent strain shared 76% identity with the M strain. A fourth strain of HEV was obtained from an outbreak in Pakistan (P) and its nucleotide sequence determined. In comparing the sequences from three isolates that have been sequenced completely (B, M, and P), the B and P strains were found to be related more closely to each other, whereas the M strain differed from both of them (Table 5). The nucleic acid sequences of HEV M, HEV B, and HEV P differed by about 23% to 24%; the amino acid sequences were 83% to 84% identical in ORF 1, 93% identical in ORF 2, and 87% identical in ORF 3 (see Table 5). The nucleotide sequences of HEV P and B were 93% to 94% similar and the amino acid sequences were 99% identical. Because only a limited number of strains have been sequenced, it is not known how much diversity exists among the HEV strains of the world, nor is it known if there are differences in the pathogenicity associated with the various strains.

TABLE 5.

Comparison of the Three Open Reading Frames for Mexico (M), Burma (B), and Pakistan (P) Strains of Hepatitis E Virus (HEV)*

		Identity (%)			
		Nucleotides		Amino Acids	
Size (Nucleotides)†		HEV (B)	HEV (P)	HEV (B)	HEV (P)
5073/5079/5079	HEV (M)	74	75	83	84
	HEV (P)	93	100	99	100
1977/1980/1980	HEV (M)	81	81	93	93
	HEV (P)	94	100	99	100
369/369/369	HEV (M)	90	91	87	87
	HEV (P)	99	100	100	100

*From Huang C-C, Nguyen D, Fernandez J, et al: *Virology* 1992; 191:550–558. Used by permission.

Although the overall sequence homology between HEV B, M, and P is about 73% to 74% across the genome, there is a region within ORF 1 between nucleotide positions 1500 and 3000 with overall sequence homology of only 67%.[234] There appears to be a hypervariable region between nucleotide positions 2121 and 2329; the sequence similarity between M and B is 58% and that between M and P is 54%.[235] The biologic function of this region and its potential are unknown.

Detection of Exposure to Hepatitis E Virus

Although there is genetic diversity among the various HEV strains, immuno-electronmicroscopy studies performed with viral-like particles and corresponding sera from various epidemics of ET-NANBH indicate that there is likely only one virus type or, alternatively, one class of serologically related viruses that causes ET-NANBH.[236] In addition, the commonality of the various strains was strengthened further by the identification of ET1.1 sequences in nonspecifically amplified complementary DNA obtained from stool extracts from various outbreaks of ET-NANBH.[224] The reactivity of antibodies to recombinant antigens of various strains of HEV also suggested that these strains shared common epitopes.[229] Exposure to HEV has been detected by analyzing serum or stool specimens for viral-like particles by electron microscopy,[225] or by detecting HEV RNA using PCR.[224, 237] Antibodies have been detected by several different techniques using the native virus in various forms (blocking immunofluorescence[238] using HEV-infected liver tissue, immunoelectronmicroscopy using semipurified stool suspensions[225]) or by using engineered antigens, including recombinant antigens (for Western blot assays[239] or enzyme-linked immunosorbent assays[229, 240]) and synthetic peptides.[240]

An increased number of studies was published in 1991 and 1992 linking exposure to HEV with acute viral hepatitis occurring in either epidemics or sporadic cases. Exposure to HEV has been linked to acute sporadic cases in regions where HEV is believed to be endemic, such as Egypt,[241] Hong Kong,[242] Sudan,[243] and areas within the former Soviet Union (Kirgizstan and Turkmentistan[244]). In addition, exposure to HEV has been detected among travelers from industrialized nations returning from HEV-endemic regions.[245–247] Recently, exposure to HEV also has been noted in outbreaks of ET-NANBH in Pakistan,[248] India,[249] and Ethiopia.[250]

Surprisingly, antibodies to HEV were detected in 1% to 2% of volunteer blood donors in the United States, where HEV is not considered to be normally endemic.[240] Although no epidemiologic factors could be identified that would have explained these results (immigration from an endemic country, travel to an endemic country, etc.), the serologic results were "confirmed" by enzyme-linked immunosorbent assays using synthetic peptides and by blocking inhibition assays.[240] It is unclear whether the detection of antibodies to epitopes encoded by HEV sequences necessarily indicates exposure to HEV or, rather, the detection of cross-reacting antibodies. There also remains the possibility that there may be an animal reservoir for HEV that could serve as a source of HEV infection in man. There has been a recent report indicating that acute viral hepatitis, complete with the icteric phase of infection, can be produced in pigs experimentally infected with HEV.[251] The potential role of animals in the transmission of HEV remains an area that has not been explored in depth.

The successful detection of antibodies or viral sequences, where infection with an ET-NANBH virus agent was suspected, provides objective data that HEV is endemic in many geographic areas and likely is responsible for a significant number of cases of acute, sporadic viral hepatitis throughout the world. These data also provide evidence, although indirect, that there are common epitopes shared by the various HEV strains in endemic regions.

Natural History of Hepatitis E Virus Infection

Although there is no evidence that HEV produces chronic liver disease, it is unclear how long the virus persists in biologic fluids (serum, fecal material), how long antibodies persist after infection, and whether antibody positivity confers immunity to reinfection. Nonhuman primates have been used successfully as an animal model in which to study HEV infection.[222] In recent reports, investigators have monitored liver enzyme levels, antibodies to HEV, and viral presence in serum, bile, or stool by PCR.[252, 253] Elevations in levels of liver enzymes often were detected in serum 15 to 30 days after inoculations and then returned to normal. In general, the virus was detected in stool, bile, or serum before liver enzyme levels became elevated and persisted for 10 to 30 days, disappearing shortly after the appearance of specific antibodies to HEV. As reported above, HEV RNA also has been detected in the stool of HEV-infected individuals.[224] Recently, this technique was applied to stool specimens obtained from epidemic and sporadic cases of non-A, non-B hepatitis in India, where PCR was used to identify the etiologic agent as being HEV.[254, 255]

Ordinarily, the natural history of HEV infection would be difficult to trace in humans. There have been two reports of volunteer transmission of HEV, however, one in 1983[225] and one in 1993.[256] In both cases, the investigators were able to detect virus in stools before the observed elevation in liver enzyme levels. In the 1993 study, HEV RNA was detected in serum on day 22 after inoculation and preceded the development of symptoms by about 1 week.[256] The virus was detected in several additional specimens before disappearing on day 46, when a peak in the alanine aminotransferase level was noted. Antibodies were detected first on day 41 and persisted for 2 years.

The first demonstration of HEV RNA in serum in a naturally occurring infection was noted in a study in Egypt in which HEV RNA was detected via PCR in four children with acute viral hepatitis (Table 6).[257] HEV RNA was not detected in subsequent serum samples (about 10, 20, or 30 days after the appearance of symp-

TABLE 6.

Anti-HEV Antibody and HEV RNA From Serial Serum Samples*†

Patient	Days After Onset	ALT (IU/L)	IgM (S/CO)‡	IgG (S/CO)	PCR
1	3	980	5	12.5	+
	13	38	2.5	10	−
	23	24	1.5	8.1	−
	33	ND	0.9	5.8	−
2	3	555	11.8	14.9	+
	13	28	3.2	14.3	−
	23	20	1.9	13.1	−
	33	ND	1	11.9	−
3	2	435	4.8	16.5	+
	12	25	2.3	14.2	−
	22	18	1.4	12.7	−
	32	ND	1	9.9	−
4	2	1,080	16.4	11.6	+
	12	30	7.1	10.3	−
	22	22	3.1	7.7	−
	32	ND	1.6	5.7	−

*From Schlauder GG, Dawson GJ, Mushahwar IK, et al: *Lancet* 1993; 341:378. Used by permission.
†HEV = hepatitis E virus; ALT = alanine aminotransferase; S/CO = XX; PCR = polymerase chain reaction; ND = not determined.
‡S/CO = sample to cutoff value; >1.0 considered positive.

toms). Using enzyme-linked immunosorbent assays employing recombinant antigens, both IgG and IgM class antibodies were noted at the time of presentation. High absorbance values were observed initially and decreased over time. HEV appears to produce a viremic stage, but it is short lived, disappearing soon after the appearance of specific antibodies. As noted in previous studies, the specific anti-HEV IgM response declines rapidly and usually becomes undetectable by 60 days after the initial appearance of symptoms.[241, 242, 244]

Although there have been reports that IgG class antibodies may become undetectable by 6 to 12 months after the initial infection,[241] other reports suggest that antibodies are long-lasting. In one study, at least one of two patients remained anti-HEV IgG–positive for 1 year after infection,[242] whereas in a second study, no significant decrease in anti-HEV IgG reactivity was seen for 2 years after the initial HEV infection.[244] In yet another investigation, only a slight decline in antibody titer occurred over 4½ years after a diagnosed infection.[247] Specific IgG against HEV was detected for more than 2 years after a volunteer was infected.[256] These data suggest that, although the immune response to HEV is short lived in some cases, it generally persists for years after the initial infection.

Hepatitis E Virus Cell Culture

There have been two reports of the cultivation of HEV in cell culture.[258, 259] In one of these studies,[259] the virus particles produced in cell culture were shown to be aggregated specifically by acute-phase sera of individuals obtained from different known cases of HEV infection. In addition, the investigators demonstrated that anti-HEV IgG identified a protein band of about 76 kd after Western blotting, which should correspond to the expected size of the ORF 2 protein. Large-scale successful propagation of HEV in culture will be very important in establishing the utility of some of the above mentioned antibody tests, which in many cases do not use infectious virions as the antigenic target. In this same study, it was demonstrated that neutralizing antibodies are produced in HEV-infected individuals. Further studies in this area will be increasingly important as vaccines are discussed for the potential protection and control of HEV.

Summary

Techniques in molecular biology were important for the discovery of HEV, and now are being used to diagnose and trace the natural history of HEV infection. Many of the convenient diagnostic assays rely on recombinant antigens as their antigenic target. In addition, the natural history of infection is being traced using nucleic acid probes.

CONCLUDING COMMENTS

As illustrated by the many examples provided in this chapter, the tools and techniques of molecular biology have provided many benefits. The genotype diversity of the various hepatotropic viruses is being studied; eventually, we may be able to ascertain the rate(s) of evolution for each of the viruses as well as to correlate genetic changes with the severity and prognosis of disease. Nucleic acid probe technology has been applied to each of the viruses and has elucidated viral presence in biologic fluids and tissues at various stages of infection and disease. It is likely that, in the near future, we may witness the widespread application of probe technology in combination with fully automated immunoassays for the diagnosis and prognosis of these infections. Recombinant antigens expressed in various host cells are being used to detect antibodies to HBV and HCV, eliminating the necessity of using blood or blood products from individuals who have been exposed to parenterally transmitted viruses. Vaccines using recombinant antigens are being used for HBV and may be used in the future for HCV, HAV, and HEV.

REFERENCES

1. Deinhardt F: Prevention of viral hepatitis A: Past, present and future. *Vaccine* 1992; 10(suppl 1):S10–14.

2. Melnick JL: Properties and classification of hepatitis A virus. *Vaccine* 1992; 10(suppl 1):S24–26.

3. Siegl G: Replication of hepatitis A virus and processing of proteins. *Vaccine* 1992; 10(suppl 1):S32–34.

4. Hollinger FB, et al: Hepatitis A virus, in Fields BN, et al (eds): *Field Virology,* 2nd ed. New York, Raven Press, 1990, pp 631–667.

5. Jewell DA et al: Hepatitis A virus 3C proteinase substrate specificity. *Biochemistry* 1992; 31:7826–7829.

6. Kusov YY, et al: Intramolecular cleavage of hepatitis A virus (HAV) precursor protein P1-P2 by recombinant HAV proteinase 3C. *J Virol* 1992; 66:6794–6796.

7. Siegl G, et al: Recent advances in hepatitis A vaccine development. *Virus Res* 1990; 17:75–92.

8. Wimmer E, et al: Hepatitis A virus and the molecular biology of Picornaviruses: A case for a new genus of the family Picornaviridae, in Hollinger FB, Lemon SM, Margolis HS (eds): *Viral Hepatitis and Liver Disease. Baltimore, Williams & Wilkins, 1991, pp 31–41.*

9. Ticehurst JR et al: Replication of hepatitis A virus: New ideas from studies with cloned cDNA, in Ehrenfeld E, Semler BL (eds): *Molecular Aspects of Picornavirus Infection and Detection* Washington, DC, ASM Press, 1989, pp 27–50.

10. Jansen RW, et al: Molecular epidemiology of human hepatitis A virus defined by an antigen-capture polymersae chain reaction. *Proc Natl Acad Sci U S A* 1990; 87:2867–2871.

11. Robertson BH, et al: Epidemiologic patterns of wild-type hepatitis A virus determined by genetic variation. *J Infect Dis* 1991; 163:286–292.

12. Lemon SM, et al: Genetic, antigenic and biological differences between strains of hepatitis A virus. *Vaccine* 1992; 10(suppl):S40–44.

13. Robertson BH, et al: Genetic relatedness of hepatitis A virus strains recovered from different geographical regions. *J Gen Virol* 1992; 73:1365–1367.

14. Ping L-H, et al: Antigenic structure of human hepatitis A virus defined by analysis of escape mutants selected against murine monoclonal antibodies. *J Virol* 1992; 66:2208–2216.

15. Nainan OV, et al: Identification of amino acids located on the antibody binding sites of human hepatitis A virus. *Virology* 1992; 91:984–987.

16. Lemon SM, et al: Immunogenicity and antigenicity of chimeric picornaviruses which express hepatitis A virus (HAV) amino terminus of VP1 of HAV. *Virology* 1992; 188:285–295.

17. Margolis HS, et al: Who should receive hepatitis A vaccine? Considerations for the development of an immunization strategy. *Vaccine* 1992; 10(suppl):S85–87.

18. Katz SL et al: Prospects for immunizing against hepatitis A virus, in *New Vaccine Development: Establishing Priorities Diseases of Importance in the United States*. Washington, DC, National Academy Press, 1985, pp 252–260.

19. Kane M: Perspectives on the control of hepatitis A virus by vaccination. *Vaccine* 1992; 10 (suppl 1):93–96.

20. Provost PJ, et al: An inactivated hepatitis A virus vaccine prepared from infected marmoset liver. *Proc Soc Exp Biol Med* 1978; 159:201–203.

21. Provost PJ, et al: Propagation of human hepatitis A virus in cell culture in vitro. *Proc Soc Exp Biol Med* 1979; 160:213–221.

22. Provost PJ: In vitro propagation of hepatitis A virus, in Gerety RJ (ed): *Hepatitis A*. Orlando, Academic Press, 1984, pp 245–261.

23. Andre FE, et al: Inactivated candidate vaccines for hepatitis A. *Prog Med Virol* 1990; 37:72–95.

24. Flehmig B, et al: Prospects of a hepatitis A virus vaccine. *Prog Med Virol* 1990; 37:56–71.

25. Werzberger A, et al: A controlled trial of a formalin-inactivated hepatitis A vaccine in healthy children. *N Engl J Med* 1992; 327:453–457.

26. Tilzey AJ, et al: Clinical trial with inactivated hepatitis A vaccine and recommendations for its use. *BMJ* 1992; 304:1272–1276.

27. Tilzey AJ, et al: Effect of hepatitis A vaccination schedules on immune response. *Vaccine* 1992; 10(suppl 1):S121–123.

28. Andre FE, et al: Clinical assessment of the safety and efficacy of an inactivated hepatitis A vaccine: Rationale and summary of findings. *Vaccine* 1992; 10(suppl 1):S160–168.

29. Theilmann L, et al: Reactogenicity and immunogenicity of three different lots of a hepatitis A vaccine. *Vaccine* 1992; 10(suppl 1):S132–134.

30. Schiff ER: Atypical clinical manifestations of hepatitis A. *Vaccine* 1992; 10(suppl):S18–20.

31. Sjoren MH, et al: Hepatitis A virus in stool during clinical relapse. *Ann Intern Med* 1987; 106:221–229.

32. Glikson M, et al: Relapsing hepatitis A: Review of 14 cases and literature survey. *Medicine (Baltimore)* 1992; 71:14–23.

33. Fagan E, et al: Persistence of hepatitis A virus in fulminant hepatitis and after liver transplantation. *J Med Virol* 1990; 30:131–136.

34. Rosenblum LS, et al: Hepatitis A outbreak in a neonatal intensive care unit: Risk factors for transmission and evidence of prolonged viral excretion among preterm infants. *J Infect Dis* 1991; 164:476–492.

35. Tiollais P, et al: The hepatitis B virus. *Nature* 1985; 317:489–495.

36. Gerlich WH, et al: Functions of hepatitis B virus protein and virus assembly, in Hollinger FB, Lemon S, Margolis H (eds): *Viral Hepatitis and Liver Disease*. Baltimore, Williams & Wilkins, 1991, pp 121–134.

37. Radiwell G, et al: Mutational analysis of the hepatitis B virus P gene product: Domain structure and RNase H activity. *J Virol* 1990; 64:613–620.

38. Rossner MT: Review: Hepatitis B virus X-gene product: A promiscuous transcriptional activator. *J Med Virol* 1992; 36:101–117.

39. Yen TSB: Regulation of hepatitis B virus gene expression. *Seminars in Virology*, 1993; 4:33–42.

40. Carman W, et al: Genetic variation in hepatitis B virus. *Gastroenterology* 1992; 102:711–719.

41. Harrison TJ, et al: Variants of hepatitis B virus. *Vox Sang* 1992; 63:161–167.

42. Carman W, et al: Viral genetic variations: Hepatitis B virus as a clinical example. *Lancet* 1993; 341:349–353.

43. Courouce AM, et al: HBs antigen subtypes. *Bibliotheca Haematologica* 1976; 42:1.

44. Norder H, et al: Molecular basis of hepatitis B virus serotype variations within the four major subtypes. *J Gen Virol* 1992; 73:3141–3145.

45. Peters M, et al: Immunology and the liver. *Hepatology* 1991; 13:977–994.

46. Davies SE, et al: Hepatitis histological findings after transplantation for chronic hepatitis B virus infection, including a unique pattern of fibrosing cholestatic hepatitis. *Hepatology* 1991; 13: 150–157.

47. Lau JV, et al: High-level expression of hepatitis B viral antigens in fibrosing cholestatic hepatitis. *Gastroenterology* 1992; 102:956–962.

48. Guilhot S, et al: Hepatitis B virus (HBV) specific cytotoxic T-cell response in humans: Production of target cells by stable expressions of HBV-encoded proteins in immortalized human B-cell lines. *J Virol* 1992; 66:2670–2678.

49. Missale G, et al: HLA-A31- and HLA-AW68-restricted cytotoxic T cell responses to a single hepatitis B virus nucleocapsid epitope during acute viral hepatitis. *J Exp Med* 1993; 177: 751–752.

50. Penna A, et al: Hepatitis B virus (HBV) specific cytotoxic T-cell (CTL) response in humans: Characterization of HLA class II-restricted CTLs that recognize endogenously synthesized HBV envelope antigens. *J Virol* 1992; 92:1193–1198.

51. Kamogawa Y, et al: Hepatitis B virus-DNA transected myeloma cell-specific cytotoxic T cells in chronic hepatitis B patients. *Virology* 1992; 191:321–326.

52. Barnaba V, et al: Recognition of hepatitis B virus envelope proteins by liver-infiltrating lymphocytes in chronic HBV infection. *J Immunol* 1989; 143:2650–2655.

53. Ando K, et al: Cytotoxic T cell induced fulminant hepatitis in HBV envelope transgenic mice (abstract), in *Molecular Biology of Hepatitis B Viruses*. University of California, San Diego, 1992; p 136.

54. Gilles PN, et aL: HBsAg sensitizes the hepatocyte to injury by physiologic concentrations of inteferon-gamma. *Hepatology* 1992; 16:655–663.

55. Robbins D, et al: Serological detection of HBeAg and anti-HBe using automated microparticle enzyme immunoassays. *J Virol Methods* 1992; 38:267–287.

56. Marayuma T, et al: Serological evidence of ongoing immune responses in asymptomatic and symptomatic hepatitis B carriers (abstract), in *Molecular Biology of Hepatitis B Viruses*. University of California, San Diego, 1992, p 132.

57. Cuthbert JA: Hepatitis B–molecular variants with clinical significance. *Am J Med Sci* 1992; 302:396–403.

58. Brunetto MR, et al: Wildtype and e antigen-minus hepatitis B viruses and course of chronic hepatitis. *Proc Natl Acad Sci U S A* 1991; 88:4186–4190.

59. Naoumov NV, et al: Pre core mutant hepatitis B virus infection and liver disease. *Gastroenterology* 1992; 102:538–543.

60. Carman WF, et al: Pre-core sequence variation in Chinese isolates of hepatitis B virus. *J Infect Dis* 1992; 165:127–133.

61. Tur-Kaspa R, et al: Hepatitis B virus pre-core mutants are identical in carriers from various ethnic origins and are associated with a range of liver disease severity. *Hepatology* 1992; 16:1338–1342.

62. Chuang WL, et al: Pre-core mutations and core clustering mutations in chronic hepatitis B virus infection. *Gastroenterology* 1993; 104:263–271.

63. Okamato H, et al: Hepatitis B viruses with pre-core region defects prevail in persistently infected hosts along with seroconversion to the antibody against e antigen. *J Virol* 1990; 64:1298–1303.

64. Xu J, Brown D, et al: Absence of hepatitis B virus pre-core mutants in patients with chronic hepatitis B responding to interferon. *Hepatology* 1992; 15:1002–1006.

65. Lo ES, Lo YM, et al: Detection of hepatitis B-pre-cores mutant by cellele specific polymerase chain reaction. *J Clin Pathol* 1992; 45:689–692.

66. Hasegawa H, et al: Lack of association of hepatitis B virus pre-core mutations with fulminant hepatitis B in the USA. *Hepatology* 1991; 14:78A.

67. Manzin A, et al: Sequence analysis of the hepatitis B virus pre-C region in hepatocellular carcinoma (HCC) and nontumoral liver tissues from HCC patients. *Virology* 1992; 188:890–895.

68. Schlicht HJ, et al: The quaternary structure, antigenicity and aggregation behavior of the secretary core protein of human hepatitis B virus are determined by its signal sequence. *J Virol* 1991; 65:6817–6825.

69. Tong SP, et al: Replication capacities of natural and artificial stop codon mutants of hepatitis B virus: Relevance of pregenome encapsidation signal. *Virology* 1992; 191:237–245.

70. Fiordalisi G, et al: High genomic variability in the pre-C region of hepatitis B virus in anti-HBe, HBV DNA positive chronic hepatitis. *J Med Virol* 1990; 31:297–300.

71. Raimando G, et al: A new hepatitis virus variant in a chronic carrier with multiple episodes of viral reactivation and acute hepatitis. *Virology* 1990; 179:64–68.

72. Ackrill AM, et al: Comparison of the pre-core/core hepatitis B virus region in liver tissue and serum from patients with chronic hepatitis B infection. *J Hepatol* 1992; 16:224–227.

73. Peterson DL, et al: Antigenic structure of hepatitis B surface antigen: Identification of the "d" subtypes determinant by chemical modification and use of monoclonal antibodies. *J Immunol* 1984; 132:920–927.

74. Carman WF, et al: Vaccine-induced escape mutant of hepatitis B virus. *Lancet* 1990; 336:325–329.

75. Okamoto H, et al: Mutations within the S gene of hepatitis-B virus transmitted from mothers to babies immunized with hepatitis-B immune globulin and vaccine. *Pediatr Res* 1992; 32:264–268.

76. McMahon G, et al: Genetic alterations in the gene encoding the major HBsAg: DNA and immunological analysis of recurrent HBsAg derived from monoclonal antibody-treated liver transplant patients. *Hepatology* 1992; 15:757–766.

77. Fujii H, et al: Gly 145 to Arg substitution in HBs antigen of immune escape mutant of hepatitis B virus. *Biochem Biophys Res Commun* 1992; 184:1152–1157.

78. Harrison TJ, et al: Independent emergence of a vaccine-induced escape mutant of hepatitis B virus. *J Hepatol* 1991; 13:5105–5107.

79. Waters JA, et al: Loss of the common "A" determinant of hepatitis B surface antigen by a vaccine induced escape mutant. *J Clin Invest* 1992; 90:2543–2547.

80. Okamoto H, et al: The loss of subtypic determinants in alleles, d/y or w/r on hepatitis B surface antigen. *Mol Immunol* 1989; 26:197–205.

81. Karthigesu V, et al: Breakthrough infections among children immunized against hepatitis B due to a novel variant (abstract), in *Molecular Biology of Hepatitis B Viruses*. University of California, San Diego, 1992, p 101.

82. Moriyama K, et al: Immunoselected hepatitis B virus mutant. *Lancet* 1991; 337:125.

83. Fernholz D, et al: Replicating and virions secreting hepatitis B mutant virus unable to produce pre S2 protein. *J Hepatol* 1991; 13:102–104.

84. Gerken G, et al: Hepatitis B defective virus with rearrangements in the pre S gene during chronic HBV infection. *Virology* 1991; 183:555–565.

85. Tran A, et al: Emergence and takeover by hepatitis B virus (HBV) with rearrangements in the preS/S and Pre-C/c genes during chronic HBV infection. *J Virol* 1991; 65:3566–3574.

86. Santantonio T, et al: Hepatitis B virus genomes that cannot synthesize pre S2 proteins occur frequently and as dominant virus populations in chronic carriers in Italy. *Virology* 1992; 188:948–952.

87. Blum HE, et al: Naturally occurring missense mutation in the polymerase gene terminating hepatitis B virus replication. *J Virol* 1992; 65:1836–1842.

88. Repp R, et al: Detection of a hepatitis B virus variant with a truncated X gene and enhancer II. *Arch Virol* 1992; 125:299–304.

89. Kim SH, et al: Replication of a mutant hepatitis B virus with a fused X-C reading frame in hepatoma cell. *J Gen Virol* 1992; 73:2421–2424.

90. Okamoto H, et al: Trans complementation among naturally occurring deletion mutants of hepatitis B virus and integrated viral DNA for the production of viral particles with mutant genomes in hepatoma cell lines. *J Gen Virol* 1993; 74:407–414.

91. Wands JR, et al: Molecular pathogenesis of liver disease during persistent hepatitis B virus infection. *Semin Liver Dis* 1992; 12:252–264.

92. Wright TL, et al: Hepatitis B virus and apparent fulminant non-A, non-B hepatitis. *Lancet* 1992; 339:952–955.

93. Sallie R, et al: Occult HBV in NANB fulminant hepatitis. *Lancet* 1993; 341:123.

94. Wang JT, et al: Detection of hepatitis B virus DNA by polymerase chain reaction in plasma of volunteer blood donors negative for hepatitis B surface antigen. *J Infect Dis* 1991; 163:397–399.

95. Courgaget P, et al: Detection of hepatitis B virus DNA by polymerase chain reaction in HBsAg negative Senegalese patients suffering from cirrhosis or primary liver cancer. *FEMS Microbiol Lett* 1991; 83:35–38.

96. Fagan EA, et al: Detection of hepatitis B virus DNA sequences in liver in HBsAg seronegative patients with liver disease with and without anti-HBc antibodies. *Q Rev Med* 1991; 78:123–134.

97. Paterlini P, et al: Polymerase chain reaction to detect hepatitis B virus DNA and RNA sequences in primary liver cancers from patients negative for hepatitis B surface antigen. *N Engl J Med* 1990; 323:80–85.

98. Rumi MG, et al: Serum hepatitis B virus DNA detects cryptic hepatitis B virus infections in multitransfused hemophilia patients. *Blood* 1990; 75:1654–1658.

99. Tanaka T, et al: Persistence of hepatitis B virus DNA after serological clearance of hepatitis B virus. *Liver* 1990; 10:6–10.

100. Kaneko S, et al: Detection of hepatitis B virus DNA in serum by polymerase chain reaction. *Gastroenterology* 1990; 99:799–804.

101. Carman WF, et al: Incidence of hepatitis B viremia, detected using the polymerase chain reaction, after successful therapy of hepatitis B virus carriers with interferon. *J Med Virol* 1991; 34:114–118.

102. Kuhns M, et al: Serum and liver hepatitis B virus DNA in chronic hepatitis B after sustained loss of surface antigens. *Gastroenterology* 1992; 103:1649–1656.

103. Gerken G, et al: Assay of hepatitis B virus DNA by polymerase chain reaction and its relationship to pre-S and S-encoded viral surface antigens. *Hepatology* 1991; 13:158–166.

104. Petit MA, et al: Pre-S antigen expression and anti-pre S response in hepatitis B virus infections: Relationship to serum HBV-DNA, intrahepatic HBcAg, liver damage and specific T-cell response. *Arch Virol Suppl* 1992; 4:105–112.

105. Zoulim F, et al: New assays for the quantitative determination of viral markers in the management of chronic hepatitis infection. *J Clin Microbiol* 1992; 30:1111–1119.

106. Budkowska A, et al: Anti-preS responses and viral clearance in chronic hepatitis B virus infection. *Hepatology* 1992; 15:26–31.

107. Budkowska A, et al: A biphasic pattern of anti-pre-S responses in acute hepatitis B virus infection. *Hepatology* 1990; 12:1271–1277.

108. Milich DR: T-cell and B-cell recognition of hepatitis B viral antigens. *Immunol Today* 1988; 9:380–386.

109. Thoma HA, et al: Does preS2 have the same effect in improving the HBV immune response as preS1?, in Hollinzer FB, et al (eds): *Viral Hepatitis and Liver Disease*. Baltimore, Williams & Wilkins, 1991, pp 736–741.

110. Neurath AR, et al: Identification and chemical synthesis of a host cell receptor binding site on hepatitis B virus. *Cell* 1986; 45:429–436.

111. Petit MA, et al: HepG2 cell binding activities of different hepatitis B virus isolates: Inhibitory effect of anti-HBs and anti-preS1(21-47). *Virology* 1991; 180:483–491.

112. Petit MA, et al: Inhibitory activity of monoclonal antibody F35.25 on the interaction between hepatocytes (HepG2 cells) and preS1-specific ligands. *Mol Immunol* 1991; 28:517–521.

113. Pontisso P, et al: Identification of an attachment site for human liver plasma membranes on hepatitis B virus particles. *Virology* 1989; 173:522–530.

114. Pontisso P, et al Human liver plasma membranes contain receptors for the hepatitis B virus pre-S1 region and, via polymerized human serum albumin, for the pre-S2 region. *J Virol* 1989; 63:1981–1988.

115. Neurath AR, et al: Search for the hepatitis B virus cell receptors reveals binding sites for interleukin 6 on the virus envelope protein. *J Exp Med* 1992; 175:461–469.

116. Neurath AR, et al: Cells transfected with human interleukin 6 cDNA acquire binding sites for the hepatitis B virus envelope protein. *J Exp Med* 1992; 175:1561–1569.

117. Petit MA, et al: PreS1 specific binding proteins as potential receptors for hepatitis B virus in human hepatocytes. *Virology* 1992; 187:211–222.

118. Petit M, et al: Identification of natural human interleukin 6 protein species as the pre S1 binding proteins involved in hepatitis B virus-hepatocyte interaction (abstract), in *Molecular Biology of Hepatitis B Viruses*. University of California, San Diego, 1992, p 56.

119. Yang X, et al: Specific binding of recombinant HBsAg particles to apolipoprotein H (abstract), in *Molecular Biology of Hepatitis B Viruses*, University of California, San Diego, 1992, p 57.

120. Gray JJ, et al: Laboratory techniques in the diagnosis and assessment of hepatitis B virus infection. *Genitourin Med* 1992; 68:263–268.

121. Eble K, et al: Improvements in anti-HBc detection by treating specimens with reducing agent in an automated microparticle enzyme immunoassay. *J Clin Microbiol* 1991; 29:611–616.

122. Spronk A, et al: Improvements in anti-HBc detection by treating specimens with reducing agent in an automated microparticle enzyme immunoassay. *J Clin Microbiol* 1991; 29:611–616.

123. Ostrow D, et al: Quantitation of hepatitis B surface antibody by an automated microparticle enzyme immunoassay. *J Virol Methods* 1991; 32:265–287.

124. Chernesky MA, et al: The diagnosis of acute viral hepatitis A or B by microparticle enzyme immunoassays. *J Virol Methods* 1992; 38:267–287.

125. Khalil OS, et al: Abbott Prism: A multichannel heterogeneous chemiluminescence immunoassay analyzer. *Clin Chem* 1991; 37:1540–1547.

126. Wolf-Rogers J, et al: A chemiluminescent microparticle-membrane capture immunoassay for the detection of antibodies to hepatitis B core antigen. *J Immunol Methods* 1990; 133:191–198.

127. Septak M, et al: VISTA® qualitative enzyme immunoassay method for detection of hepatitis B surface antigen in serum and plasma samples. *Clin Chem* 1992; 38:S0723.

128. Bouveresse E, et al: A chemiluminescent enzyme immunoassay for the detection of hepatitis B surface antigen (HBsAg). *Clin Chem* 1992; 38:S0669.

129. Perrillo R, et al: Monitoring of antiviral therapy by the quantitative evaluation of hepatitis B e antigen: A comparison to HBV DNA testing. *Hepatology* 1993; 18:1306–1312.

130. Hadziyannis SJ, et al: Serum anti-HBc IgM levels in establishing the etiology of liver cell damage in anti-HBe positive chronic hepatitis B virus infection. *Hepatology* 1991; 14:83A.

131. Gerken G, et al: Clinical evaluation of ligase chain reaction (LCR) assay for detection of HBV DNA in hepatitis B virus (HBV) infection. *Hepatology* 1992; 16:66A.

132. Jeffers LJ, et al: Evaluation of an assay for quantitative detection of HBV DNA in human sera. *Hepatology* 1992; 16:105A.

133. Choo Q-L, et al: Isolation of a cDNA clone derived from a blood-borne non-A, non-B viral hepatitis genome. *Science* 1989; 244:359–362.

134. Bradley DW: The agents of non-A, non-B viral hepatitis. *J Virol Methods* 1985; 10:307–319.

135. Bradley DW, et al: Posttransfusion non-A, non-B hepatitis: Physiochemical properties of two distinct agents. *J Infect Dis* 1983; 48:254–264.

136. He L-F, et al: Determining the size of non-A, non-B hepatitis virus by filtration. *J Infect Dis* 1978; 156:636–640.

137. Feinstone SM, et al: Inactivation of hepatitis B virus and non-A, non-B hepatitis by chloroform. *Infect Immun* 1983; 41:816–823.

138. Miyamoto H, et al: Extraordinarily low density of hepatitis C virus estimated by sucrose density gradient centrifugation and the polymerase chain reaction. *J Gen Virol* 1992; 73:715–718.

139. Carrick RJ, et al: Examination of the buoyant density of hepatitis C virus by the polymerase chain reaction. *J Virol Methods* 1992; 39:279–290.

140. Choo Q-L, et al: Genetic organization and diversity of the hepatitis C virus. *Proc Natl Acad Sci U S A* 1991; 88:2451–2455.

141. Houghton M, et al: Molecular biology of the hepatitis C viruses: Implications for diagnosis, development and control of viral disease. *Hepatology* 1991; 14:381–388.

142. Han JH, et al: Characterization of the terminal regions of hepatitis C virus RNA: Identification of conserved sequences in the 5′ untranslated region and poly(A) tails at the 3′ end. *Proc Natl Acad Sci U S A* 1991; 88:1711–1715.

143. Okamoto H, et al: Detection of hepatitis C virus RNA by a two-stage polymerase chain reaction with two pairs of primers deduced from the 5′-noncoding region. *Jpn J Exp Med* 1990; 60:215–222.

144. Okamoto H, et al: Full-length sequence of a hepatitis C virus genome having poor homology to reported isolates: Comparative study of four distinct genotypes. *Virology* 1992; 188:331–341.

145. Bukh J, et al: Sequence analysis of the 5′ noncoding region of hepatitis C virus. *Proc Natl Acad Sci U S A* 1992; 89:4942–4946.

146. Tsukiyama-Kohara K, et al: Internal ribosome entry site within hepatitis C virus RNA. *J Virol* 1992; 66:1476–1483.

147. Yoo BJ, et al: Regulation of gene expression by the 5′ and 3′ regions of hepatitis C viral RNA (abstract), in *Hepatitis C Virus and Related Viruses: Molecular Virology and Pathogenesis First Annual Meeting.* Venice, Italy, 1992, p 26.

148. Han J, et al: Group specific sequences and secondary structures at the 3′ end of HCV genome and its implication for viral replication. *Nucleic Acids Res* 1992; 20:3520.

149. Miller RH, et al: Hepatitis C virus shares amino acid sequence similarity with pestiviruses and flaviviruses as well as members of two plant virus supergroups. *Proc Natl Acad Sci U S A* 1990; 87:2057–2061.

150. Takamizawa A, et al: Structure and organization of the hepatitis C virus genome isolated from human carriers. *J Virol* 1991; 65:1105–1113.

151. Weiner AJ, et al: Variable and hypervariable domains are found in the regions of HCV corresponding to the flavivirus envelope and NS1 proteins and the pestivirus envelope glycoproteins. *Virology* 1991; 180:842–848.

152. Hijikata M, et al: Gene mapping of the putative structural region of the hepatitis C virus genome by *in vitro* processing analysis. *Proc Natl Acad Sci U S A* 1991; 88:5547–5551.

153. Manabe S, et al: Expression of the entire HCV genome in tissue culture cells (abstract), in *Hepatitis C Virus and Related Viruses: Molecular Virology and Pathogenesis First Annual Meeting.* Venice, Italy, 1992, p 16.

154. Grakoui A, et al: Hepatitis C virus polyprotein processing (abstract), in *Hepatitis C Virus and Related Viruses: Molecular Virology and Pathogenesis First Annual Meeting.* Venice, Italy, 1992, p 27.

155. Takeuchi K, et al: The putative nucleocapsid and envelope protein genes of hepatitis C virus determined by comparison of the nucleotide sequences of two isolates derived from an experimentally infected chimpanzee and healthy human carriers. *J Gen Virol* 1990; 71:3027–3033.

156. Weiner AJ, et al: Evidence of immune selection of hepatitis C putative envelope glycoprotein variants: Potential role in chronic HCV infections. *Proc Natl Acad Sci U S A* 1992; 89:3468–3472.

157. Kato N, et al: Molecular structure of the Japanese hepatitis C viral genome. *FEBS Lett* 1991; 280:325–328.

158. Choo Q-L, et al: The NS3 domain of HCV encodes a serine protease responsible for cleavage of nonstructural proteins from the polyprotein precursor (abstract), in *Hepatitis C Virus and Related Viruses: Molecular Virology and Pathogenesis First Annual Meeting.* Venice, Italy, 1992, p 25.

159. Chambers TJ, et al: Evidence that the N-terminal domain of nonstructural protein NS3 from yellow fever virus is a serine protease responsible for site specific cleavages in the viral polyprotein. *Proc Natl Acad Sci U S A* 1990; 87:8898–8902.

160. Okayama H, et al: European Patent Application No. 91305717.0, 1992, p 11.

161. Argos P: A sequence motif in many polymerases. *Nucleic Acids Res* 1988; 16:9909–9916.

162. Poch O, et al: Identification of four conserved motifs among the RNA-dependent polymerase encoding elements. *EMBO J* 1989; 8:3867–3874.

163. Inchauspe G, et al: Genomic structure of the human prototype strain H of hepatitis C virus: Comparison with American and Japanese isolates. *Proc Natl Acad Sci U S A* 1991; 88:10292–10296.

164. Cha T-A, et al: At least five related, but distinct hepatitis C viral genotypes exist. *Proc Natl Acad Sci U S A* 1992; 89:7144–7148.

165. Nakao T, et al: Typing of hepatitis C virus by restriction fragment length polymorphism. *J Gen Virol* 1991; 72:2105–2112.

166. Martell M, et al: Hepatitis C virus (HCV) circulates as a population of different but closely related genomes: Quasispecies nature of HCV genome distribution. *J Virol* 1992; 66:3225–3229.

167. Murakawa K, et al: Heterogeneity within the nonstructural protein 5-encoding region of hepatitis C viruses from a single patient. *Gene* 1992; 117:229–232.

168. Hijikata M, et al: Hypervariable regions in the putative glycoprotein of hepatitis C virus. *Biochem Biophys Res Commun* 1991; 175:220–228.

169. Kato N, et al: Marked sequence diversity in the putative envelope proteins of hepatitis C viruses. *Virus Res* 1992; 22:107–123.

170. Kato N, et al: Sequence diversity of hepatitis C viral genomes. *Mol Biol Med* 1990; 7:495–501.

171. Lesniewski RR, et al: The hypervariable 5′-terminus of HCV E2/NS1 encodes antigenically distinct variants. *J Med Virol,* in 1993; 40:150–156.

172. Okamoto H, et al: Genetic drift of hepatitis C virus during an 8.2 year infection in a chimpanzee: Variability and stability. *Virology* 1992; 190:894–899.

173. Farci P, et al: Lack of protective immunity against reinfection with hepatitis C virus. *Science* 1992; 258:135–140.

174. Houghton M, et al: Vaccine approaches to HCV (abstract), in *Hepatitis C Virus and Related Viruses: Molecular Virology and Pathogenesis First Annual Meeting.* Venice, Italy, 1992, p 144.

175. Schlauder GG, et al: Detection of the hepatitis C virus genome in acute and chronic experimental infection in chimpanzees. *J Clin Microbiol* 1991; 29:2175–2179.

176. Farci P, et al: The natural history of infection with hepatitis C virus (HCV) in chimpanzees: Comparison of serologic responses measured with first- and second-generation assays and relationship to HCV viremia. *J Infect Dis* 1992; 165:1006–1011.

177. Young KK, et al: Detection of hepatitis C virus RNA by a combined reverse transcription-polymerase chain reaction assay. *J Clin Microbiol* 1993; 31:882–886.

178. Seelig R, et al: PCR in the diagnosis of viral hepatitis. *Ann Med* 1992; 124:225–230.

179. Schlauder GG, et al: Detection of hepatitis C viral RNA by the polymerase chain reaction in serum of patients with post-transfusion non-A, non-B hepatitis. *J Virol Methods* 1992; 37:189–200.

180. Alter MJ, et al: The natural history of community-acquired hepatitis C in the United States. *N Engl J Med* 1992; 327:1899–1905.

181. Sherlock S, et al: Hepatitis C virus updated. *Gut* 1991; 32:965–967.

182. Aach RD, et al: Hepatitis C virus infection in post transfusion hepatitis. An analysis with first- and second-generation assays. *N Engl J Med* 1991; 325:1325–1329.

183. Weiland O, et al: Hepatitis C: Virology, epidemiology, clinical course, and treatment. *Scand J Gastroenterol* 1992; 27:337–342.

184. Gitnick G: Hepatitis C: What progress? *Scand J Gastroenterol* 1992; 27(suppl 192):50–54.

185. Clemens JM, et al: IgM antibody response in acute hepatitis C viral infection. *Blood* 1992; 79:169–172.

186. Chen PJ, et al: Transient immunoglobulin M response to hepatitis C virus capsid antigen in post-transfusion hepatitis C: Putative serological marker for acute viral infection. *Proc Natl Acad Sci U S A* 1992; 89:5971–5975.

187. Chau KH, et al: IgM-antibody response to hepatitis C virus antigens in acute and chronic post-transfusion non-A, non-B hepatitis. *J Virol Methods* 1991; 35:343–352.

188. Purcell RH, et al: Hepatitis delta virus in Fields BN (ed): *Virology,* 2nd ed. New York, Raven Press, 1990, pp 2275–2287.

189. Sharmeen L, et al: The antigenomic RNA of human hepatitis delta virus can undergo self cleavage. *J Virol* 1988; 62:2674–2679.

190. Perrotta AT, et al: The self cleaving domain from the genomic RNA of hepatitis delta virus: Sequence requirements and the effects of denaturants. *Nucleic Acids Res* 1990; 18:6821–6827.

191. Ryu WS, et al: Analysis of ribonucleoproteins of hepatitis delta virus (abstract), in *Molecular Biology of Hepatitis B Virus.* University of California, San Diego, 1992, p 122.

192. Chao M, et al: The antigen of hepatitis delta virus: Examination of in vitro RNA binding specificity. *J Virol* 1991; 65:4056–4062.

193. Sureau C, et al: Cloned hepatitis delta virus cDNA is infectious in the chimpanzee. *J Virol* 1992; 63:4292–4297.

194. Kuo MY, et al: Initiation and replication of the human hepatitis delta virus genome from cloned DNA: Role of delta antigen. *J Virol* 1989; 63:1945–1950.

195. Glenn JS, et al: In vitro synthesized hepatitis delta virus RNA initiates genome replication in cultured cells. *J Virol* 1990; 64:3104–3107.

196. Wu JC, et al: Production of hepatitis delta virus and suppression of helper hepatitis B virus in a human hepatoma cell line. *J Virol* 1991; 65:1099–1104.

197. Sureau C, et al: Tissue culture system for infection with human hepatitis delta virus. *J Virol* 1992; 65:3443–3450.

198. Sureau C, et al: Production of infectious hepatitis delta virus in vitro and neutralization with antibodies directed against hepatitis B virus pre S antigens. *J Virol* 1992; 66:1241–1245.

199. Davies S, et al: Evidence that hepatitis D virus needs hepatitis B virus to cause hepatocellular damage. *Am J Clin Pathol* 1992; 98:554–558.

200. Crain JR: Hepatitis delta virus: No longer a defective virus. *Am J Clin Pathol* 1992; 98:552–553.

201. Ottobrelli A, et al: Patterns of hepatitis delta virus reinfection and disease in liver transplantation. *Gastroenterology* 1991; 101:1649–1655.

202. Mason WS, et al: Liver transplantation: A model for the transmission of hepatitis delta virus. *Gastroenterology* 1991; 101:1741–1743.

203. Lee CM et al: Evolution of hepatitis delta virus RNA during chronic infection. *Virology* 1992; 188:265–273.

204. Imazeki F, et al: Heterogeneity and evolution rates of delta virus RNA sequences. *J Virol* 1990; 64:5594–5599.

205. Wu HN et al: Mutagenic analysis of the self cleavage domain of hepatitis delta virus antigenome RNA. *Nucleic Acids Res* 1992; 20:5937–5941.

206. Thill G, et al: Self cleavage: The 71 nucleotide long ribozyme derived from hepatitis delta virus genomic RNA. *Nucleic Acids Res* 1992; 19:6519–6525.

207. Branch AD: Efficient trans cleavage and a common structural motif for the ribozymes of the human hepatitis agent. *Proc Natl Acad Sci U S A* 1991; 88:10163–10167.

208. Been MD, et al: Secondary structure of the self-cleaving RNA of hepatitis delta virus: Applications to catalytic RNA designs. *Biochemistry* 1992; 31:11843–11852.

209. Huey-Nan W, et al: Sequence and structure of the catalytic RNA of hepatitis delta virus genomic RNA. *J Mol Biol* 1992; 223:233–245.

210. Casey JL, et al: Structural requirements for RNA editing in hepatitis delta virus: Evidence for a uridine-to-cytidine editing mechanism. *Proc Natl Acad Sci U S A* 1992; 89:7149–7153.

211. Zheng H, et al: Editing on the genomic RNA of human hepatitis delta virus. *J Virol* 1992; 66:4693–4697.

212. Zheng H, et al: Specific in vitro editing of HDV RNA by nuclear extracts (abstract), in *Molecular Biology of Hepatitis B Viruses*. University of California, San Diego, 1992, p 121.

213. Xia YP, et al: Characterization of nuclear targeting signal of hepatitis delta antigen, nuclear transport as a protein complex. *J Virol* 1992; 66:914–921.

214. Xia YP, et al: Oligomerization of hepatitis delta antigen is required for both the trans-activating and trans-dominant inhibitory activities of the delta antigen. *J Virol* 1992; 66:6641–6648.

215. Hwang SB, et al: Hepatitis delta antigen expressed by recombinant baculoviruses: Comparison of biochemical properties and post-translational modifications between the large and small forms. *Virology* 1992; 190:413–422.

216. Chen PJ, et al: Functional study of hepatitis delta virus large antigen in packaging and replication inhibition: Role of the amino-terminal leucine zipper *J Virol* 1992; 66:2853–2859.

217. Glenn JS, et al: Identification of a prenylation site in delta virus large antigen. *Science* 1992; 256:1331–1333.

218. Chang FI, et al: The large form of hepatitis antigen is crucial for assembly of hepatitis virus. *Proc Natl Acad Sci U S A* 1991; 88:8490–8494.

219. Ryu WS, et al: Assembly of hepatitis delta virus particles. *J Virol* 1992; 66:2310–2315.

220. Taylor JM, et al: Structure and replication of hepatitis delta virus, in Hollinger FB, et al (eds): *Viral Hepatitis and Liver Disease*. Baltimore, Williams & Wilkins, 1991, pp 460–463.

221. Hollinger FB: Non-A, non-B hepatitis viruses, in Fields BN, et al (eds): *Virology,* 2nd ed. New York, Raven Press, 1990, pp 2239–2271.

222. Bradley DW: Hepatitis non-A, non-B viruses become identified as hepatitis C and E viruses. *Prog Med Virol* 1990; 37:101–135.

223. Gust ID, et al: Report of a workshop: Waterborne non-A, non-B hepatitis. *J Infect Dis* 1987; 156:630–635.

224. Reyes GR, et al: Isolation of cDNA from the virus responsible for enterically transmitted non-A non-B hepatitis. *Science* 1990; 247:1335–1339.

225. Balayan MS, et al: Evidence for a virus in non-A, non-B hepatitis transmitted via the fecal-oral route. *Intervirology* 1990; 20:23–31.

226. Andjaparidze AG, et al: Fecal-orally transmitted non-A, non-B hepatitis induced in monkeys. *Vopr Virusol* 1990; 1:73–80.

227. Bradley DW, et al: Virus of enterically transmitted non-A, non-B hepatitis. *Lancet* 1988; 1:819.

228. Reyes GR, et al: Molecular biology of non-A, non-B hepatitis agents: Hepatitis C and hepatitis E viruses. *Adv Virus Res* 1991; 40:57–102.

229. Yarbough PO, et al: Hepatitis E virus: Identification of type-common epitopes. *J Virol* 1991; 65:5790–5797.

230. Reyes GR, et al: Sequence-dependent, single-primer amplification (SISPA) of complex DNA populations. *Mol Cell Probes* 1991; 5:473–481.

231. Tam AW, et al: Hepatitis E virus (HEV): Molecular cloning and sequencing of the full-length viral genome. *Virology* 1991; 185:120–131.

232. Huang C-C, et al: Molecular cloning of the Mexico isolate of hepatitis E virus. *Virology* 1992; 191:550–558.

233. Fry KE, et al: Hepatitis E virus (HEV): Strain variation in the nonstructural region encoding consensus motifs site. *Virus Genes,* 1992; 6:173–185.

234. Tsarev SA, et al: Characterization of a prototype strain of hepatitis E virus. *Proc Natl Acad Sci USA* 1992; 89:559–563.

235. Koonin EV, et al: Computer assisted assignment of functional domains in the nonstructural polyprotein of hepatitis E virus: Delineation of an additional group of positive strand RNA plant and animal viruses. *Proc Natl Acad Sci U S A* 1992; 9:8259–8263.

236. Bradley D: Aetological agent of enterically transmitted non-A, non-B hepatitis. *J Gen Virol* 1988; 69:731–738.

237. McCaustland KA, et al: Application of two RNA extraction methods prior to amplification of hepatitis E virus nucleic acid by the polymerase chain reaction. *J Virol Methods* 1991; 35:331–342.

238. Krawczynski K, et al: Identification of virus-associated antigen in experimentally infected cynomolgul macaques. *J Infect Dis* 1989; 159:1042–1049.

239. Purdy MA, et al: Expression of a hepatitis E virus (HEV) trpE fusion protein containing epitopes recognized by antibodies in sera from human cases and experimentally infected primates. *Arch Virol* 1992; 123:335–349.

240. Dawson GJ, et al: Solid-phase enzyme-linked immunosorbent assay for hepatitis E virus IgG and IgM antibodies utilizing recombinant antigens and synthetic peptides. *J Virol Methods* 1992; 38:175–186.

241. Goldsmith R, et al: Enzyme-linked immunosorbent assay for diagnosis of acute sporadic hepatitis E in Egyptian children. *Lancet* 1992; 339:328–331.

242. Lok ASF, et al: Seroepidemiological survey of hepatitis E in Hong Kong by recombinant-based enzyme immunoassays. *Lancet* 1992; 340:1205–1208.

243. Hyams KC, et al: Acute sporadic hepatitis E in Sudanese children: Analysis based on a new Western blot assay. *J Infect Dis* 1992; 165:1001–1005.

244. Favorov MO, et al: Serologic identification of hepatitis E virus infection in epidemic and endemic settings. *J Med Virol* 1992; 36:246–250.

245. Skidmore SJ, et al: Imported hepatitis E in UK. *Lancet* 1991; 337:1541.

246. Herrera JL, et al: Hepatitis E among U.S. travelers. *Morbidity and Mortality Weekly Review.* 1993; 42:1–4.

247. Dawson GJ, et al: Long lasting antibodies in hepatitis E virus infection. *Lancet* 1992; 340:427.

248. Ticehurst J, et al: Association of hepatitis E virus with an outbreak of hepatitis in Pakistan: Serologic response and pattern of virus excretion. *J Med Virol* 1992; 36:84–92.

249. Skidmore SJ, et al: Hepatitis E virus: The cause of a waterborne epidemic. *J Med Virol* 1992; 37:58–60.

250. Tsega E, et al: Outbreak of acute hepatitis E virus infection among military personnel in northern Ethiopia. *J Med Virol* 1991; 34:232–236.

251. Balayan MS, et al: Brief report: Experimental hepatitis E infection in domestic pigs. *J Med Virol* 1990; 32:58–59.

252. Uchida T, et al: Virulence of hepatitis E virus with serial passage to cynomolgus monkeys and identification of viremia, in Hollinger FB, et al (eds): *Viral Hepatitis and Liver Disease*. Baltimore, Williams & Wilkins, 1991, p 526–527.

253. Jameel S, et al: Enteric non-A, non-B hepatitis: Epidemics, animal transmission, and hepatitis E virus detection by the polymerase chain reaction. *J Med Virol* 1992; 37:263–270.

254. Ray R, et al: Hepatitis E virus genome in stools of hepatitis patients during large epidemic in north India. *Lancet* 1991; 338:783–784.

255. Chauhan A, et al: Common aetiological agent for epidemic and sporadic non-A, non-B hepatitis. *Lancet* 1992; 339:1509–1510.

256. Chauhan A, et al: Hepatitis E virus transmission to a volunteer. *Lancet* 1993; 341:149–150.

257. Schlauder GG, et al: Viremia in Egyptian children with hepatitis E virus infection. *Lancet* 1993; 341:378.

258. Kazachkov YA, et al: Hepatitis E virus in cultivated cells. *J Arch Virol* 1992; 127:399–402.

259. Huang RT, et al: Isolation and identification of hepatitis E virus in Xinjiang, China. *J Gen Virol* 1992; 73:1143.

CHAPTER 4

Drug-Induced Liver Disease

Dev Samarasinghe, M.B., Ch.B., F.R.A.C.P.

Australian National Health and Medical Research Council Medical Postgraduate Research Scholar, Department of Medicine, University of Sydney, Sydney, Australia; Westmead Hospital, Westmead, New South Wales, Australia

Jacob George, M.B., B.S., F.R.A.C.P.

Australian National Health and Medical Research Council Medical Postgraduate Research Scholar, Department of Medicine, University of Sydney, Sydney, Australia; Westmead Hospital, Westmead, New South Wales, Australia

Geoffrey C. Farrell, M.D., F.R.A.C.P.

Professor in Hepatic Medicine, University of Sydney, Sydney, Australia; Head, Department of Gastroenterology and Hepatology, Westmead Hospital, Westmead, New South Wales, Australia

An adverse drug reaction should be considered part of the differential diagnosis in most cases of hepatobiliary disease. Information about the hepatotoxic potential of individual drugs, the types of liver injury that they cause, the latent interval to onset, and other clinical features may help the clinician to identify or exclude a drug-related etiology. With the constant stream of new therapeutic agents being developed, novel adverse hepatic drug reactions doubtless will occur. It also is increasingly apparent that drugs may cause liver injury through multiple mechanisms, including direct and metabolite-induced toxicity, systemic hypersensitivity, and, possibly, tissue-specific immune responses to adducts formed from interactions between drug metabolites and tissue proteins. As it has in previous volumes of *Current Hepatology*,[1-3] this chapter focuses on newly recognized forms of drug-induced liver disease. Particular emphasis also is given to advances in our understanding of the mechanisms of adverse hepatic reactions to particular drugs.

DOSE-DEPENDENT HEPATOTOXINS

Acetaminophen

Acetaminophen remains the most common cause of drug-induced acute liver injury and fulminant hepatic failure.[4] Furthermore, the incidence of acetaminophen self-poisoning does not appear to be declining.[5, 6] A recent Australian study indicated that hospital admissions for acetaminophen overdose remained constant from 1985 to 1990, with an annual incidence of at least 6 cases per 100,000 population.[6] The study also emphasized the way in which the appropriate use of antidote therapy has reduced in-hospital mortality to negligible levels: no fatalities occurred among more than 300 cases.

Mechanism of Liver Injury

As discussed in earlier volumes of *Current Hepatology*,[2, 7] hepatocellular necrosis results from the cytochrome P-450 (P-450) 2E1–catalyzed formation of N-acetyl-p-benzoquinonemine (NAPQI). NAPQI is a highly electrophilic metabolite that binds to and is reduced by reduced glutathione (GSH). Poisoning by acetaminophen depletes hepatic stores of GSH. This allows NAPQI to bind covalently to macromolecules (alkylation); NAPQI also produces severe oxidant stress.

Alkylation and oxidation of protein thiol groups may damage Ca^{2+}-adenosine triphosphatases (ATPases), thereby impairing microsomal sequestration and plasma membrane extrusion of calcium.[8, 9] This leads to the disruption of intracellular calcium homeostasis. Oxidative stress also alters the redox state of the reduced and oxidized forms of nicotinamide-adenine dinucleotide phosphate (NADPH/ $NADP^+$), which facilitates the release of Ca^{2+} from the mitochondrial calcium pool.[10] This exacerbates the rise in cytoplasmic Ca^{2+} concentrations ($[Ca^{2+}]_i$). Sustained increases in $[Ca^{2+}]_i$ activate such catabolic enzymes as phospholipases, proteases, and endonucleases[11, 12]; these could contribute to the production of hepatocellular necrosis. Recently, nuclear accumulation of Ca^{2+} was observed in cultured mouse hepatocytes exposed to toxic (5mM to 25mM) concentrations of acetaminophen.[13] This was associated with the activation of endonuclease and the fragmentation of DNA. The endonuclease inhibitor aurintricarboxylic acid, as well as the chelation of Ca^{2+} with ethyleneglycolbis-(aminoethyl-ether) tetra-acetic acid (EGTA), decreased DNA fragmentation at 6 and 12 hours; this abrogated cytotoxicity. The results resemble those found in apoptosis and with redox-cycling quinones.[1] They provide further evidence that oxidative stress and disordered calcium homeostasis may be relevant to the mechanism of acetaminophen-induced hepatic necrosis.

Levels of thromboxane B_2 (TXB) increase soon after the acetaminophen-induced rise in $[Ca^{2+}]_i$ and reach a maximum 14 hours after acetaminophen administration.[14, 15] This occurs presumably because Ca^{2+} activates phospholipase A_2. In turn, this hydrolyzes membrane phospholipids to release arachidonic acid, which facilitates the synthesis of eicosanoids. Thromboxane may act as an intermediary in calcium-mediated injury and cell death, possibly acting through TXB receptors on hepatocytes.[16] Recently, Horton and Wood[17] studied the effects of Sulotroban (BM 13177), an inhibitor of thromboxane action, on acetaminophen hepatotoxicity. When it was administered to rats 7 hours after acetaminophen, Sulotroban prevented the loss of membrane integrity and the development of hepatocellular necrosis, as assessed by alanine aminotransferase (ALT) activity, trypan blue uptake, and histologic examination. Sulotroban does not inhibit eicosanoid synthesis. The mechanism by which it prevents the cytotoxic effects of thromboxane is unclear, but could be by inhibition of the TXB receptor.

Risk Factors for Severe Liver Injury

More women than men are seen with acetaminophen self-poisoning, but the frequency of significant hepatotoxicity is greater in men.[5, 6, 18] This presumably is because men tend to take larger doses, seek medical assistance later, and have a higher prevalence of alcoholism.[6]

Recent publications have reinforced the importance of suspecting acetaminophen toxicity in the chronic alcoholic, particularly when aminotransferase levels are elevated more than fivefold.[19, 20] Chronic excessive ingestion of alcohol is an important risk factor for acetaminophen hepatotoxicity.[6, 19, 21-25] Ethanol-mediated induction of P-450 2E1 or reduced hepatic GSH levels[25, 26] are partially responsible for this susceptibility. Bray and colleagues[27] investigated the level of alcohol consumption that increases the risk of acetaminophen-induced hepatotoxicity. In a retrospective study of patients with severe liver damage after acetaminophen overdose, mortality was greater among high consumers of alcohol (more than 168 g of ethanol per week in men or 112 g of ethanol per week in women)[28] than among those who drank less (67% vs. 34%, $P < .01$). Unlike other reports, heavy drinkers were not seen late in this study; therefore, this does not explain their higher mortality. The frequency of raised serum creatinine and low arterial pH (<7.30) levels was higher in individuals who consumed alcohol regularly. The authors were unable to determine whether the efficacy of N-acetylcysteine (NAC) was altered by previously increased alcohol consumption.

Thus, alcoholics not only appear to be more susceptible to acetaminophen-induced liver injury, they also have a worse prognosis when such injury occurs, primarily because of late presentation.[6, 23] Individuals who consume alcohol to excess should take no more than 2 g of acetaminophen daily. It is not known whether similar dose restriction is necessary in patients taking drugs that are known to induce hepatic P-450 1A or 2E, such as omeprazole or isoniazid,[29-32] or in those taking anticonvulsants. The King's College Hospital group also investigated (retrospectively) whether long-term anticonvulsant therapy worsens the outcome of acetaminophen poisoning.[33] Among 15 patients taking anticonvulsants who had acetaminophen-induced fulminant hepatic failure but did not receive NAC, 14 (93%) died. Among those not taking anticonvulsant therapy (who also were not given NAC), the mortality rate was 65% ($P < .025$). Only 3 patients taking anticonvulsants received NAC, 2 of whom survived. There were trends toward more severe coma, acidosis, and coagulopathy in those receiving anticonvulsant therapy, but none of these changes were significant. Other case reports have suggested a heightened risk and severity of hepatotoxicity after acetaminophen overdose among patients taking anticonvulsants.[34, 35] This is in keeping with the effect of phenobarbital, which has enhanced acetaminophen-induced liver injury in most, but not all, animal studies.[36-38] Although the induction of P-450 would explain the effect of multiple doses, a single dose of phenobarbital given 1 hour before acetaminophen ingestion also enhances hepatotoxicity.[38] This may result from competition with the glucuronidation of acetaminophen, thereby favoring enhanced oxidation of acetaminophen to NAPQI. Among patients taking anticonvulsants (phenytoin, carbamazepine), there also have been deaths from acetaminophen-induced liver damage in individuals who had nontoxic blood levels of acetaminophen.[39-41]

Prediction of Outcome

The following factors are associated with a poor prognosis after acetaminophen-induced hepatotoxicity: systemic acidosis (arterial pH <7.30) at hospital admission, development of grade III hepatic encephalopathy, serum creatinine level greater than 300 μmol/L, and prothrombin time (PT) greater than 100 seconds.[42] A more precise indicator would be valuable, however. Recently, the ratio of factor VIII/V has been shown to be related to prognosis.[43] Among 22 patients, the ratio of factor VIII/V at hospital admission was less than 30 (median, 17) in all those who survived, while 10 of 11 patients who died had values greater than 30 (median, 39). A factor V level of 10% or less on admission to the hospital also was a sensitive predictor of adverse outcome (it identified 10 of the 11 fatal cases), but by itself had poor specificity (55%).

The early administration of antidote therapy overrides the importance of all the criteria outlined above in determining the outcome of acetaminophen-induced hepatotoxicity. When it is given within 16 hours of acetaminophen ingestion, NAC is so effective that severe liver injury now is rare after acetaminophen self-poisoning.[5, 6] Conversely, late presentation is the most important determinant of a poor prognosis. The main drawback to NAC therapy is the risk of hypersensitivity. When it is given intravenously, adverse reactions to NAC occur in at least 10% of recipients.[6, 44-46] Severe reactions may include angioedema and anaphylaxis, as well as rash, nausea, hypotension, and bronchospasm. Fatalities have been reported, although usually when more than twice the recommended dose has been used.[47] Thus, NAC should be given only when acetaminophen blood levels are in the toxic range.

Novel Approaches to Therapy

The possibility that voltage-dependent calcium channel blockers could protect against acetaminophen-induced liver injury has been of some interest. Nifedipine reduced hepatic necrosis in rats when it was given before and after treatment with acetaminophen.[48] In mice, diltiazem reduced liver damage when it was given 20 minutes after acetaminophen, but was less effective at 3 hours.[49] In contrast, Deakin and associates[50] found in mice that the administration of diltiazem at 6 hours showed no efficacy and that toxicity appeared to be greater (although not statistically significant) in the treated group at 12 and 24 hours. At 9 hours after acetaminophen ingestion, the administration of diltiazem significantly reduced the plasma aspartate aminotransferase (AST) level and tended to reduce mortality, although no reduction in liver injury was evident histologically.[50] The presence of increased mitotic figures at 30 hours in the diltiazem group was suggestive of enhanced efficacy of hepatocellular regeneration. Further experiments are required to verify the role of voltage-dependent calcium channel blockers in acetaminophen toxicity. We note, however, that there is scant evidence for the existence of voltage-dependent calcium channels on normal hepatocytes.[51, 52] As was discussed in an earlier volume in relation to $FeCl_3$-induced liver injury,[3] conventional voltage-dependent calcium channel blockers also prevented the entry of extracellular Ca^{2+} after lipid peroxidation. This suggests that oxidative injury may open nifedipine-sensitive channels through which Ca^{2+} enters the hepatocyte. It also should be noted that voltage-dependent calcium channels recently have been identified on Kupffer cells.[53]

Treatment of acetaminophen overdose with NAC is highly effective when it is given within 16 hours of self-poisoning. Recently, late administration of NAC (36 to 80 hours after poisoning) also has been shown to be useful.[54, 55] A recent study in rats led the authors to suggest that glutamine may augment host antioxidant protection.[56] These authors found that depletion of hepatic GSH in acetaminophen-poisoned rats occurred rapidly if the animals were receiving standard total parenteral nutrition. Supplementation of total parenteral nutrition with glutamine rendered rats resistant to this decrease and replenished GSH stores rapidly. The glutamine-treated group also had less elevation in hepatic enzyme levels and reduced mortality (4 of 26 compared with 13 of 28 patients; $P < .05$).

In another study, cysteine isopropylester, a novel, highly lipophilic cysteine ester, was shown to be equally efficacious as NAC in reducing mortality among acetaminophen-poisoned mice.[57] Likewise, *S*-adenosylmethionine (SAM) prevented death in mice when it was given within 1 hour of a toxic dose of acetaminophen; mortality also was reduced if SAM was given within 2 to 5 hours.[58] This protective effect was abolished by buthionine sulfoximine, an inhibitor of glutathione synthesis.[58] This indicates that the protective effect of SAM was mediated through its metabolism to GSH, thereby replenishing the GSH pool. SAM also may provide protection by increasing adenosine triphosphate (ATP) synthesis,[59] stimulating the methylation of phospholipid (thereby stabilizing cell membranes),[60] or facilitating the sulfation of acetaminophen and thereby reducing NAPQI formation.[61] SAM can be administered orally or intravenously. Although the intravenous route carries a theoretic risk of precipitating encephalopathy in patients with fulminant hepatic failure, this did not occur in this study.[58] Because SAM was useful at 5 hours after acetaminophen administration to mice, it may have a role in the late treatment of acetaminophen overdose in humans when NAC is tolerated poorly.

The design of mechanism-based prevention of acetaminophen-induced hepatotoxicity recently has been reviewed.[62] The possibility of providing acetaminophen in formulations with a built-in antidote (such as *N*-acetylmethionine or another GSH precursor) was considered. Another approach is the development of alkyl-substituted derivatives of acetaminophen, such as the 3,5-dimethyl derivative, which retain analgesic efficacy but are less able to be metabolized into hepatotoxic metabolites.[62]

Methotrexate

Frequency and Clinical Significance of Hepatic Fibrosis

Hepatic fibrosis is a potential complication of long-term methotrexate (MTX) therapy. The risk is increased with higher incremental dose, daily therapy, high cumulative dose, preexistent liver disease, alcoholism, diabetes mellitus, renal insufficiency, and advancing age. The extent to which low-dose MTX therapy causes liver damage is controversial, as discussed previously.[2, 3] Most earlier studies addressing this issue were retrospective and did not include pretreatment liver biopsies. The problem is complicated by the fact that hepatic histologic abnormalities may be present in as many as two thirds of patients with rheumatoid arthritis or psoriasis who never have received MTX.[63–65]

Hall and coworkers[66] recently used a microcomputer image analysis system to measure hepatic collagen deposition in liver biopsy specimens. This analytic approach correlated well with semiquantitative histologic methods, and had the advantage of objectivity. Among patients with rheumatoid arthritis who were receiving low-dose MTX, there was no correlation between the cumulative dose of MTX and increased collagen deposition. This is consistent with the proposition that factors other than MTX may contribute to liver injury.

The frequency of clinically significant MTX-induced cirrhosis is not known. Even in the presence of cirrhosis, the risks of continuing low-dose MTX are unclear. Zachariae and Soggard[67] prospectively studied 25 patients taking MTX who had established cirrhosis with serial biopsies for 1 to 13 years; none had progression of hepatic fibrosis or liver failure. It should be noted that earlier regimens of high-dose MTX were associated with end-stage chronic liver disease and even hepatocellular carcinoma.[68] Recently, three patients treated for psoriasis with MTX for 5, 10, and 12 years, respectively, required liver transplantation for progressive liver failure.[69] Unfortunately, no information was provided regarding other etiologic factors for liver disease. The cumulative doses of MTX in these patients were 9.5 g, 26 g, and an unspecified but likely high dose in a patient who self-medicated. Thus, in each case, the dose considerably exceeded recommended levels. In contrast to older regimens, however, the evidence incriminating low-dose pulse MTX therapy as a cause of significant hepatic fibrosis is unimpressive. It remains possible that MTX may enhance the progression of fibrotic liver disease in the presence of other etiologic factors, such as alcohol and preexistent liver disease.

Prevention of Hepatic Fibrosis

The optimal surveillance strategy for patients treated with low-dose MTX is controversial. Serum levels of hepatic enzymes correlate poorly with histologic changes.[70] The serum aminoterminal peptide of type III procollagen has been suggested as a marker of hepatic fibrosis, but it has poor specificity.[71] Liver biopsy remains the only reliable gauge of hepatotoxicity in patients taking MTX. Whiting-O'Keefe and associates[72] suggested that liver biopsy be performed after every 4 g of MTX, and that the biopsy interval be shortened for patients with persistent abnormalities in liver test results. Others have suggested biopsy performance at lower cumulative doses of MTX.[69, 73] Kremer[74] recently presented the following detailed guidelines for liver monitoring among patients with rheumatoid arthritis who are taking MTX:

1. Baseline liver biopsy is required only if there is a history of significant alcohol intake or preexistent liver disease.
2a. AST values should be determined monthly. Liver biopsy is recommended if 6 of 12 AST values are elevated, if the serum albumin concentration falls to <3.3 g/dL, or . . .
2b. If 3 to 5 of the monthly AST values are abnormal per year for 3 consecutive years.
3. The biopsy result should be considered a "benign outcome" if the liver shows Roenigk[75] class I, II, or IIIA changes (minimal fibrosis). In this situation,

another liver biopsy need be performed only if the circumstances in 2a or 2b occur. Conversely, the presence of Roenigk class IIIB (significant fibrosis) or IV (cirrhosis) would be cause for discontinuing MTX therapy.

Watson and Smallwood[76] also considered liver biopsy to be indicated only if liver test result abnormalities raise suspicion for liver injury. These appear to be practical guidelines, notwithstanding the previously mentioned poor correlation between liver test result abnormalities and MTX-induced hepatic fibrosis. The recommendation that heavy users of alcohol should not receive long-term MTX[72] also is consistent with the available data.

Mechanism

To date, it is unclear how MTX or its metabolites damage the liver. Neither is it apparent whether acute and chronic toxicity share a common mechanism. Recently, Bremnes and colleagues[77] assessed the acute hepatotoxic effects of MTX (10 to 1,000 mg/kg) in male Wistar rats. At 1,000 mg/kg of MTX, four of eight rats had acute hepatotoxicity with cholestasis and severe liver injury as assessed morphologically and by aminotransferase release. The remaining four rats had minor morphologic changes with no rise in liver enzyme levels. The major metabolite of MTX is 7-hydroxy-MTX.[78, 79] Immediately before the onset of cholestasis in affected rats, biliary excretion of this metabolite was increased threefold compared to rats without cholestasis; these raised levels were equivalent to the threshold concentration for the precipitation of 7-hydroxy-MTX in rat bile in vitro.[80] Ninety-five percent of the drug in the precipitate was in the form of 7-hydroxy-MTX. The authors suggest, therefore, that 7-hydroxy-MTX has a role in precipitate formation after high doses of MTX.

Ahern and associates[81] showed that concentrations of MTX, 2,4 diamino-N-10-methylpteroic acid and MTX-polyglutamate were raised markedly in liver biopsy specimens from three patients with severe fibrosis. There was no linear relationship between the accumulation of MTX or its metabolites, however, and lesser degrees of hepatic fibrosis. Whether hepatic fibrosis is related to hepatic retention of MTX or its metabolites has yet to be clarified.

Sex Steroids

Case reports over the past year have continued to highlight the association between sex steroids and cholestasis,[82] hepatic vascular abnormalities,[83] and liver tumors.[84, 85] Of particular interest, several authors emphasized the severe and prolonged course of cholestasis that rarely may follow the intake of oral contraceptive steroids (OCS). Lieberman and coworkers[86] described a patient whose symptoms and serum bilirubin level worsened progressively for almost 3 months after the discontinuation of OCS. Results of biochemical tests of liver function normalized over 6 months. Another case of possible OCS-associated prolonged cholestasis has been reported recently by Weden and colleagues.[82] They noted biochemical features of cholestasis incidentally in a previously healthy 35-year-old woman who had received OCS for the preceding 14 years. Liver test results indicating cholestasis persisted for a further 10 years after the termination of drug therapy! Serial liver biopsies performed over 2 years showed gradual resolution of histologic evidence of cholestasis. The patient remained essentially asymptomatic during this entire period. Test results for antimitochondrial, smooth muscle, and antinuclear antibodies were negative, as were serum globulin concentrations and serology for hepatitis A, B, and C viruses. An intravenous cholangiogram revealed normal biliary anatomy.[82]

Prolonged use of OCS is associated with the development of hepatocellular adenomas.[87] Transformation of these adenomas to carcinoma has been reported in several instances.[88-90] A report by Korula and associates[85] noted the coexistence of hepatic adenoma and hepatocellular carcinoma in an asymptomatic woman who had received long-term OCS. These and other reports of hepatocellular dysplasia in hepatic adenomas[91] emphasize the importance of early diagnosis and resection of hepatic adenomas, especially in patients who have taken OCS for more than 5 years.

Nicotinic Acid

Nicotinic acid (3-pyridinecarboxylic acid, or niacin), is used to treat hypercholesterolemia and is a widely available over-the-counter vitamin. Sustained-release (SR) products have been developed in an attempt to minimize the common side effect of cutaneous flushing. Both unmodified[92-98] and SR forms of nicotinic acid[98-100] can cause hepatotoxicity. Mild and transient elevations in AST levels and jaundice (presumed to result from cholestasis) are the most frequent abnormalities.[94, 97] Fulminant hepatic failure has been reported with both forms of nicotinic acid[97, 100, 101]; one patient required liver transplantation.[101] Hepatotoxicity usually has been associated with a dose of more than 3 g/day.[101] Hodis,[100] however, described a case of fulminant hepatic failure in a patient receiving only 500 mg/day of SR niacin.

It has been suggested that SR niacin is more hepatotoxic than is the unmodified compound.[102, 103] In a trial comparing unmodified and SR niacin, Knopp and coworkers[104] found slightly higher AST and alkaline phosphatase levels in patients taking SR preparations, although the possibility that this was a chance finding does not appear to have been excluded. Among recently reported cases of SR niacin–associated hepatotoxicity,[105, 106] a change from unmodified to SR niacin had been made in most cases, sometimes inadvertently. In the majority of cases, however, the dose of the SR preparation was the same as that of the unmodified agent, but greatly exceeded the maximum recommended dose (0.25 to 1.00 g of SR niacin per day).[107, 108] There is a sixfold difference in the recommended maximal doses of SR niacin (1 g/day) and unmodified niacin (6 g/day).[107, 108] Henkin and colleagues[105] reported three further cases of hepatitis among patients treated with SR niacin; the SR niacin doses in these patients also were higher than recommended. It is of interest, however, that rechallenge with equal or higher doses of unmodified niacin did not produce recurrent hepatotoxicity in these cases.

Niacin is metabolized in a complex fashion. The products include nicotinamide, nicotinamide N-oxide, nicotinuric acid (the glycine conjugate of nicotinic acid), two isomeric carboxamides, and several methylated derivatives. The ratios of these metabolites differ significantly with the dose of niacin.[109] The mechanism by which niacin or one of its metabolites induces injury is unknown; a dose-related direct toxic effect is most likely. SR niacin may prolong hepatic exposure to the drug, and this may favor the accumulation of a toxic metabolite. Further pharmacologic and toxicologic studies are required to determine the differences between various preparations. SR niacin preparations should be used with caution, particularly because they have a limited (if any) benefit in relation to reduced flushing, but appear to have a greater potential to cause severe liver injury. Considering the widespread availability of niacin without prescription in some countries and its potential for unmonitored use, awareness of this rare but significant toxicity should be increased.

IDIOSYNCRATIC HEPATOTOXINS

3-Hydroxy-3-Methylglutaryl-Coenzyme A (HMG CoA) Reductase Inhibitors

The 3-hydroxy-3-methylglutaryl-coenzyme A (HMG CoA) reductase inhibitors are cholesterol-lowering agents that recently have been introduced into clinical practice. They now are in widespread use, as indicated by U.S. data. Lovastatin was released in 1987 and, by December 1988, more than 750,000 individuals were taking it on a daily basis. The HMG CoA reductase inhibitors appear to be relatively safe compounds, although a mild form of myopathy may occur in as many as 10% of patients. Abnormal liver test results have been noted in about 2% of patients taking lovastatin, but the risk of jaundice or other manifestations of significant hepatic injury is rare and not well documented.[110, 111] It has been recommended that patients be monitored with liver tests every 4 to 6 weeks during the initial 12 months of lovastatin therapy, and "periodically" thereafter.[112] After discontinuation of the drug, liver test result abnormalities resolve relatively slowly, raising the possibility that this is a metabolic form of liver injury rather than drug-induced hepatitis.

Simvastatin also has been associated with persistent but mildly abnormal aminotransferase levels in 1.5% of patients.[113] Values that exceed threefold the upper limit of normal are observed in only 0.1% of individuals.[114] Reversible hepatitis has been noted; it was symptomatic in one case.[115, 116] In these cases, ALT abnormalities were less than fivefold elevated, but a mild zone 3 lobular hepatitis was documented in one instance.[116] Other causes of hepatitis were excluded and the abnormalities resolved after discontinuation of simvastatin. It seems reasonable to predict that, with the widespread prescription of HMG CoA inhibitors, more will be written on this subject.

Antimicrobial Agents and Liver Injury

Amoxicillin and Clavulanic Acid (Augmentin)

As highlighted in a previous volume of *Current Hepatology*,[2] Augmentin (amoxicillin and the β-lactamase inhibitor clavulanic acid) is a well-recognized, though infrequent, cause of liver injury. The frequency of symptomatic hepatitis ranges from 1 to 5/1 million treated patients.[117] Fifteen cases of Augmentin-associated hepatitis that either were diagnosed in liver units or were reported to regional centers of the French National Drug Surveillance Network and Beecham Laboratories between January 1987 and June 1990 were reported recently.[117] This information extends our understanding of the spectrum of liver disease associated with Augmentin. The illness is either a cholestatic hepatitis or drug-induced cholestasis with minimal hepatic inflammation.[117, 118] Granulomatous hepatitis rarely has been seen.[119] Hepatitis may develop during Augmentin therapy or be seen as long as 1 to 5 weeks after the completion of treatment.[117, 118]

Several factors increase the likelihood of Augmentin hepatitis. Men appear to be more susceptible than women, with a male:female sex ratio of 2 to 4:1[117, 118]; this difference has been noted despite similar prescription rates. Older patients are affected more frequently; 9 of 15 patients in the series by Larrey and associates[117] were more than 60 years of age. Prolonged treatment also may increase the risk of hepatotoxicity. Thirty-three percent of patients with hepatitis in this study had received Augmentin for more than 15 days compared with less than 1% of all treated patients.[117]

The mechanism of Augmentin-associated cholestasis is uncertain. An immunoallergic mechanism has been suggested by the presence of eosinophilia, rash, and autoantibodies in a few patients. Despite 15 years of extensive use, amoxicillin rarely has been associated with hepatitis. Moreover, reports of negative rechallenge with amoxicillin, and instances of previous exposure to amoxicillin being unassociated with hepatitis in patients in whom hepatitis developed after exposure to Augmentin suggest that the clavulanic acid moiety is responsible for liver injury.[117, 118] Two reports of Timentin (ticarcillin-clavulanic acid)–associated jaundice support this hypothesis, although in both instances, other complicating factors may have been responsible for the liver injury.[120, 121]

The prognosis of Augmentin-associated jaundice is variable. In the majority of cases, jaundice resolves within 1 to 8 weeks and liver test results become normal in 2 to 4 months.[117] A single case of prolonged cholestatic hepatitis with progression to liver failure (as evidenced by the onset of hepatic encephalopathy) and death has been reported.[122] The possibility that concomitant estradiol therapy increased the susceptibility to or modified the course of the hepatitis cannot be excluded, however. Estrogens are known to alter the physical properties of liver cell membranes,[123] and their concomitant use previously has been implicated in cases of prolonged cholestasis from other hepatotoxic drugs.[2]

Flucloxacillin

Severe and prolonged cholestatic hepatitis is a well-recognized feature of liver injury associated with the oxacillin derivatives, cloxacillin, dicloxacillin, and flucloxacillin. Olsson and coworkers[124] have reported a case of severe flucloxacillin-induced hepatitis that persisted for 7½ years. The development of cirrhosis resulted in liver failure that ultimately required orthotopic liver transplantation. In serial biopsies, the histologic features were unusual, with the predominant finding being large bile duct thrombi (microliths) rather than canalicular cholestasis. Extrahepatic biliary obstruction was excluded by appropriate imaging.

In a review of hepatic drug reactions reported to the Swedish Adverse Drug Reactions Advisory Committee between 1981 and 1990, the authors noted 77 cases of cholestatic hepatitis that probably or possibly were related to oxacillin derivatives.[124] The frequency of liver injury was estimated to be 1.6 to 1.9 cases per 1 million defined daily doses. An additional case of liver failure attributed to flucloxacillin was noted in these 77 patients, and we are aware of several such cases in Australia. One hundred seventy-nine instances of this problem had been reported to the Australian Adverse Drug Reactions Advisory Committee as of June 1992, and 255 had been reported to the World Health Organization.[125] In 71 of the Australian cases, flucloxacillin was the only drug to which the patient had been exposed. There were 11 deaths.

Among reported cases of flucloxacillin hepatitis, women predominate (sex ratio, 2:1). The mean age of affected individuals is 59 years. A case-control study has identified increasing age as an independent risk factor, with the odds ratio for age greater than 55 years vs. age less than 30 years being 18.[125] The dose and route of flucloxacillin therapy were not related to the risk of liver injury, but the duration of therapy was; thus, the odds ratio for the intake of flucloxacillin for more than 14 days vs. 14 days or less was 7.[125] Based on reports to drug monitoring authorities, it has been estimated that the risk of flucloxacillin-induced liver injury is 1 case reported per 10,000 to 30,000 prescriptions in Sweden,[124] 1 report per 500,000 prescriptions in the United Kingdom, and 1 report per 12,000 to 100,000 prescriptions in Australia.[125]

The identification of age greater than 55 years and duration of therapy more than 2 weeks as independent risk factors suggests that consideration should be given to the use of alternative agents under these circumstances. It has been calculated that this would reduce the number of cases by about one third.[125] It is noteworthy that many cases of flucloxacillin-induced hepatitis have occurred in patients who had been given the drug for inadequate indications; indeed, the vast number of prescriptions written for flucloxacillin also suggest that this is the case. Careful assessment of the risk-benefit ratio is crucial for the appropriate use of a potentially hepatotoxic agent such as flucloxacillin.

Nitrofurantoin

Liver disease induced by nitrofurantoin was first reported in 1961. This commonly used urinary antiseptic may cause acute cholestatic hepatitis or acute hepatocellular liver injury, and chronic active hepatitis also has been associated with long-term therapy. The majority of hepatic reactions probably are cases of acute hepatitis.[1] Reports of hepatitis associated with nitrofurantoin continue to appear.[126, 127] Some cases were fatal, or the patient required orthotopic liver transplantation.[126] These reports serve to highlight the potentially serious nature of nitrofurantoin-induced liver disease. Patients taking this drug should be informed of the need to report symptoms that might be attributable to liver injury. Close monitoring of liver test results in patients receiving long-term nitrofurantoin therapy also may serve to remind physicians of the possible occurrence of hepatotoxicity, although it has not been demonstrated that this reduces the incidence of clinically significant hepatic drug reactions.

Antifungal Agents

About 5% to 10% of patients exposed to ketoconazole have minor, reversible elevations in liver enzyme levels without clinical features of hepatotoxicity. Symptomatic hepatitis has been estimated to affect only 1 in 15,000 exposed individuals, but it can be fatal.[128, 129]

Newer antifungal agents, such as fluconazole and itraconazole, have been implicated less often as the cause of hepatic dysfunction. Asymptomatic elevations of liver enzyme levels have been reported in less than 5% of patients treated with fluconazole.[130, 131] Holmes and associates[132] reported a case of mixed cholestatic and hepatocellular injury in a patient being treated with ketoconazole; liver biopsy showed focal necrosis. The patient was infected with the human immunodeficiency virus (HIV) and had hemophilia. Liver test results continued to deteriorate after therapy was changed to fluconazole, but resolved when fluconazole was discontinued. The time course of the enzyme abnormalities with respect to the antifungal therapy and their resolution after drug withdrawal make it possible that ketoconazole and fluconazole were the likely hepatotoxins. The authors hypothesized that fluconazole may have aggravated ketoconazole-associated hepatotoxicity, perhaps by acting through a similar mechanism. The presence of concomitant HIV infection, an episode of presumed non-A non-B hepatitis 5 years previously, and the failure to report hepatitis C virus serology, however, make the issue less clear-cut.

Another report suggests that fluconazole indeed may be hepatotoxic. In this case, liver test results deteriorated as the dose of fluconazole was increased in a patient with the acquired immunodeficiency syndrome (AIDS). Furthermore, abnormalities recurred on two occasions when fluconazole was reintroduced.[133] The liver biopsy showed centrilobular cholestasis without fibrosis or inflammation.

Asymptomatic minor elevations in liver test results also have been noted in patients treated with itraconazole.[134, 135] Three cases of symptomatic liver injury (two cholestatic, one mixed) were attributed to this agent.[136] The time course of the reaction was suggestive of drug-induced liver injury, although biopsy data were not available. The paucity of immunoallergic features and the long latent period (5 to 6 weeks) before the appearance of abnormal liver test results suggest that the basis for liver injury may be metabolic idiosyncrasy. Additional well-documented cases of hepatic dysfunction after therapy with the newer antifungal agents, together with adequate exclusion of other possible causes for hepatic injury, will serve to clarify this issue.

Minocycline

Fulminant hepatic failure with microvesicular steatosis is a recognized reaction to high-dose intravenous tetracycline. The mechanism for toxicity is uncertain. Impaired mitochondrial β-oxidation of fatty acids and reduced synthesis of very–low-density lipoprotein with decreased hepatocellular secretion of triglycerides may contribute to steatosis. Adverse reactions to the semisynthetic tetracycline minocycline are rare. A single case of acute hepatitis has been reported after 5 days of intravenous minocycline therapy (400 mg/day).[137] The clinical syndrome was analogous to that seen with tetracycline, and the liver biopsy showed diffuse macrovesicular and microvesicular steatosis.

In contrast, *oral* minocycline-associated hepatitis appears to be characterized by a hypersensitivity syndrome similar to that seen with sulfonamides and the aromatic anticonvulsants (phenytoin, phenobarbital, and carbamazepine). In four reported cases,[138–140] hepatitis developed 4 weeks after minocycline therapy and was associated with high fever, generalized exfoliative dermatitis, lymphadenopathy, and peripheral blood leukocytosis with eosinophilia. In two cases, fulminant hepatic failure developed; one case resolved and the other led to death despite liver transplantation.[139, 140] Liver biopsy was not performed in any of the patients. The similar mode of presentation with a hypersensitivity syndrome and the reappearance of this syndrome after inadvertent rechallenge in one patient,[138] however, suggest that minocycline was the responsible agent.

Valproic Acid Hepatotoxicity

Valproic acid (VPA) is a widely used anticonvulsant drug that rarely can cause fatal hepatic injury. To date, at least 100 cases have been reported. The reaction is thought to be idiosyncratic. In a review of the United States experience from 1978 to 1984, the overall frequency of fatal cases of VPA-associated hepatotoxicity was 1 per 10,000 patients exposed.[141] Age less than 2 years and anticonvulsant drug polytherapy were highlighted as important risk factors. The risk of hepatic fatality among individuals receiving polytherapy was 1 per 500 patients exposed, compared with 1 per 7,000 patients exposed among those receiving monotherapy.[141] Individuals aged more than 2 years had a lower fatality rate, 1 in 12,000 for polytherapy vs. 1 in 45,000 for monotherapy.[141] After awareness of these risk factors increased, changes in prescribing patterns led to a major decrease in the overall incidence of VPA-associated mortality from hepatotoxicity to a current level of 1 in 39,000.[142]

Although much is known about the metabolic fate of VPA (Fig 1), less is known about the precise mechanism for its toxicity. The major routes of VPA metabolism are glucuronidation and fatty acid β-oxidation. The latter occurs in mitochondria and leads to the formation of 3-keto-VPA and the unsaturated metabolite, 2-(en)-valproic acid.[143, 144] Subsequent biotransformation of 2-(en)-VPA can occur to 3-(en)-VPA and 2,3-(dien)-VPA.[143] Minor pathways involve microsomal ω, $\omega 1$, δ, and γ oxidation reactions and conjugation to carnitine and glycine.[144] Impaired β-oxidation was evident in all reported cases of VPA hepatitis for which sufficient biochemical data were available.[144–146] In various reports, however, the site of impaired β-oxidation varied. Eadie and colleagues[144] studied three patients with VPA-associated hepatotoxicity and showed impaired β-oxidation at the following enzymatic steps: acyl CoA dehydrogenase, enoyl CoA hydratase, and 3-hydroxy acyl CoA dehydrogenase.

There are several mechanisms by which VPA may inhibit β-oxidation: (1) competition with endogenous fatty acids; (2) induction or exacerbation of carnitine deficiency by the sequestration of free carnitine, in the form of valproylcarnitine; (3) sequestration of free CoA by the formation of valproyl-CoA, thereby decreasing CoA availability for free fatty acid metabolism; and (4) inhibition of β-oxidative enzymes by certain metabolites of VPA, especially 4-en-VPA.[147–149]

It also is unclear how impaired β-oxidation of fatty acids leads to hepatotoxicity. Eadie and coworkers[144] have drawn attention to the similarity between VPA hepatotoxicity and certain disorders of branched chain amino acid metabolism. Unsaturated metabolites, including 4-en-VPA, have been suggested as potential hepatotoxins.[150, 151] 4-en-VPA is structurally similar to methylenecyclopropylacetic acid, the hepatotoxic metabolite of hypoglycin A that causes Jamaican vomiting sickness.[152] 4-en-VPA is present in low concentrations in all patients taking VPA, however, so its presence in serum does not indicate abnormal VPA metabolism or the development of severe hepatic injury.[153] A recent study of 106 patients receiving VPA showed a negative correlation between patient age and the serum ratio of 4-(en)-VPA/VPA.[153] This indicates that young children form increased amounts of 4-(en)-VPA. This could explain in part their unusual susceptibility to VPA-induced hepatotoxicity.

In patients receiving VPA as monotherapy, there was a positive correlation between serum valproate levels and the 4-(en)-VPA/VPA ratio, whereas the 3-(en)-

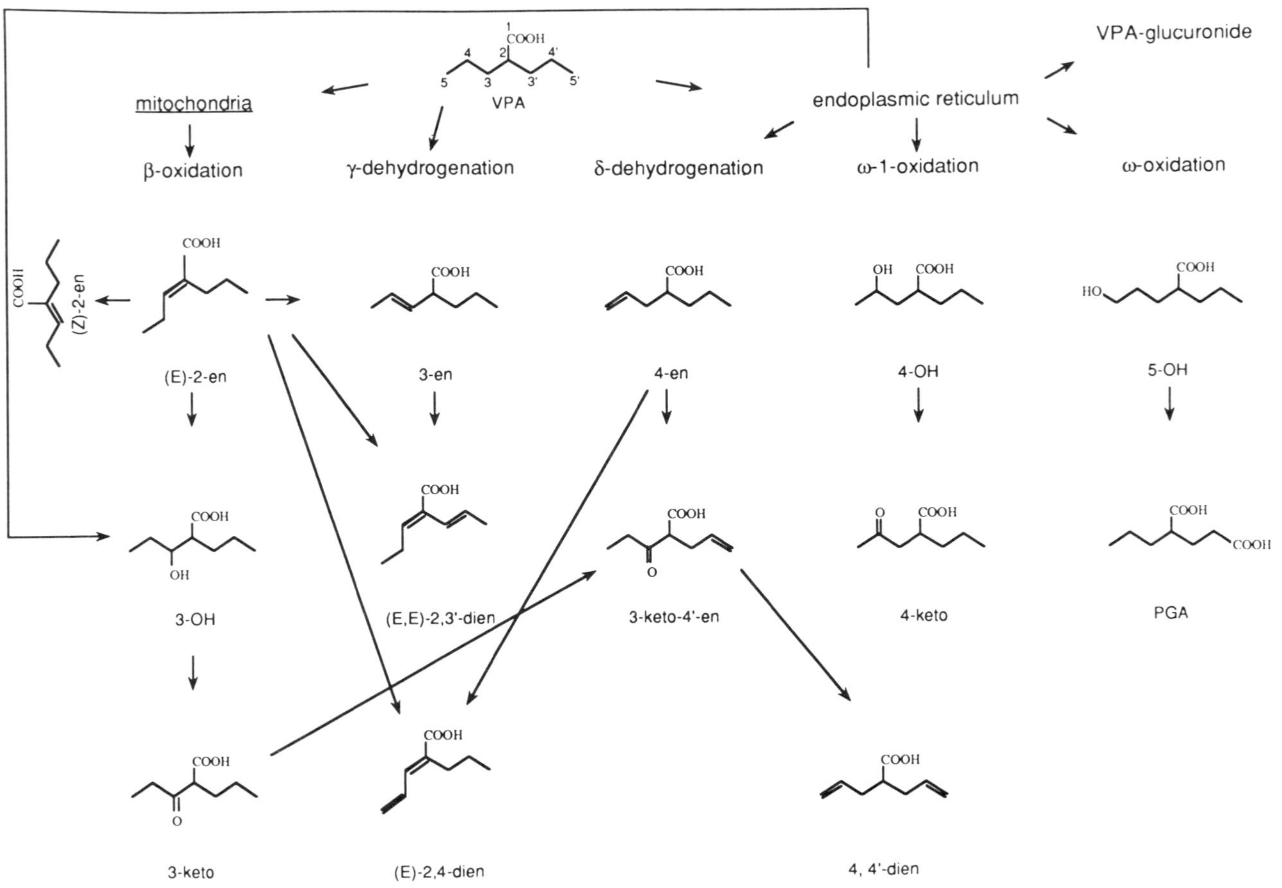
VPA-glucuronide
VPA
mitochondria
endoplasmic reticulum
β-oxidation
γ-dehydrogenation
δ-dehydrogenation
ω-1-oxidation
ω-oxidation
(Z)-2-en
(E)-2-en
3-en
4-en
4-OH
5-OH
3-OH
(E,E)-2,3'-dien
3-keto-4'-en
4-keto
PGA
3-keto
(E)-2,4-dien
4, 4'-dien

VPA/VPA and 2-(en)-VPA/VPA ratios showed significant negative correlations with the serum VPA level. Among individuals aged more than 10 years who were taking VPA as part of multidrug therapy, the 4-(en)-VPA/VPA ratio was higher than in the monotherapy group, whereas the 3-(en)-VPA/VPA ratio was lower. Surprisingly, a similar profile could not be demonstrated in the younger patients taking polytherapy.[153]

Most cases of VPA-associated hepatic failure occur within the first 4 months of drug administration,[141, 142, 154] although deaths rarely have occurred after treatment for as long as 5 years.[155] The initial presentation often is with prodromal symptoms such as nausea, vomiting, lethargy, confusion, or loss of seizure control.[141, 142, 154] At biopsy or necropsy, the liver usually has microvesicular steatosis in zones 3 and 2, together with submassive necrosis in zone 3.[156] A fatal outcome is common, although full recovery is possible after cessation of the drug.

Predicting acute idiosyncratic hepatic drug reactions has proved difficult. Abnormal liver test results are indicative of minor dose-dependent toxicity and may not necessarily precede severe VPA-induced hepatotoxicity.[157] Some authors have advocated regular laboratory monitoring of liver enzyme levels,[158] but the difficulties of interpreting abnormalities and the need to repeat tests that show minor abnormalities are limitations of this approach. Moreover, VPA sometimes may be discontinued inappropriately in response to unimportant laboratory findings. On the other hand, clinical monitoring is limited because the clinical features of liver damage occur late in the disease. A novel suggestion is that the initial stages of hepatotoxicity may be accompanied by changes in VPA metabolism; it is possible that early detection of such changes may reduce the risk of severe liver injury. In a prospective study, Fisher and associates[143] noted transiently altered β-oxidation with increases in 2-en-VPA, 2,3-dien-VPA, and 3-en-VPA in two children infected with adenovirus and *Escherichia coli,* respectively. These abnormal metabolic profiles were associated with abnormal liver test results and hepatomegaly. The biochemical and clinical abnormalities were reversed after the VPA dosage was reduced. The significance of this abnormal metabolic profile is unclear; it may have been a nonspecific response to infection.

Because of the unpredictability of acute idiosyncratic hepatic drug reactions, deaths are likely to occur in rare cases until specific markers are available that identify susceptible individuals. Notwithstanding the above reservations, routine moni-

---

FIG 1.
Metabolites of valproic acid. *VPA* = valproic acid (2-propylpentanoic acid); *2-en* = 2-propyl-(E)-2-pentenoic acid; *3-en* = 2-propyl-3-pentenoic acid; *4-en* = 2-propyl-4-pentenoic acid; *2,3'-dien* = 2-((E)-1'propenyl)-(E)-2-pentenoic acid; *2-4-dien* = 2-propyl-(E)-2,4,-pentadienoic acid; *3-keto-4'-en* = 2-(2'-propenyl)-3-oxo-pentanoic acid; *3-OH* = 3-hydroxy-2-propylpentanoic acid; *4-OH* = 4-hydroxy-2-propylpentanoic acid; *5-OH* = 5-hydroxy-2-propylpentanoic acid; *3-keto* = 3-oxo-2-propylpentanoic acid; *4-keto* = 4-oxo-2-propylpentanoic acid; *PGA* = 2-propylglutaric acid. (From Fisher E, Siemes H, Pund R, et al: *Epilepsia* 1992; 33:165–171. Used by permission.)

toring of liver tests may be prudent, especially during the first 6 months of treatment. Minor abnormalities should not necessarily be an indication to discontinue VPA, but treatment probably should be modified in individuals with AST levels exceeding three times the upper limit of normal. The onset of prodromal features, especially lethargy, somnolence, anorexia, and vomiting are important indications for the discontinuation of VPA. Dreifuss and colleagues[142] have suggested the following precautions to reduce the incidence of VPA-induced hepatotoxicity: (1) avoidance of polytherapy in children less than 3 years of age, (2) avoidance of VPA when there is a family history of childhood hepatic disease, (3) avoidance of fasting and salicylates with intercurrent illness, (4) use of the minimal effective dose, and (5) careful vigilance for prodromal symptoms of liver injury.

Haloalkane Anesthetics

Halothane

Halothane and the fluorinated ethers enflurane and isoflurane are the most widely used inhalational anesthetic agents. Halothane-associated liver injury has been reviewed in a previous volume of *Current Hepatology*.[3] To date, halothane has been associated with more than 1,000 reported cases of liver injury.[159, 160] Minor hepatotoxicity, characterized by transiently abnormal liver test results in asymptomatic patients, may occur in as many as 25% of patients exposed to halothane.[160] The severe form of halothane hepatitis is rare, with a mortality rate of 20% to 50%. The risk of halothane hepatitis increases from 1 in 35,000 after single exposure to 1 in 700 after multiple exposures to halothane, especially when reexposure occurs within a short interval.[160, 161] Other risk factors are age greater than 40 years, female gender, and obesity.

The mechanism of hepatic necrosis after haloalkane exposure is uncertain. Halothane is metabolized through oxidative and reductive pathways, with the latter generating free radical metabolites. Oxidative metabolism of halothane generates the trifluoroacetyl (TFA) halide. This can react with free amines of proteins or phospholipids to yield the corresponding amides.[162, 163] Protein binding of TFA forms adducts that appear to act as neoantigenic epitopes. Antibodies directed against these epitopes are found in some (but not all) patients with halothane hepatitis.[164] If a cytotoxic immune response to TFA adducts is the mechanism for halothane hepatitis, antibodies should bind to TFA adducts on the surface of the hepatocyte. This is an attractive hypothesis, the main drawback to which is that neoantigens are microsomal proteins and are not generated on the cell surface. Recently, Trudell and associates[165] showed that antibodies raised against TFA-modified proteins cross-react strongly with the respective TFA-modified phospholipid. This cross-reactivity is important, because the exchange of phospholipids between cellular membranes could make TFA-modified phospholipid the major antigenic structure on the cell surface. It has been proposed, therefore, that the initial exposure to halothane allows TFA to react with free amino groups of proteins and phospholipids. When TFA-altered hepatocytes lyse because of acute toxicity or cell turnover, the modified proteins migrate to mesenteric lymph nodes, where they invoke antiadduct IgG and activate T lymphocytes. These antiadduct antibodies then could react with phospholipid adducts on the cell surface.[165] Alternatively, Kupffer cells, which are naturally competent antigen-presenting cells, may participate in processing or presenting TFA adducts or fragments thereof to immune-competent cells. In support of the latter hypothesis, TFA adducts similar to those found in hepatocytes recently have been demonstrated within Kupffer cells from rats exposed to halothane.[166]

Enflurane

Hepatic injury is even rarer with enflurane. In one study, hepatotoxicity after enflurane anesthesia was associated with features similar to halothane and methoxyflurane-associated hepatitis.[167] Eger and coworkers[168] reevaluated the same data, however, and found inconclusive evidence for a syndrome of "enflurane hepatitis."

Isoflurane

Last on the clinical scene, with recently increased use as litigation-conscious anesthetists abandon halothane, is isoflurane. There is minimal convincing evidence that isoflurane can cause hepatotoxicity, despite recent case reports. Most of these have been confounded by the presence of viral infections,[169, 170] other medications,[171, 172] concomitant surgery, and the existence of concurrent disease. A subcommittee of the Food and Drug Administration analyzed 45 reports of possible isoflurane-associated liver injury and found the evidence that isoflurane causes hepatic dysfunction to be weak.[173] Recently, a prospective study in 11 infants and children exposed daily to isoflurane for at least 2 weeks showed no change in liver test results.[174] The children were given an average of 24 ± 11 isoflurane anesthetics, with an exposure time of 15 to 30 minutes each day. We remain convinced that isoflurane is nothing more than a possible, and possibly an unlikely, cause of drug-induced liver disease.

Sevoflurane

Sevoflurane is a fluorinated haloalkane anesthetic that currently is undergoing clinical trials. It is biotransformed to inorganic fluoride and hexafluoroisopropanol; the latter is conjugated and excreted in the urine. In humans, only 1% to 4% of the absorbed dose of sevoflurane undergoes biotransformation. In rats and dogs, frequent exposure to sevoflurane over a period of 2 weeks failed to cause hepatotoxicity.[175] In contrast, studies in guinea pigs showed biochemical and histologic evidence for liver injury[176]; the latter may be attributable to hepatic ischemia. Sevoflurane produced only minimal toxicity in the form of depressed protein synthesis when added to guinea pig liver slices.[177] This is consistent with in vivo studies in which minimal or no hepatotoxicity has been observed. To date, no liver test abnormalities have been noted among human volunteers.[178, 179]

Desflurane

Desflurane (formerly I-653) is another volatile anesthetic. It differs from isoflurane by the substitution of a fluorine for a chlorine atom. This results in a compound that is less soluble and more stable, thereby permitting rapid recovery from anesthesia. To date, studies in rats[180] and healthy human volunteers[181, 182] suggest that it is free of hepatotoxicity.

Antiandrogens

The potent, orally active, nonsteroidal antiandrogens flutamide and nilutamide exhibit no androgenic, estrogenic, progestational, glucocorticoid, or other hormonal activity. These agents are used commonly in combination with luteinizing hormone-releasing hormone (LH-RH) agonists and are extremely beneficial for the palliative treatment of metastatic carcinoma of the prostate. Newer indications for their use include hirsutism, benign prostatic hyperplasia, and acne. Flutamide-associated hepatotoxicity has been noted, but is not well documented.[183–185]

Gomez and colleagues[186] recently published a detailed analysis of flutamide-associated liver injury. The cohort comprised 1,091 patients with stage C or D adenocarcinoma of the prostate treated with flutamide and the LH-RH agonist [D-Trp^6 des-Gly-NH$_2$^{10}] LH-RH ethylamide. Patients were treated for at least 2 months with a standard dose of flutamide (250 mg three times daily). The overall frequency of hepatic dysfunction in this group was 0.36%, and the proportion with symptomatic hepatitis was 0.18%. Pretreatment liver test results did not exceed 20% of the upper limit of normal. During therapy, serial enzyme estimations were within normal limits or revealed only minor asymptomatic elevations of serum ALT levels (less than four times the upper limit of normal) in the majority of patients.

Four patients had acute flutamide-associated hepatitis within 4 weeks of commencing therapy, 2 of whom were symptomatic.[186] ALT levels ranged between 4 and 20 times the upper limit of normal. The pattern of enzyme elevations was hepatocellular in three cases and cholestatic in the remainder. Liver biopsy in the latter case revealed cholestatic hepatitis with canalicular bile plugs, spotty necrosis, and a lymphocytic infiltrate in the portal tracts. In all patients, liver test result abnormalities resolved within 8 weeks of the discontinuation of flutamide, despite continuation of the LH-RH agonist. In two cases, rechallenge with half the dose of flutamide resulted in a greater than twofold elevation of aminotransferase levels within 3 days. The authors recommended that liver tests be performed in patients taking flutamide to avoid the risk of significant liver injury.[186] This seems justified, because all cases of hepatotoxicity during flutamide therapy could be detected by performing liver tests at 2 and 4 weeks after initiation of therapy with the drug.

Hart and Stricker[187] reported a similar case of cholestatic liver injury that began 5 weeks after the commencement of flutamide. Another case of fulminant hepatic failure associated with a 6-month course of flutamide therapy has been published.[188] This was unlike previous reports, especially in the time course for the reaction, and may represent a case of fulminant hepatic failure of unknown etiology.

Nilutamide, an analogue of flutamide, also has been shown by Gomez and colleagues[189] to be associated with liver injury. In their report, a 69-year-old man treated with nilutamide and an LH-RH agonist for prostatic carcinoma had dyspnea and abnormal liver test results within 2 months of starting therapy. The respiratory findings were compatible with interstitial pneumonitis and fibrosis, whereas the liver enzyme elevations indicated a hepatocellular reaction. Cessation of nilutamide therapy for 2 months (with continuation of the LH-RH agonist) resulted in normalization of liver test results and improvement in lung function. No cross-reactivity was observed when therapy subsequently was altered to flutamide.

The mechanism of hepatotoxicity associated with the oral antiandrogens is uncertain. Immunoallergic features such as peripheral blood eosinophilia have been noted, but appear to be rare.[187] It is of interest that these agents increase blood testosterone concentrations, giving rise to the possibility that the cholestatic type of liver injury associated with flutamide may be an androgen-related effect.[190]

Sulfasalazine and Melsalazine

Friis and Andreasen[191] noted the increasing importance of sulfasalazine as a cause of drug-induced liver disease in Denmark. On the basis of consumption data, the increase was shown to result from increased utilization of sulfasalazine for rheumatoid arthritis, but it was unclear whether sulfasalazine hepatotoxicity is more or less common in patients with rheumatoid arthritis or inflammatory bowel disease. Side effects of sulfasalazine usually are ascribed to the sulfapyridine moiety, although Friis and Andreasen[191] commented that the pattern of liver injury associated with sulfasalazine differs from the frequently cholestatic forms observed with sulfonamides. Thus, a recent case report from Belgium is of considerable interest.[192] A rash developed in a patient with Crohn's disease after 3 weeks of treatment with sulfasalazine and resolved within 4 days of its discontinuation. Three days later (7 days after the discontinuation of sulfasalazine), melsalazine therapy was begun. Within 2 days, the patient had a generalized pruritic rash, a high fever, and gastrointestinal symptoms. Liver tests indicated cholestasis and increasing aminotransferase levels until melsalazine was discontinued. The AST level peaked at 5,622 IU/L and the nadir of the international normalized ratio was 0.18, indicating very severe hepatitis. Liver biopsy showed marked degenerative changes in virtually all hepatocytes and a mixed-cell type of portal inflammatory infiltrate; cholestasis was minimal. The patient eventually recovered. It seems likely that melsalazine was responsible for hepatotoxicity in this case because of the definite exacerbation of drug allergy after melsalazine therapy was initiated, even though some types of drug hepatitis may not become evident until days or weeks after discontinuation of the causative agent. Because melsalazine contains only 5-aminosalicylic acid, this case raises the question as to whether this moiety, rather than sulfapyridine, could be responsible for the apparently immunoallergic reactions to sulfasalazine. In accord with this possibility, one case of possible mild olsalazine hepatitis also has been described.[193]

Drug-Induced Chronic Cholestasis

The number of drugs reported as causes of chronic cholestasis continues to increase. Two cases of chronic cholestasis recently were reported as a sequel to co-trimoxazole–induced cholestatic hepatitis.[194] Because trimethoprim has been associated with only a single reported instance of liver injury.[195] it seems likely that the sulfonamide moiety was responsible for these cases, although sulfonamides previously have not been well documented as a cause of prolonged cholestasis.

At least 20 cases of clinically significant carbamazepine-induced liver disease have been reported. Granulomatous hepatitis was the principal lesion in three fourths of these.[196–198] Acute cholangitis also was present in some cases. In two patients, this was the predominant feature,[199] and in one recently reported case, it resulted in the vanishing bile duct syndrome.[200]

Oncotherapeutic Drugs

Cytotoxic agents may cause acute or chronic hepatocellular and endothelial cell damage.[201] In addition, azathioprine, which also is used for immunosuppression, may cause cholestatic hepatitis,[1, 202] nodular regenerative hyperplasia,[203] and perivenous fibrosis.[203, 204]

Veno-occlusive Disease After Busulfan and Cyclophosphamide Treatment

High-dose busulfan and cyclophosphamide, without total body irradiation, has become a popular conditioning regimen before bone marrow transplantation. It is reported to have a lower incidence of toxicity, particularly for hepatic veno-occlusive disease (VOD).[205] The risk of VOD with this conditioning regimen remains controversial, however.[206] Recently, Kasai and colleagues[207] noted that the frequency of VOD after busulfan/cyclophosphamide treatment was 25%. All patients died within 1 to 2 months of bone marrow transplantation; the diagnosis of VOD was confirmed at autopsy.

The occurrence of VOD was dependent on the dose of busulfan/cyclophosphamide. Because the dose was calculated on real body weight, patients with VOD had received 1.22-fold (range, 1.16- to 1.29-fold) more drug than they would have had the dose been calculated on ideal body weight. For patients without VOD, this ratio was 0.96 ($P < .05$). As a result of these observations, it has been recommended that the dose for busulfan and cyclophosphamide be based on ideal body weight, or real body weight if this is less than ideal weight.

Methotrexate and Veno-occlusive Disease After Graft-vs.-Host Disease Prophylaxis

Regimens used as prophylaxis against graft-vs.-host disease (GVHD) also may contribute to the development of VOD. Lower rates of VOD (2.0% to 10.8%) have been reported using cyclosporin A/methylprednisolone for GVHD prophylaxis in combination with busulfan/cyclophosphamide conditioning therapy.[208, 209] Essell and associates[210] described 87 patients who received conditioning therapy with busulfan and cyclophosphamide for allogenic bone marrow transplantation. Sixty-seven patients received cyclosporin A and methylprednisolone (historical controls) and 20 patients received cyclosporin A and MTX for GVHD prophylaxis. All other supportive measures were similar between the two groups. The frequency of clinically apparent VOD increased from 18% for those given methylprednisolone to 70% for those given MTX ($P = .0001$). Moreover the use of MTX increased the risk of VOD-related death from 4.5% to 25% ($P = .02$). Overall survival, however, was not significantly different because of the higher non-VOD death rate among the historical control patients.

Cyclosporin A/MTX is effective for GVHD prophylaxis and has been shown to have acceptable toxicity when it is used after cyclophosphamide/total body irradiation conditioning. The interaction between busulfan and MTX needs further investigation, and physicians using busulfan-containing preparative regimens must be aware of the potential for serious liver toxicity if cyclosporin A/MTX is used for GVHD prophylaxis.

Veno-occlusive Disease and Disordered Coagulation

A recent case report of VOD in a child with rhabdomyosarcoma once again emphasizes the hepatotoxicity of actinomycin D and vincristine.[211] Similar occurrences have been noted in patients with Wilms' tumor treated with these two agents, with or without radiation.[3, 212] Interestingly, enhanced coagulation and fibrinolysis were noted before any signs of liver damage appeared. Several authors have alluded to this phenomenon previously and suggested that it may be a harbinger of VOD.[213, 214] In early VOD, Shulman and coworkers[215] demonstrated dense deposits in the terminal hepatic and sublobular central venules that immunostained with anti-factor VIII and antifibrinogen antibodies.

The role of anticoagulant therapy in VOD remains uncertain. Although gabexate mesylate was used in the case reported by Adachi and Matsuda,[211] its usefulness in the prevention and treatment of VOD is unclear. Gluckman and colleagues[216] used prostaglandin E_1 prophylactically in patients undergoing allogenic bone marrow transplantation and reported a decrease in the incidence of VOD from 39% to 13%. The pathogenesis of VOD may be related to the initial injury to the endothelium and subsequent activation of the coagulation cascade. Further studies are required to determine the role of anticoagulation therapy in the prevention and treatment of this problem.

Thioguanine Toxicity

Thioguanine can cause a wide spectrum of liver disease.[1, 201] When it was used in combination with busulfan as maintenance therapy in patients with chronic myeloid leukemia, it was associated with a higher incidence of noncirrhotic portal hypertension, whereas patients receiving busulfan alone had none.[217] This was the result of nodular regenerative hyperplasia, perisinusoidal fibrosis, and, in some cases, associated minor portal sclerosis. Unfortunately, liver histology was obtained in only a few cases, making the results somewhat inconclusive. Unlike other trials using thioguanine (e.g., Medical Research Council, acute leukemia trial), the increased frequency of VOD in this trial may be related to regular and extended administration of the drug and interactive toxicity with busulfan. Because combined therapy with these agents did not prolong survival, it no longer is recommended for long-term maintenance therapy in chronic myeloid leukemia.

A "New Syndrome" After N-Phosphonoacetyl-L-Aspartate and Fluorouracil Treatment

A "new syndrome" of ascites, increased total bilirubin levels, and hypoalbuminemia recently has been described among patients receiving low-dose N-phosphonoacetyl-L-aspartate and high-dose bolus fluorouracil for metastatic colorectal carcinoma.[218] The biochemical features included mild elevation of the AST level and prolongation of the prothrombin time, but no significant change in serum alkaline phosphatase (SAP). These abnormalities were more frequent among patients who responded to chemotherapy. N-phosphonoacetyl-L-aspartate inhibits de novo pyrimidine synthesis.[219] The subsequent decrease in the size of the uridine pool increases the incorporation of fluorouracil into RNA and thereby inhibits protein synthesis.[220] The defect in bilirubin secretion also may be explained by the decrease in the uridine pool; this could impair bilirubin glucuronidation because of the requirement for uridine 5'-diphosphate as a cosubstrate in this reaction.[221] Clinicians must be aware of this "syndrome" to recognize it as being secondary to the chemotherapeutic drugs and not to hepatic complications of the underlying malignant disease.

Tumor Necrosis Factor

Recombinant human tumor necrosis factor-α (TNF) currently is an investigational antitumor agent. Mild elevations of bilirubin and aminotransferase levels have been reported after the administration of TNF.[222] A case of severe hepatic dysfunction with a 40-fold increase in the ALT level after TNF infusion has been described recently.[223] The patient remained asymptomatic. After the discontinuation of TNF, liver test results returned toward normal within 6 days. Further reports of hepatic abnormalities in association with this agent are awaited, particularly given the considerable interest in the role of TNF in alcoholic liver disease,[224] ischemia-reperfusion injury,[225] and experimental hepatotoxicity.[226]

Fipexide Hepatotoxicity

Fipexide, a drug that activates dopaminergic receptors, has been used in Europe since 1973 for the treatment of asthenia and memory disorders. Mion and coworkers[227] reported a single case of acute hepatitis associated with fipexide. Recently, three more cases of fulminant hepatic failure necessitating orthotopic liver transplantation have been reported in patients taking fipexide.[228] Two of the three patients survived transplantation. In all four reported cases of fipexide-associated liver disease,[227, 228] the drug had been administered for 1 to 2 months before the appearance of jaundice. The subsequent course was one of rapid progression to fulminant liver failure. Histologic examination in all cases revealed massive, predominantly centrilobular (acinar zone 3) liver cell necrosis with a moderate inflammatory cell infiltrate in the portal tracts. Although these changes are consistent with severe drug-induced hepatotoxicity, it is unfortunate that no evidence was presented to exclude hepatitis C virus infection. The mechanism of fipexide-induced liver injury is unknown, although immunoallergy would be consistent with the lack of a relationship between the dose and the severity of liver injury, and with the presence of a rash in one patient. Awareness of the association between fipexide and fulminant hepatic failure mandates more cautious prescription of this drug.

Omeprazole

Omeprazole is a substituted benzimidazole that inhibits the hydrogen-potassium ATPase and thereby profoundly inhibits gastric acid secretion. It has become a valuable agent for the treatment of refractory reflux esophagitis and the Zollinger-Ellison syndrome. Trivial and reversible elevations in aminotransferase levels previously have been described with this agent.[229] The first case of fulminant hepatic failure attributed to omeprazole has been described recently.[230] It occurred in a 62-year-old man with reflux esophagitis who was taking 20 mg/day of omeprazole. He had no previous liver disease or risk factors for hepatitis, but also had been taking atenolol, diltiazem, and aspirin for at least 1 year (these agents all have been described as rare hepatotoxins, but their effect would be expected within 3 months). Seventeen days after the commencement of omeprazole, the patient was admitted to the hospital with hepatic failure; he died 5 days later. Histologic examination of the liver revealed massive zone 3 necrosis and hemorrhage with proliferation of bile ducts. No vascular, obstructive, or metabolic cause for liver injury was found, and infectious causes were excluded by serology and viral immunoperoxidase stains. The patient denied taking other drugs, but a drug screen was not performed.

We previously have commented on the difficulty of ascribing causality to drugs based on isolated case reports of fulminant hepatic failure,[1, 3] particularly knowing that the majority of cases of fulminant hepatic failure appear to be viral-like in etiology, but are not associated with markers of any known hepatitis virus.[4] Additional case reports, particularly with note of any more persuasive features of drug etiology (especially rechallenge), are required before omeprazole can be regarded as a potential cause of drug-induced liver disease.

Nonsteroidal Anti-inflammatory Drugs

Although hepatic drug reactions are uncommon with currently used nonsteroidal anti-inflammatory drugs (NSAIDs), the enormous consumption of these agents has ensured that they feature prominently among present causes of drug-induced liver disease.[3, 231] Some recent publications have quantified the magnitude of the problem. In Denmark,[232] the average consumption of NSAIDs in the period 1969 to 1985 was equivalent to a permanent intake by 2.2% of the population. Furthermore, the total sales of NSAIDs quadrupled during this period. Among 3,521 adverse drug reactions to NSAIDs, 3% involved the liver. Practically all types of NSAIDs were implicated; the only fatal cases were associated with indomethacin (one case) and benoxaprofen (two cases). With the exception of benoxaprofen, only sulindac (see below) and fenbrufen (like benoxaprofen, a propionic acid derivative) were reported more often than once per million defined daily doses (both 1.2, compared with benoxaprofen 12.6, phenylbutazone 0.2, indomethacin 0.2, diclofenac 0.4, piroxicam 0.3, and tolmetin 0.3).[232]

The conclusion that the overall risk of NSAIDs causing acute liver injury is extremely low is well supported by a Canadian study.[233] The study was retrospective, but involved 228,392 adults and 645,456 person-years from the health records of a provincial data base in Saskatchewan. The size and comprehensive nature of the data base, as well as the incorporation of a crossover design, strengthen the validity of the findings. The main end point was admission to the hospital for newly diagnosed acute liver injury. The incidence rate among current users of NSAIDs was 9 (95% confidence interval, 6 to 15) per 100,000 person-years, compared with 2.3 (1.1 to 4.9) in those not currently using NSAIDs. Thus, the age- and sex-adjusted risk ratio was 1.7 (0.8 to 3.7), and the excess risk of having acute liver disease attributable to the use of NSAIDs was 5 per 100,000 person-years. The strength of the association between NSAIDs and acute liver disease increased when only cases with no concomitant use of other potentially hepatotoxic drugs were considered. There was no increased risk with longer duration of treatment. The clinical features leading to hospital admission were similar in the two groups, except that there was a predominance of cholestatic liver disease among NSAID users. This is a very useful study because it affirms the fact that NSAIDs unequivocally contribute to morbidity from drug-induced liver disease and it quantifies the very low level of that risk.

The strength of epidemiologic studies that utilize health records linked to community-based data bases is that incidence data relevant to the general population can be obtained. A weakness is that clinicopathologic aspects of illnesses are less well defined. Thus, it is not clear from the Canadian study how many cases of "acute liver injury" were attributable to known causes, such as viral hepatitis and acute cholangitis resulting from biliary disease. This type of information requires perusal of the case record. This point was emphasized by another study that examined the feasibility of using Medicaid data in Michigan and Florida to study drug-induced hepatitis.[234] The medical records were examined of patients receiving Medicaid who were aged 20 years or older and had an *International Classification of Diseases-9-CM (ICD-9-CM)* in patient billing code that was consistent with acute hepatitis. Cases were excluded by "computerized diagnosis" if there was a concurrent diagnosis of hepatitis A or B, or an alcohol-related diagnosis at any time before the study. The medical records of 414 cases were retrieved, representing 53% of potential cases. They comprised 15.9% alcoholics, 31.9% patients with acute hepatitis A or B, 13.5% intravenous drug abusers, 8.2% patients with acute biliary tract disease, and 4.1% patients who had received a blood transfusion within the preceding 6 months. No evidence to support a diagnosis of liver disease was found in 10.6% of patients, whereas 5.7% had chronic liver disease. This left 169 patients with "idiopathic acute liver disease." Many of these had very mild liver disease and were hospitalized for other reasons. Drug-induced liver disease was thought by attending physicians to account for liver disease in 26.6% of cases. Agents that were incriminated on more than one occasion were phenytoin (10 cases), α-methyldopa (6 cases), isoniazid (5 cases), erythromycin (4 cases), VPA (3 cases), carbamazepine (3 cases), chlorpromazine (2 cases), co-trimoxazole (2 cases), and erythromycin (2 cases). This series illustrates the importance of obtaining the medical record to validate coded diagnostic information, and of understanding the relative importance of adverse hepatic drug reactions in relation to other clinical problems. Limitations of this approach also are evident, such as the 10.6% misclassification rate, the low retrieval rate (53%), and the inadequacy of recorded information in medical records.

NSAIDs were not an important cause of acute drug-induced liver disease in the Medicaid data survey.[234] Is this because these agents are not an important cause of acute liver injury in the United States, or because cases were not recognized or were classified incorrectly? Perusal of reports of adverse reactions made to monitoring authorities indicates the former explanation. In Denmark, between 1978 and 1987, about 9% of all hepatic drug reactions were attributable to NSAIDs.[235] The two most often incriminated agents were sulindac (18 of 1,100 cases of drug-induced liver disease) and ibuprofen (17 cases). Consumption data were available for these two drugs, allowing calculation of the relative frequency of adverse hepatic reactions to each agent. On this basis, sulindac was nearly 20-fold more likely to be associated with liver injury than was ibuprofen. Both drugs were associated with cytotoxic ("hepatocellular") reactions and with cholestatic reactions.

Sulindac

A more detailed assessment of the pattern of liver injury associated with individual agents is afforded by examining reports of adverse drug reactions made to drug monitoring authorities. A limitation of this approach is case selection and inadequate recording of data. Thus, among 338 reports of suspected sulindac-associated hepatic injury that had been submitted to the Food and Drug Authority, 247 were considered inadequate or unconvincing for sulindac toxicity.[236] The remaining 91 cases were analyzed, including histologic examination of the 15 for which material was available. There were 4 fatal cases; death was attributable to fulminant hepatic failure in 1 case and to severe generalized hypersensitivity in the other 3 cases. The ratio of women to men of 3.5:1 is likely to be greater than for drug utilization, although the relevant data were not available in this study. Two thirds of affected patients were older than 50 years of age. Features of drug hypersensitivity have been prominent in earlier reports of sulindac hepatitis and were noted in two thirds of cases in the Food and Drug Authority series. Among the 91 selected cases, hepatotoxicity was relatively severe, as indicated by the fact that jaundice was noted in 67%; whether this reflects case selection or is indicative of the usual type of reaction to sulindac is one of the difficulties of this type of survey.

The clinicopathologic pattern of liver injury was cholestatic in 43% of cases, hepatocellular in 25%, and mixed or otherwise indeterminant in the remaining 32%. A point of note was that eosinophilia was more common (40%) among patients with a cholestatic profile of liver tests than among those with hepatocellular injury (0%). There are several explanations for this, however, other than the authors' contention that different pathogenetic mechanisms may operate to produce the various clinicopathologic patterns of liver test result and histologic abnormalities. It is well known that many infectious, neoplastic, and immunologic disorders can produce protean manifestations of hepatic disease. Hence, we prefer not to interpret clinicopathologic data in mechanistic terms until further information that has a more direct bearing on etiopathogenesis is forthcoming. As an example, pancreatitis without recognized hepatic involvement may be caused by sulindac and was the possible cause of cholestasis in 4 cases in the present study. In most cases, however, the generalized nature of adverse reactions to sulindac, which include a high frequency of fever, rash (including the Stevens-Johnson syndrome), and nephrotoxocity, is suggestive of an immunologically mediated form of hypersensitivity.

Piroxicam

Piroxicam is an oxicam, structurally unrelated to most other NSAIDs. It is possibly the most widely used NSAID on a world scale.[237] Last year, we mentioned a report of severe cholestasis attributed to piroxicam.[238] Sherman and Jones[239] have drawn attention to another case of piroxicam-induced hepatitis in a 61-year-old woman. The onset occurred 12 days after the initiation of piroxicam, but the drug was not discontinued for another 2 weeks. Clinical features were those of cholestatic hepatitis, but ALT levels peaked at 2,000 IU/L 2 weeks after piroxicam was discontinued. The patient made a slow recovery over 3 months. Two other cases of severe piroxicam-associated hepatitis have been reported recently from Brisbane, Queensland.[240] One patient, who had been taking piroxicam for 15 months, died. The other had submassive hepatic necrosis and was treated with orthotopic liver transplantation. This brings the total reported number of cases of piroxicam-induced liver injury to seven.[238, 239, 241–243] The reported cases have been characterized by severe reactions, with subacute hepatic necrosis and features of cholestasis in some cases. Two patients have been treated with corticosteroids with no beneficial response, and two others have received a successful liver transplant. We agree with the comment by Paterson and associates[240] that hepatic transplantation should be considered in cases of drug-induced liver injury with a deteriorating course.

"Street Drugs"

In previous volumes of *Current Hepatology*,[2, 3] we discussed the association between cocaine intoxication and liver injury and failure. Several possible mechanisms for this have been proposed, including chemical hepatotoxicity, hepatic ischemia (which we favor), and hyperthermia. Phencyclidine is another popular "recreational" drug; its "street" names include "angel dust," "crystal," and "peace pill." It is a stimulant that has been associated with aggressive behavior, convulsions, autonomic dysfunction, hyperthermia, and rhabdomyolysis, occasionally complicated by renal failure. Liver injury also has been described in cases of phencyclidine-induced malignant hyperthermia in which there was associated respiratory failure and coma.[244] The clinical and laboratory features of severe hepatic injury, together with rhabdomyolysis, are similar to those resulting from hyperthermia produced by heatstroke[245] and to the syndrome observed in some cases of cocaine intoxication.

5-Methoxy-3,4-methylenedioxymethamphetamine (MDMA) is another psychedelic agent, similar to lysergic acid, the street name of which is "ecstasy." It was patented in 1914 as an appetite suppressant, then was investigated as a mood-altering drug, but was banned in 1985 because of neurotoxicity, cardiac arrhythmias, and the propensity for misuse. MDMA currently is popular in some countries, notably the United Kingdom, for its stimulant effects that facilitate all-night dancing or "rave" parties.[246] Several cases of heatstroke now have been attributed to the combined effects of severe MDMA poisoning and prolonged exertion in hot nightclubs. The features of the cases included convulsions, rhabdomyolysis, myoglobinuria, and disseminated intravascular coagulation. These complications are similar to those of the malignant hyperthermia syndrome that occurs after the use of several anesthetic agents, and which has a heterogeneous genetic predisposition. The essential pathogenetic feature of malignant hyperthermia is an abnormality in muscle metabolism that leads to disordered regulation of myoplasmic Ca^{2+} homeostasis.[247]

Hyperpyrexia is a rare complication of MDMA abuse. It has been hypothesized to result from the presence of underlying abnormalities of muscle metabolism, similar to those of the malignant hyperthermia syndrome.[248] This would accord with the observation that the reaction appears to be independent of dose; fatalities have occurred after 1 to 3 tablets of MDMA.[249] Although the hyperthermic action of MDMA is ascribed to a central effect on serotonin receptors, dantrolene, the action of which is thought to be on the sarcoplasmic reticulum, apparently has therapeutic benefit. It should be noted that agents such as "ecstasy" and "angel dust" frequently are contaminated with other hallucinogens and a variety of potentially toxic agents (fish tank oxygenating tablets have been mentioned); the role of these contaminants in organ toxicity is unknown.

Hepatocellular necrosis is a recently reported feature of MDMA toxicity. Among seven cases (6 in men, all aged between 19 and 29 years), one died and another survived after orthotopic liver transplantation.[249] Alcohol and viral hepatitis were excluded and the authors believed that hyperthermia-induced liver injury was an unlikely factor in these cases. Several individuals had taken MDMA repeatedly, and recurrent episodes of jaundice after reexposure were noted in one case. The clinical and biochemical features of liver injury included hepatomegaly, jaundice, pruritus, severe hyperbilirubinemia, and disproportionate increase in the AST compared with the ALT level. Unexplained liver test result abnormalities and hepatomegaly in young people should prompt inquiry into illicit drug use.

Drug-Induced Autoantibodies

In an earlier volume of *Current Hepatology*,[2] we discussed drug-induced autoantibodies. Dihydrallazine-induced hepatitis has been associated with antibodies that exhibit an unusual pattern of liver microsomal immunofluorescence. For this reason, they have been termed antiliver microsomal (anti-LM) antibodies. Bourdi and colleagues[250] have characterized the anti-LM antibodies as being directed toward P-450 1A2, but not the closely related P-450 1A1. In rats, and in human hepatocytes treated in vitro, dihydrallazine specifically induced P-450 1A–catalyzed activities. Anti-LM was shown to be specific for dihydrallazine-induced hepatitis. Moreover, these autoantibodies were present at high titer during the illness, but titers waned and eventually disappeared during clinical recovery. Thus, as for neoantigen-directed antibodies in halothane hepatitis,[3] it still remains to be determined whether drug-induced autoantibodies are mediators of hepatotoxicity. It does seem possible, as suggested by the authors, that the highly variable expression of drug-metabolizing enzymes, such as P-450 1A, could be one reason for individual predisposition to idiosyncratic types of drug hepatitis. The induction of the enzyme responsible for metabolism of the inciting drug, in this case P-450 1A, may increase further the risk of hepatotoxicity by causing the formation of reactive metabolites and enhancing expression of the target antigen for autoantibodies and cytotoxic T cells.

We also previously have reviewed potential mechanisms by which aromatic anticonvulsants may produce liver injury.[2] It is of interest, therefore, that anti–P-450 antibodies recently have been detected in nine patients with hypersensitivity hepatitis caused by carbamazepine, phenytoin, and phenobarbital.[251] Serum from the patients contained an IgG antibody that recognized a 53-kilodalton protein in rat liver microsomes; this protein was constitutively expressed and phenobarbital-inducible. The rat protein was shown to be a P-450 3A subfamily member (P-450 3A1). To date, the human protein has not been identified; it is not P-450 3A4, but other human P-450 3A proteins should be examined. In human liver, a 53-kilodalton microsomal protein was expressed to a greater extent in one patient with fatal phenytoin-induced hepatotoxicity. Identification of the relevant human P-450 should lead to a better understanding of individual susceptibility to drug-induced liver injury, as well as of the relationships between drug metabolism, the production of drug-induced autoantigens, and their role in idiosyncratic drug-induced hepatitis.

Environmental Hepatotoxins

Monochlorobenzene and Interaction With Chronic Alcohol Ingestion

Toxicity from environmental agents is an aspect of clinical hepatology that is of increasing interest. Epidemiologic studies have delineated likely causal associations between exposure to environmental agents and hepatotoxicity. These studies also have measured the risks of low-level but long-term exposure to hepatotoxins, especially within the work environment. In this regard, previous volumes have highlighted the growing number of data on interactive hepatotoxicity between environmental agents and alcohol ingestion.[2, 3] These data have formed the basis for industrial safeguards designed to prevent hepatotoxicity.

Babany and coworkers[252] reported a case of severe hepatic necrosis after suicidal ingestion of the benzene derivative, monochlorobenzene, in a man who had regularly consumed 200 g of ethanol per day. Over 3 days after poisoning, AST and ALT levels rose to 345 and 201 times the upper limit of normal, respectively, while the prothrombin time and factor V levels declined to 25% and 14% of control levels. Liver biopsy revealed extensive zone 2 and 3 necrosis without inflammation. Liver test results returned to normal by day 18.

Benzene derivatives, such as hexachlorobenzene and bromobenzene, are hepatotoxic in man and other animals.[253, 254] Benzene (and its halogenated derivatives) is metabolized by cytochrome P-450 2E1,[255] the same P-450 isoform that is inducible by and responsible, in part, for the oxidation of ethanol. In rats, chronic ethanol administration increases the biotransformation of benzene to benzene-3,4-epoxide.[256] Bromobenzene-3,4-epoxide is the reactive metabolite that depletes GSH and causes liver injury.[257–259] It is likely that monochlorobenzene metabolism proceeds in an analogous manner, with toxicity being mediated by the reactive epoxide.[252] The authors speculated, therefore, that chronic ethanol consumption may have exaggerated the hepatotoxicity of monochlorobenzene in this case via enhanced oxidation of monochlorobenzene and also by the depletion of GSH that occurs in chronic alcoholism.[252, 260]

Herbal Remedies and Hepatotoxicity

Hepatitis has been associated with the ingestion of a wide range of herbal preparations, including asafetida, hops, gentian,[261] mistletoe,[262] chaparral leaf,[263] senna extract,[264] and chinese herbs.[265] Abnormal liver test results are common in patients who regularly consume herbal preparations.[266] Seven cases of acute hepatitis followed the ingestion of germander *(Teucrium chamaedrys)*, an herbal preparation used to facilitate weight loss, as reported by Larrey and colleagues.[267] Liver injury developed an average of 9 weeks after the initiation of therapy with germander. It was characterized by jaundice and elevated aminotransferase levels. Liver biopsy showed acute cytolytic hepatitis in two cases and chronic active hepatitis in another.

In all patients, the withdrawal of germander was followed by resolution of the symptoms, signs, and biochemical features of liver injury. Moreover, rechallenge in three cases led to a recurrence of hepatitis. The mechanism of germander-associated hepatotoxicity is uncertain. The chemical composition of this preparation is complex; it contains flavonoids, tannins, diterpenes, and polyphenol derivatives.[267] On the basis of the authors' recommendations, the manufacturers ceased the production of germander in capsule and teabag form.[267] These cases serve to illustrate the importance of obtaining an adequate history of "over-the-counter" preparation use when dealing with liver injury of uncertain etiology.

Industrial Solvents and Fatty Liver Disease

In a previous volume of *Current Hepatology*,[2] we cited the report of four cases of macrovesicular steatosis that had been attributed to 1,1,1-trichloroethane exposure.[268, 269] Guzelian[270] has called into question the association between 1,1,1-trichloroethane and fatty liver disease in two of these cases. One patient was diabetic. In the other, serial liver biopsies showed questionable evidence of improvement, despite withdrawal from toxin exposure.

Fatty liver disease most often is related to obesity, hyperlipidemia, diabetes, or excessive ethanol consumption. In a case-control study from western Pennsylvania, Hodgson and coworkers[271] compared 19 cases of fatty liver disease with matched controls. Logistic regression suggested that obesity and exposure to known hepatotoxic agents, or to agents that were thought to be potentially hepatotoxic on the basis of structure-activity relationships, were independent risk factors for the development of fatty liver disease.[271]

A similar study from Taiwan examined the relationship in paint workers between liver test result abnormalities and exposure to solvents, especially xylene and toluene.[272] Applying a multivariate model that controlled for alcohol consumption, age, medications, and hepatitis B infection, the authors found increasing serum gamma-glubamyl transpeptidase (γGT) activity to be associated with the severity of exposure to solvents.[272] Jie and colleagues[273] noted that persistent ethanol consumption increased the frequency of liver injury induced by exposure to trinitrotoluene among workers in a munitions plant in China. Such studies of occupational exposure to toxic chemicals emphasize the importance of close monitoring of the work environment for potential toxins and the need for vigilance by clinical hepatologists.

Angiosarcoma

Angiosarcoma of the liver is a rare tumor associated with exposure to agents such as Thorotrast, arsenic, and vinyl chloride monomer. The most important approach to vinyl chloride–induced angiosarcoma is primary prevention through improved ventilation, a cleaner work environment, and monitoring of air to reduce occupational exposure. Although these measures now are usual, if not universal, an outstanding difficulty is that the latent period for the development of angiosarcoma is 20 to 40 years. Thus, secondary prevention (i.e., early detection of cases) also will remain important for some time. Serum levels of von Willebrand's factor (vWf), a glycoprotein synthesized by megakaryocytes and endothelial cells, are increased in cases of endothelial damage or vascular proliferation. The use of vWf as a marker of vinyl chloride–induced liver endothelial cell injury was studied in 107 exposed workers by Froment and colleagues.[274] The vWf level was slightly, but significantly, higher in the exposed group when compared to that of a control population, although overlap of values was considerable. In 17 vinyl chloride workers with a vWf level above the 90th percentile, there were no biochemical signs of hepatic dysfunction. In 3 patients with hepatic angiosarcoma, serum vWf levels were elevated above the 90th percentile.[274] Whether vWf levels will serve as an early marker of liver injury associated with vinyl chloride is uncertain and needs to be evaluated in longitudinal studies.

Thorotrast

Thorotrast (thorium dioxide) was used widely as a radiographic contrast medium until 1955. Because of the retention of thorium in the reticuloendothelial system (including Kupffer cells) and its long biologic half-life (more than 200 years), this agent is associated with a reduced life expectancy and excess mortality from cirrhosis, hepatic malignancy, and leukemia. The latent period for the development of hepatic fibrosis is more than 15 years; for hepatic tumors, it is greater than 25 years. Thus, a recent report of two cases of hepatic malignancy and a further case of macronodular cirrhosis in patients exposed to Thorotrast many years previously is a timely reminder that this agent is likely to be a cause of liver disease until the end of this decade.[275]

Pyrrolizidine Alkaloids

Pyrrolizidine alkaloids are found in numerous plants, including *Senecio, Heliotropium,* and *Crotalaria* species. They have been associated with epidemics and with an endemic incidence of hepatic VOD in several parts of the world, notably Jamaica and the Indian subcontinent. The hepatotoxic alkaloids, such as monocrotaline, contain a 1,2 unsaturated bond (Fig 2); it has been assumed that hepatic metabolism bioactivates this type of alkaloid to a reactive alkylating intermediate. Mattocks[276] proposed that pyrrolic dehydroalkaloids are formed initially, but direct evidence in support of this concept has been lacking. A novel approach was to incubate hepatic microsomes with monocrotaline using the sulfhydryl-containing resin, thiopropyl sepharose 6B, as a trapping agent.[277] Control experiments demonstrated how toxic, chemically reactive, alkylating pyrroles, such as dehydromonocrotaline, bound covalently to the resin via a thioether bond, whereas less toxic, poorly alkylating pyrroles did not. The authors then showed that hepatic microsomes metabolized monocrotaline to a pyrrole that bound via a thioether linkage to the resin.[277] The product released from the resin-bound pyrrole was 7-ethoxy-1-hydroxymethyl-6,7-dihydro-5H-pyrrolizidine. This establishes that dehy-

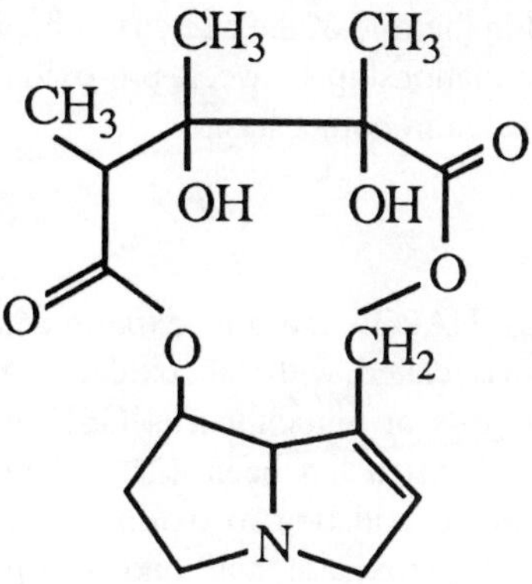

FIG 2.
Monocrotaline *(I)* and dehydromonocrotaline *(II)*. (From Glowaz SL, Michnika M, Huxtable RJ: *Toxicol Appl Pharmacol* 1992; 115:168–173. Used by permission.)

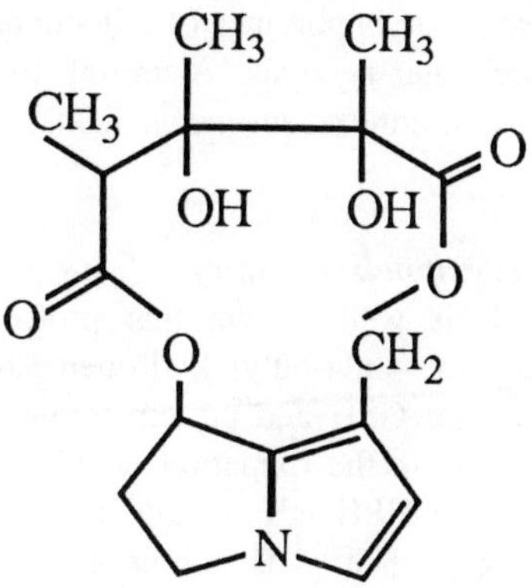

dromonocrotaline (see Fig 2), which has a half-life in water of only a few seconds,[278] is the critical intermediate in the metabolism of monocrotaline.

Summary

A review of the past year's reports on environmental hepatotoxins has shown new cases of toxicity related to chemicals (monochlorobenzene) and preparations previously considered to be harmless (e.g., germander), as well as reports of well-known but unusual forms of hepatotoxicity (e.g., Thorotrast). Epidemiologic studies have highlighted factors that should alert the physician to the possibility of liver injury from environmental or occupational toxins, such as an AST/ALT ratio of less than 1,[279] isolated elevations in γGT, and instances of fatty liver disease; the difficulties of ascribing causality to nonspecific types of liver disease, such as fatty liver disease, again have been brought to notice. The role of interactive hepatotoxicity, particularly between alcohol and solvents, has been emphasized further. Given the protean manifestations of liver injury induced by environmental agents and the preventable nature of such disorders, physicians should remain alert to this form of hepatotoxicity.

Experimental Hepatotoxicity

In recent volumes of *Current Hepatology*,[1-3] we have traced developments in the field of mechanistic hepatotoxicity. Emerging topics include heightened interest in the importance of mitochondrial injury and in the role of the nucleus in hepatocellular necrosis. A uniting theme is the interrelationship between pro-oxidant stress, antioxidant mechanisms, and disordered calcium homeostasis.

Mitochondrial Injury

It is well known that pro-oxidants, such as NAPQI and the experimental hepatotoxin *t*-butyl hydroperoxide (TBH), are associated with the oxidation of cellular GSH and protein thiols. This causes the loss of mitochondrial GSH and results in the oxidation of pyridine nucleotides.[3] It often has been assumed that loss of GSH is consequent to its direct and indirect oxidation to oxidized GSH (e.g., when it is acting as a cofactor for GSH peroxidase and phospholipid peroxidase), as well as to its consumption in conjugation reactions (either spontaneous or catalyzed by GSH S-transferases). A recent study in isolated hepatocytes has demonstrated that these may not be the only mechanisms by which toxicants deplete the hepatocytes and mitochondria of GSH.[280] Three nonoxidant inhibitors of mitochondrial function, antimycin A, potassium cyanide (KCN), and 1-methyl-4-phenylpyridium all produced extensive depletion of GSH. This effect correlated with the depletion of cellular ATP and preceded cytotoxicity. There was no increased oxidation of GSH to oxidized GSH, but about 40% of the loss of GSH was attributable to efflux from the cells. The addition of 10mM of fructose (to stimulate the formation of ATP through enhanced glycolysis) provided protection against GSH depletion, although it was not indicated whether this protected the cells against lethal injury. Fructose recently has been demonstrated to protect isolated rat hepatocytes from anoxic injury.[281] Extension of these studies to other toxicants and to more physiologic systems than freshly isolated hepatocytes[1] should help to substantiate whether mitochondrial injury and cellular "deenergization" is an important pathway leading to cell death.

In the most recent volume of *Current Hepatology*,[3] we discussed recent studies into the mechanism by which NAPQI releases Ca^{2+} from mitochondrial stores. More work in this area was published this year.[282] There is increasing evidence that cyclosporin A can provide protection against toxicant-induced mitochondrial Ca^{2+} release, and that, under selected circumstances, this may protect against cellular injury. Mitochondria have a low affinity but a high capacity for Ca^{2+}. Therefore, they may participate in Ca^{2+} homeostasis, particularly under conditions of elevated $[Ca^{2+}]_i$. Richter and colleagues[283] have shown that cyclosporin A can inhibit the release, but not the uptake of, Ca^{2+} by mitochondria. Ca^{2+} enters energized mitochondria through a ruthenium red–sensitive site in an electrophoretic response to the mitochondrial membrane potential (negative inside). The release of Ca^{2+} is electroneutral and probably is regulated by protein mono(adenosine diphosphate-ribosylation). The authors[283] showed that cyclosporin A prevented Ca^{2+} release from mitochondria by inhibiting the intramitochondrial hydrolysis of nicotinamide-adenine dinucleotide to adenosine diphosphate-ribose and nicotinamide. It has been proposed that this mechanism could interfere with cellular Ca^{2+}

homeostasis and could be related to both the immunosuppressive and the cytotoxic properties of cyclosporin A.

Broekemeier and colleagues[284] studied the putative protective effect of cyclosporin A on hepatocytes subjected to TBH-induced oxidative stress. TBH and other pro-oxidants induce a permeability transition in Ca^{2+}-loaded mitochondria that results in the loss of coupled function and Ca^{2+} release.[285] This would diminish greatly the effectiveness of mitochondria in "buffering" cells against the raised $[Ca^{2+}]_i$ associated with oxidative stress, and also may be a process that contributes directly to cell injury. Recently, cyclosporin A was found to inhibit the calcium transition with high potency and selectivity.[285] Cyclosporin A protected isolated hepatocytes from TBH toxicity when the medium Ca^{2+} concentration was 10mM, but not when it was 2.5mM. The higher Ca^{2+} concentration was associated with mitochondrial Ca^{2+} loading within the cells and the inhibition of TBH-dependent lipid peroxidation. The findings were interpreted as evidence for a peroxidation-independent mechanism for TBH toxicity in addition to the well-characterized peroxidative mechanism. Mitochondrial permeability transition and resultant deenergization are likely components of the peroxidation-independent mechanism.

Kass and associates[286] also reported that cyclosporin A was protective against pro-oxidant stress (Fig 3), although protection varied with the type and concentration of toxicant. The inhibition of mitochondrial Ca^{2+} release and abrogation of permeability transition were thought to be the protective mechanisms of cyclosporin A. These fascinating studies not only provide novel insights into how chemicals kill cells, but also open the possibility for new approaches to cytoprotection against oxidative stress.

Nuclear Injury

There is increasing interest in the possibility that the stimulation of Ca^{2+}-dependent endonucleases within the nucleus may be a critical step not only in programmed cell deletion (apoptosis), but also in oxidative stress and other toxic processes.[1] In vivo, DNA fragmentation and single strand breaks appear well in advance of cell death caused by acetaminophen, dimethylnitrosamine, and other alkylating agents. Moreover, agents such as aurintricarboxylic acid (which inhibits endonucleases) and inhibitors of poly(adenosine diphosphate-ribose) polymerase modulate cell injury in experimental systems in vitro and in vivo. The role of the nucleus and other subcellular compartments in toxic cell death produced by alkylating liver toxicants recently has been the subject of a comprehensive review.[287]

If cellular reductants are important in protecting DNA and other nuclear structures from chemical injury, one might expect to find abundant GSH in the nuclear compartment. Conventional cell fractionation studies have failed to demonstrate the existence of functionally distinct pools of GSH in subcellular locations within hepatocytes other than in the cytosol and mitochondria. Bellomo and colleagues[288] investigated the distribution of GSH within cultured hepatocytes by using the com-

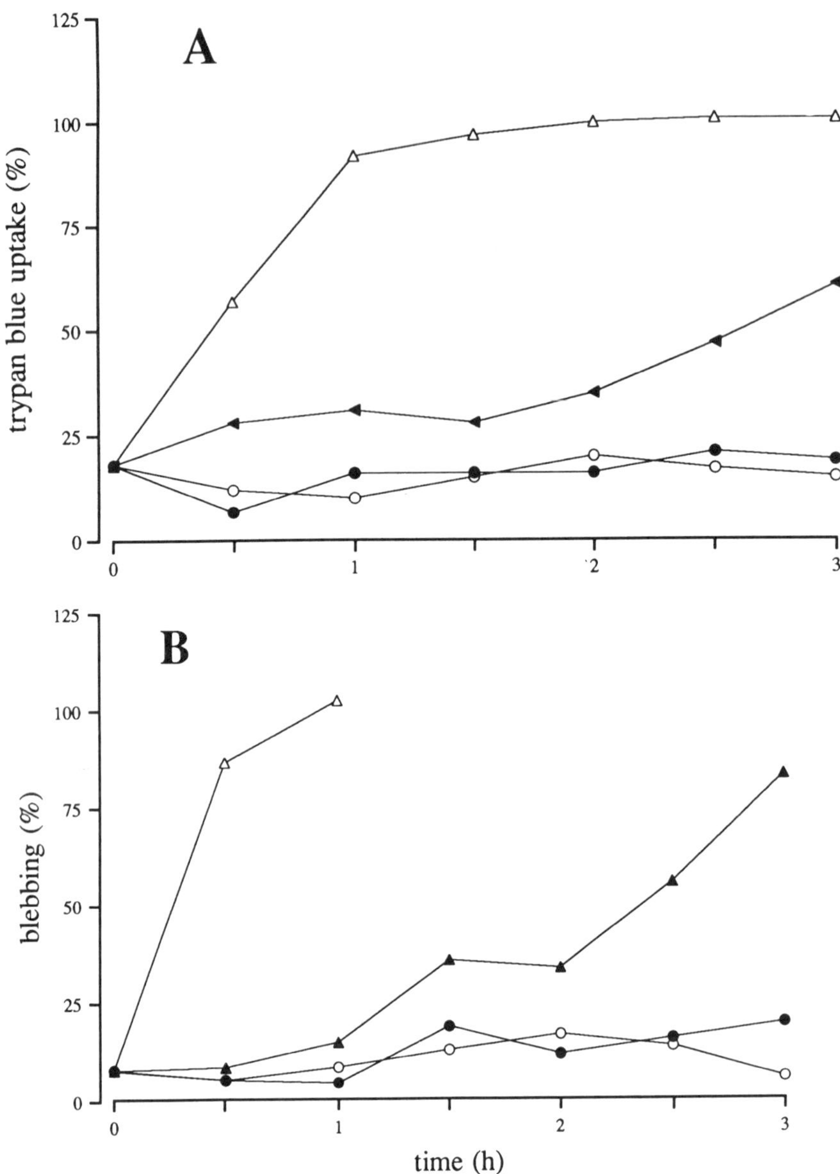

FIG 3.

A and **B,** cyclosporin A protects hepatocytes from TBH-induced cell killing. After the pretreatment of hepatocytes with cyclosporin A (500nM; *closed symbols*) or carrier solvent (ethanol; *open symbols*) for 20 minutes, the pro-oxidant or carrier solvent (Me$_2$SO) was added. The final concentrations of ethanol and Me$_2$SO did not exceed 0.15% and 0.2%, respectively. Cytotoxicity was scored by examining the cells for the appearance of plasma membrane blebs (expressed as percent of trypan blue–excluding cells with plasma membrane blebs) and trypan blue uptake (expressed as percent of the cells that had taken up the dye). Each end point is the mean plus or minus standard error of four separate experiments conducted on different hepatocyte preparations. *Open circles* indicate controls; *open triangles* indicate TBH (200µM). (From Kass GEN, Juedes MJ, Orrenius S: *Biochem Pharmacol* 1992; 44:1995–2003. Used by permission.)

pound monochlorobimane (BmCl); this interacts specifically with GSH to form a fluorescent adduct. Image analysis of BmCl-labeled hepatocytes localized BmCl fluorescence to the nucleus. The strong concentration gradient between the nucleus and cytosol (about threefold) was abolished by the depletion of ATP. Control experiments tended to refute possible reasons for localization of the fluorescent probe in the nucleus other than its specific interaction with GSH. Using the BmCl probe, it was demonstrated that the nuclear pool of GSH was more resistant to depletion by agents such as buthionine sulfoximine (which inhibits GSH synthesis), menadione (which promotes oxidative stress), and diethylmaleate (which depletes GSH by enzymatic conjugation). This initial demonstration of a specific nuclear compartment of GSH supports the concept that GSH is essential in protecting DNA and other nuclear structures from chemical injury.

SUMMARY

It always is challenging to summarize important advances in a medical field. In the area of drug-induced liver disease, it is common to observe cases of hepatic drug reactions emerging for the first time after marketing has begun. Thus, hepatotoxicity associated with newer agents such as the antiandrogens, antimycotics, and HMG CoA reductase inhibitors is not altogether surprising. For these important new drugs, severe types of hepatotoxicity thus far seem unlikely to be common enough to curtail seriously their application. More problematic are the very serious forms of liver injury that are associated with the commonly used NSAID, piroxicam. This must be one of the rarest of all idiosyncratic drug reactions, yet the few reported cases have had devastating outcomes. The field of drug-induced liver disease always produces a few surprises. This year, the award for novelty is shared between the hitherto-benign herbal tea, germander and melsalazine; the latter observation erodes earlier assumptions that it is the sulfonamide moiety of sulfasalazine that is responsible for its hepatotoxicity.

Although mechanistic studies of hepatotoxicity continue to produce new insights into liver injury and potential approaches to hepatoprotection, practical advances in the field of drug-induced liver injury also are coming from epidemiologic studies. Prevention now is partly attainable for several types of drug-induced liver disease. In this chapter, we emphasized this in relation to MTX, VPA, sex steroids, nicotinic acid, busulfan, and flucloxacillin. Appropriate prescribing, attention to defining safe dose regimens for direct hepatotoxins, and careful monitoring of patients who are receiving agents that have been associated with hepatic injury potentially can reduce the incidence and severity of drug-induced liver disease.

REFERENCES

1. Farrell GC: Drug-induced liver disease, in Gitnick G (ed): *Current Hepatology,* vol 11. St Louis, Mosby-Year Book, 1991, pp 89–132.

2. George J, et al: Drug-induced liver disease, in Gitnick G (ed): *Current Hepatology*, vol 12. St Louis, Mosby-Year Book, 1992, pp 131–168.

3. George J, et al: Drug-induced liver disease, in Gitnick G (ed): *Current Hepatology*, vol 13. St Louis, Mosby-Year Book, 1993.

4. Multimer DJ, et al: Liver transplantation for hepatic failure, in Boyer JL, Ockner RK (eds): *Progress in Liver Disease*, vol 10. Philadelphia, Saunders, 1992, pp 349–367.

5. Smilkstein MJ, et al: Efficacy of oral N-acetylcysteine in the treatment of acetaminophen overdose. Analysis of the national multicenter study (1976 to 1985). *N Engl J Med* 1988; 319:1557–1562.

6. Brotodihardjo AE, et al: Hepatotoxicity from paracetamol self-poisoning in Western Sydney: A continuing challenge. *Med J Aust* 1992; 157:382–385.

7. Lu S, et al: Drug-induced hepatotoxicity, in Gitnick G (ed): *Current Hepatology*, vol 9. St Louis, Mosby-Year Book, 1989, pp 105–140.

8. Moore M, et al: The toxicity of acetaminophen and N-acetyl-p-benzoquinoneimine in isolated hepatocytes is associated with thiol depletion and increased cytosolic calcium. *J Biol Chem* 1985; 260:13035–13040.

9. Tsokos-Kuhn JO, et al: Alkylation of liver plasma membrane and inhibition of the Ca^{2+} ATPase by acetaminophen. *Biochem Pharmacol* 1988; 37:2125–2131.

10. Moore GA, et al: Role of sulfhydryl groups in benzoquinone-induced Ca^{2+} release by rat liver mitochondria. *J Biol Chem* 1988; 267:539–550.

11. Orrenius S, et al: Ca^{2+}-activated mechanisms in toxicity and programmed cell death. *ISI Atlas of Science: Pharmacology, Philadelphia, Institute for Scientific Information*, 1988, pp 319–323.

12. Thomas CE, et al: Current status of calcium in hepatocellular injury. *Hepatology* 1989; 10:375–384.

13. Shen W, et al: Acetaminophen-induced cytotoxicity in cultured mouse hepatocytes: Effects of Ca^{2+}-endonuclease, DNA repair, and glutathione depletion inhibitors on DNA fragmentation and cell death. *Toxicol Appl Pharmacol* 1992; 112:32–40.

14. Horton AA, et al: Effects of inhibitors of phospholipase A2, cyclooxygenase and thromboxane synthase on paracetamol hepatotoxicity in the rat. *Eicosanoids* 1989a; 2:123–129.

15. Horton AA, et al: Prevention of Ca^{2+}-induced hepatocyte plasma membrane bleb formation by inhibitors of eicosanoid synthesis. *J Lipid Mediat* 1989b; 1:231–242.

16. Horton AA, et al: Prevention of thromboxane B2-induced hepatocyte plasma membrane bleb formation by certain prostaglandins and a proteinase inhibitor. *Biochim Biophys Acta* 1990; 1022:319–324.

17. Horton AA, et al: Prevention of paracetamol induced hepatotoxicity in the rat by the thromboxane receptor antagonist, Sulotroban (BM 13177). *J Lipid Mediat* 1991; 4:245–248.

18. Prescott LF, et al: The treatment of acetaminophen poisoning. *Annu Rev Pharmacol Toxicol* 1983; 23:87–101.

19. Kumar S, et al: Failure of physicians to recognize acetaminophen hepatotoxicity in chronic alcoholics. *Arch Intern Med* 1991; 151:1189–1191.

20. Rex DK, et al: Recognizing acetaminophen hepatotoxicity in chronic alcoholics. *Postgrad Med* 1992; 91:241–245.

21. Licht H, et al: Apparent potentiation of acetaminophen hepatotoxicity by alcohol. *Ann Intern Med* 1980; 92:511.

22. Seeff LB, et al: Acetaminophen hepatotoxicity in alcoholics. A therapeutic misadventure. *Ann Intern Med* 1986; 104:399–404.

23. Denison H, et al: Paracetamol medication and alcohol abuse: A dangerous combination for the liver and the kidney. *Scand J Gastroenterol* 1987; 22:701–704.

24. Maddrey WC: Hepatic effects of acetaminophen. Enhanced toxicity in alcoholics. *J Clin Gastroenterol* 1987; 9:180–185.

25. Lauterberg BH, et al: Glutathione deficiency in alcoholics: Risk factor for paracetamol hepatotoxicity. *Gut* 1988; 29:1153–1157.

26. Wootton FT, et al: Acetaminophen hepatotoxicity in the alcoholic. *South Med J* 1990; 83:1047–1049.

27. Bray GP, et al: The effect of chronic alcohol intake on prognosis and outcome in paracetamol overdose. *Hum Exp Toxicol* 1991; 10:435–438.

28. Royal College of Physicians: *A Great and Growing Evil: Medical consequences of alcohol abuse,* London, New York, Travistock, 1987, pp 1–19.

29. Diaz D, et al: Omeprazole is an aryl hydrocarbon-like inducer of human cytochrome P450. *Gastroenterology* 1990; 99:37–47.

30. Burk RF, et al: Isoniazid potentiation of acetaminophen hepatotoxicity in the rat and 4-methylpyrazole inhibition of it. *Res Commun Chem Pathol Pharmacol* 1990; 69:115–118.

31. Moulding TS, et al: Acetaminophen, isoniazid, and hepatic toxicity. *Ann Intern Med* 1991; 114:431.

32. Murphy R, et al: Severe acetaminophen toxicity in a patient receiving isoniazid. *Ann Intern Med* 1990; 113:799–800.

33. Bray GP, et al: Long-term anticonvulsant therapy worsens outcome in paracetamol-induced fulminant hepatic failure. *Hum Exp Toxicol* 1992; 11:265–270.

34. Pirotte JH: Apparent potentiation by phenobarbital of hepatotoxicity from small doses of acetaminophen. *Ann Intern Med* 1984; 101:403.

35. McClements BM, et al: Management of paracetamol poisoning complicated by enzyme induction due to alcohol or drugs. *Lancet* 1990; 335:1526.

36. Mitchell JR, et al: Acetaminophen-induced hepatic necrosis. 1. Role of drug metabolism. *J Pharmacol Exp Ther* 1973; 187:185–194.

37. Pessayre D, et al: Additive effects of inducers and fasting on acetaminophen hepatotoxicity. *Biochem Pharmacol* 1980; 29:2219–2223.

38. Douidar SM, et al: A novel mechanism for the enhancement of acetaminophen hepatotoxicity by phenobarbital. *J Pharmacol Exp Ther* 1987; 240:578–583.

39. Wright N, et al: Potentiation by previous drug therapy of hepatotoxicity following paracetamol overdosage. *Scott Med J* 1973; 18:56–58.

40. Smith JAE, et al: Paracetamol toxicity; is enzyme induction important? *Hum Toxicol* 1986; 5:383–385.

41. Minton NA, et al: Fatal paracetamol poisoning in an epileptic. *Hum Toxicol* 1988; 7:33–34.

42. O'Grady JG, et al: Early indicators of prognosis in fulminant hepatic failure. *Gastroenterology* 1989; 94:1186–1192.

43. Pereira LMMB, et al: Coagulation factor V and VII/V ratio as predictors of outcome in paracetamol induced fulminant hepatic failure: Relation to other prognostic factors. *Gut* 1992; 33:98–102.

44. Bateman DN, et al: Adverse reactions to N-acetylcysteine. *Hum Toxicol* 1984; 3:393–398.

45. Dawson AH, et al: Adverse reactions to N-acetylcysteine during treatment for paracetamol poisoning. *Med J Aust* 1989; 150:329–331.

46. Editorial: Acetylcysteine. *Lancet* 1991; 337:1069–1070.

47. Mant TG, et al: Adverse reactions to acetylcysteine and effects of overdose. *BMJ* 1984; 289:217–219.

48. Landon EJ, et al: Effects of calcium channel blocking agents on calcium and centrilobular necrosis in the liver of rats treated with hepatotoxic agents. *Biochem Pharmacol* 1986; 35:697–705.

49. Kobusch AB, et al: Effect of diltiazem on acetaminophen and phalloidine hepatotoxicity. *Res Commun Chem Pathol Pharmacol* 1990; 68:143–157.

50. Deakin CD, et al: Delayed calcium channel blockade with diltiazem reduces paracetamol hepatotoxicity in mice. *Hum Exp Toxicol* 1991; 10:119–123.

51. Mauger J-P, et al: Calcium channels in hepatocytes. *J Hepatol* 1988; 7:278–282.

52. Kass GEN, et al: Receptor-operated calcium influx in rat hepatocytes. Identification and characterization using manganese. *J Biol Chem* 1990; 265:17486–17492.

53. Hijioka T, et al: Kupffer cells contain voltage-dependent calcium channels. *Mol Pharmacol* 1992; 41:435–440.

54. Harrison PM, et al: Improved outcome of paracetamol-induced fulminant hepatic failure by late administration of acetylcysteine. *Lancet* 1990; 335:1572–1573.

55. Keays R, et al: Intravenous acetylcysteine in paracetamol induced fulminant hepatic failure. A prospective controlled trial. *BMJ* 1991; 303:1026–1029.

56. Hong RW, et al: Glutamine preserves liver glutathione after lethal hepatic injury. *Ann Surg* 1992; 215:115–119.

57. Butterworth M, et al: Cysteine isopropylester protects against paracetamol-induced toxicity. *Biochem Pharmacol* 1992; 43:483–488.

58. Bray GP, et al: S-adenosylmethionine protects against acetaminophen hepatotoxicity in two mouse models. *Hepatology* 1992; 15:297–301.

59. Montero C, et al: S-adenosylmethionine increases erythrocyte ATP *in vitro* by a route independent of adenosine kinase. *Biochem Pharmacol* 1990; 40:2617–2623.

60. Schreiber AJ, et al: Estrogen-induced cholestasis: Clues to pathogenesis and treatment. *Hepatology* 1983; 3:607–613.

61. Vandemiale G, et al: S-adenosylmethionine (SAMe) improves acetaminophen metabolism in cirrhotic patients (abstract). *J Hepatol* 1989; 9:S240.

62. Vermeulen NPE, et al: Molecular aspects of paracetamol-induced hepatotoxicity and its mechanism-based prevention. *Drug Metab Rev* 1992; 24:367–407.

63. Weinstein G, et al: Psoriasis-liver-methotrexate interactions. Cooperative study. *Arch Dermatol* 1973; 108:36–42.

64. Nyfors A, et al: Liver biopsies from psoriatics related to methotrexate therapy. 1. Findings in 123 consecutive non-methotrexate treated patients. *Acta Pathol Microbiol Scand [A]* 1976; 84:253–261.

65. Zachariae H, et al: Liver biopsy in psoriasis. A controlled study. *Dermatologica* 1973; 146:149–155.

66. Hall PM, et al: Two methods of assessment of methotrexate hepatotoxicity in patients with rheumatoid arthritis. *Ann Rheum Dis* 1991; 50:471–476.

67. Zachariae H, et al: Methotrexate-induced liver cirrhosis. A follow-up. *Dermatologica* 1987; 175:178–182.

68. Ruymann FB, et al: Hepatoma in a child with methotrexate-induced hepatic fibrosis. *JAMA* 1977; 238:2631–2633.

69. Gilbert SC, et al: Methotrexate-induced cirrhosis requiring liver transplantation in three patients with psoriasis. A word of caution in light of the expanding use of this 'steroid sparing' agent. *Arch Intern Med* 1990; 150:889–891.

70. Newman M, et al: The role of liver biopsies in psoriatic patients receiving long term methotrexate treatment. *Arch Dermatol* 1989; 125:1218–1224.

71. Zachariae H, et al: Serum aminoterminal propeptide of type III procollagen in psoriasis and psoriatic arthritis: Relation to liver fibrosis and arthritis. *J Am Acad Dermatol* 1991; 25:50–53.

72. Whiting-O'Keefe QE, et al: Methotrexate and histologic hepatic abnormalities: A meta-analysis. *Am J Med* 1991; 90:711–716.

73. Roenigk HH, et al: Methotrexate in psoriasis: Revised guidelines. *J Am Acad Dermatol* 1988; 19:145–156.

74. Kremer JM: Liver biopsies in patients with rheumatoid arthritis receiving methotrexate: Where are we going? *J Rheumatol* 1992; 19:189–191.

75. Roenigk HH, et al: Methotrexate guide lines: Revised. *J Am Acad Dermatol* 1982; 6:145–155.

76. Watson RGP, et al: Low-dose methotrexate therapy and hepatotoxicity. The view of the hepatologist. *Med J Aust* 1991; 155:428–430.

77. Bremnes RM, et al: Acute hepatotoxicity after high dose methotrexate administration to rats. *Pharmacol Toxicol* 1991; 69:132–139.

78. Slordal L, et al: Pharmacokinetics of methotrexate and 7-hydroxymethotrexate after high-dose (33.6 g/m^2) methotrexate therapy. *Pediatr Hematol Oncol* 1986; 3:127–134.

79. Borsi JD, et al: Comparative study of the pharmacokinetics of 7-hydroxy-methotrexate after administration of methotrexate in the dose range 0.5–33.6 g/m^2 to children with acute lymphoblastic leukemia. *Med Pediatr Oncol* 1990; 18:217–224.

80. Bremnes RM, et al: Dose-dependent pharmacokinetics of methotrexate and 7-hydroxymethotrexate in the rat in vivo. *Cancer Res* 1989b; 49:6359–6364.

81. Ahern MJ, et al: Hepatic methotrexate content and progression of hepatic fibrosis: Preliminary findings. *Ann Rheum Dis* 1991; 50:477–480.

82. Weden M, et al: Protracted cholestasis probably induced by oral contraceptive. *J Intern Med* 1992; 231:561–565.

83. Oligny LL, et al: Hepatic sinusoidal ectasia. *Hum Pathol* 1992; 23:953–956.

84. Kahn H, et al: Danazol-induced hepatocellular adenomas. A case report and review of the literature. *Arch Pathol Lab Med* 1991; 115:1054–1057.

85. Korula J, et al: Hepatocellular carcinoma coexisting with hepatic adenoma. Incidental discovery after long-term oral contraceptive use. *West J Med* 1991; 155:416–418.

86. Lieberman DA, et al: Severe and prolonged oral contraceptive jaundice. *J Clin Gastroenterol* 1984; 6:145–148.

87. Shortell CK, et al: Hepatic adenoma and focal nodular hyperplasia. *Surg Gynecol Obstet* 1991; 173:426–431.

88. Gordon SC, et al: Resolution of a contraceptive-steroid-induced hepatic adenoma with subsequent evolution into hepatocellular carcinoma. *Ann Intern Med* 1986; 105:547–549.

89. Tesluk H, et al: Hepatocellular adenoma: Its transformation to carcinoma in a user of oral contraceptives. *Arch Pathol Lab Med* 1981; 105:296–299.

90. Gyorffy EJ, et al: Transformation of hepatic cell adenoma to hepatocellular carcinoma due to oral contraceptive use. *Ann Intern Med* 1989; 110:489–490.

91. Tao LC: Are oral contraceptive-associated liver cell adenomas premalignant. *Acta Cytol* 1992; 36:338–344.

92. Rivin AU: Jaundice occurring during nicotinic acid therapy for hypercholesterolemia. *JAMA* 1959; 170:2088–2089.

93. Pardue WO: Severe liver dysfunction during nicotinic acid therapy. *JAMA* 1961; 175:137–138.

94. Winter SL, et al: Hepatic toxicity from large doses of vitamin B3 (nicotinamide). *N Engl J Med* 1973; 289:1180–1182.

95. Sugarman AA, et al: Jaundice following the administration of niacin. *JAMA* 1974; 228:202.

96. Patterson DJ, et al: Niacin hepatitis. *South Med J* 1983; 76:239–241.

97. Clementz GL, et al: Nicotinic acid-induced fulminant hepatic failure. *J Clin Gastroenterol* 1989; 9:582–584.

 98. Rader JI, et al: Review: Hepatic toxicity of unmodified and time-release preparations of niacin. *Am J Med* 1992; 92:77–81.

 99. Kohn RM, et al: Hepatic fibrosis following long acting nicotinic acid therapy: A case report. *Am J Med Sci* 1969; 258:94–99.

100. Hodis HN: Acute hepatic failure associated with the use of low-dose sustained release niacin. *JAMA* 1990; 264:181.

101. Mullin GE, et al: Fulminant hepatic failure after ingestion of sustained-release niacin. *Ann Intern Med* 1989; 111:253–255.

102. Jungnickel PW, et al: Comment: Adverse effect profile of sustained-release niacin. *Ann Pharmacotherapy* 1991; 25:1014.

103. Malloy MJ, et al: Niacin—the long and the short of it. *West J Med* 1991; 155:424–426.

104. Knopp RH, et al: Contrasting effects of unmodified and time-release forms of niacin on lipoproteins in hyperlipidemic subjects: Clues to mechanism of action of niacin. *Metabolism* 1985; 34:642–650.

105. Henkin Y, et al: Rechallenge with crystalline niacin after drug-induced-hepatitis from sustained-release niacin. *JAMA* 1990; 264:241–243.

106. Etchason JA, et al: Niacin-induced hepatitis: A potential side effect with low-dose time-release niacin. *Mayo Clin Proc* 1991; 66:23–28.

107. U.S. Pharmacopoeia: Drug information for the health care professional, in *United States Pharmacopoeial Convention*. Rockville, Maryland, 1989, pp 1739–1740.

108. *Physician's Desk Reference,* 45th ed. Ordell, New Jersey, Medical Economics Company, 1991, p 1785.

109. McCreanor GM, et al: The metabolism of high intake of tryptophan, nicotinamide and nicotinic acid in the rat. *Br J Nutr* 1986; 56:577–586.

110. Tobert JA, et al: Clinical experience with lovastatin. *Am J Cardiol* 1990; 65:23F–26F.

111. Mantell G, et al: Extended clinical safety profile of lovastatin. *Am J Cardiol* 1990; 66:11B–15B.

112. Brown MS, et al: Drugs used in the treatment of hyperlipoproteinemias, in Goodman Gilman A, Rall TW, Nies AS, et al (eds): *Goodman and Gilman's The Pharmacological Basis of Therapeutics,* 8th ed. New York, Pergamon Press, 1990, pp 874–896.

113. Capron JP: Augmentation modérée et prolongée de l'activité sérique des transaminases. Conduite à tenir. *Presse Med* 1989; 18:913–916.

114. Boccuzzi SJ, et al: Long-term safety and efficacy profile of simvastatin. *Am J Cardiol* 1990; 68:1127–1131.

115. Feydy P, et al: Un cas d'hépatite à la simvastatine (letter). *Gastroenterol Clin Biol* 1991; 15:94–95.

116. Roblin X, et al: Hépatite à la simvastatine (letter). *Gastroenterol Clin Biol* 1992; 16:101.

117. Larrey D, et al: Hepatitis associated with amoxycillin-clavulanic acid combination: Report of 15 cases. *Gut* 1992; 33:368–371.

118. Wong FS, et al: Augmentin-induced jaundice. *Med J Aust* 1991; 154:698–701.

119. Silvain C, et al: Granulomatous hepatitis due to combination of amoxycillin and clavulanic acid. *Dig Dis Sci* 1992; 37:150–152.

120. Ryan J, et al: Cholestasis with ticarcillin-potassium clavulanate (Timentin). *Med J Aust* 1992; 156:291.

121. Van Der Auwera P, et al: Ticarcillin-clavulanic acid therapy in severe infections. *Drugs Exp Clin Res* 1985; (suppl) 11:805–813.

122. Hebbard GS, et al: Augmentin-induced jaundice with a fatal outcome. *Med J Aust* 1992; 156:285–286.

123. Schreiber AJ, et al: Estrogen-induced cholestasis: Clues to pathogenesis and treatment. *Hepatology* 1983; 3:607–613.

124. Olsson R, et al: Liver injury from flucloxacillin, cloxacillin and dicloxacillin. *J Hepatol* 1992; 15:154–161.

125. Fairley CK, et al: Risk factors for development of flucloxacillin associated jaundice. *BMJ* 1993; 306:233–235.

126. Mollison LC, et al: Hepatitis due to nitrofurantoin. *Med J Aust* 1992; 156:347–349.

127. Reinhart HH, et al: Combined nitrofurantoin toxicity to liver and lung. *Gastroenterology* 1992; 102:1396–1399.

128. Lewis JH, et al: Hepatic injury associated with ketoconazole therapy. Analysis of 33 cases. *Gastroenterology* 1984; 86:503–513.

129. Stricker BHC, et al: Ketoconazole associated hepatic injury: A clinicopathological study of 55 cases. *J Hepatol* 1986; 3:399–406.

130. Saag MS, et al: Azole antifungal agents: Emphasis on new triazoles. *Antimicrob Agents Chemother* 1988; 32:1–8.

131. De Wit S, et al: Comparison of fluconazole and ketoconazole for oropharyngeal candidiasis in AIDS. *Lancet* 1989; 1:746–748.

132. Holmes J, et al: Jaundice in HIV positive haemophiliac. *Lancet* 1989; 1:1027.

133. Wells C, et al: Dose-dependent fluconazole hepatotoxicity proven on biopsy and rechallenge. *J Infect* 1992; 24:111–112.

134. Restrepo A, et al: Itraconazole therapy in lymphangitic and cutaneous sporotrichosis. *Arch Dermatol* 1986; 122:413–417.

135. Legendre R, et al: Itraconazole in the treatment of tinea capitis. *J Am Acad Dermatol* 1990; 23:559–560.

136. Lavrijsen APM, et al: Hepatic injury associated with itraconazole. *Lancet* 1992; 340:251–252.

137. Burette A, et al: Acute hepatic injury associated with minocycline. *Arch Intern Med* 1984; 144:1491–1492.

138. Chatham WW, et al: Leukemoid blood reaction to tetracycline. *South Med J* 1983; 76:1195–1196.

139. Davies MG, et al: Acute hepatitis and exfoliative dermatitis associated with minocycline. *BMJ* 1989; 2998:1523–1524.

140. Min DI, et al: Acute hepatic failure associated with oral minocycline: A case report. *Pharmacotherapy* 1992; 12:68–71.

141. Dreifuss FE, et al: Valproic acid hepatic fatalities: A retrospective review. *Neurology* 1987; 37:379–385.

142. Dreifuss FE, et al: Valproic acid hepatic fatalities. 11. US experience since 1984. *Neurology* 1989; 39:201–207.

143. Fisher E, et al: Valproate metabolites in serum and urine during antiepileptic therapy in children with infantile spasms: Abnormal metabolite pattern associated with reversible hepatotoxicity. *Epilepsia* 1992; 33:165–171.

144. Eadie MJ, et al: Valproate metabolism during hepatotoxicity associated with the drug. *Q J Med* 1990; 77:1229–1240.

145. Kochen W, et al: Abnormal metabolism of valproic acid in fatal hepatic failure. *Eur J Pediatr* 1983; 141:30–35.

146. Matsumoto I, et al: Differential diagnosis for hepatopathy in five patients with valproate therapy, in *Proceedings of the 34th Annual Conference on Mass Spectrometry and Allied Topics*. Cincinnati, Ohio, 1986, pp 925–926.

147. Bjorge SM, et al: Studies on the β-oxidation of valproic acid in rat liver mitochondrial preparations. *Drug Metab Dispos Biol Fate Chem* 1991; 19:823–829.

148. Porubek DJ, et al: The covalent binding to protein of valproic acid and its hepatotoxic metabolite, 2-n-propyl-4-pentenoic acid, in rats and in rat hepatocytes. *Drug Metab Dispos Biol Fate Chem* 1989; 17:123–130.

149. Coulter DL: Carnitine, valproate and toxicity. *J Child Neurol* 1991; 6:7–14.

150. Baillie TA: Metabolic activation of valproic acid and drug-mediated hepatotoxicity. Role of the terminal olefin, 2-n-propyl-4-pentenoic acid. *Chem Res Toxicol* 1988; 1:195–199.

151. Rettie AE, et al: Cytochrome P-450 catalyzed formation of 4-en-valproate, a toxic metabolite of valproic acid. *Science* 1987; 235:890–893.

152. Tanaka K, et al: Disorders of branched chain amino acid and organic acid metabolism, in Stanbury JB, Wyngaarden JB, Fredrickson DS, et al (eds): *The Metabolic Basis of Inherited Disease,* 5th ed. New York, McGraw Hill, 1983, pp 440–473.

153. Kondo T, et al: Associations between risk factors for valproate hepatotoxicity and altered valproate metabolism. *Epilepsia* 1992; 33:172–177.

154. Zimmerman HJ, et al: Valproate-induced hepatic injury: Analysis of 23 fatal-cases. *Hepatology* 1982; 2:591–597.

155. Egmond H, et al: A suspected case of late-onset sodium valproate-induced hepatic failure. *Neuropediatrics* 1987; 18:96–98.

156. Hautekeete ML, et al: Microvesicular steatosis of the liver. *Acta Clin Belg* 1990; 45:311–326.

157. Eadie MJ, et al: Valproate-associated hepatotoxicity and its biochemical mechanisms. *Med Toxicol Adverse Drug Exp* 1988; 3:85–106.

158. Loyning Y, et al: Cases of serious/fatal hepatotoxicity due to valproate: Recommended monitoring scheme and preliminary results, in Oxley J, Janz D, Meinardi H (eds): *Chronic Toxicity of Antiepileptic Drugs.* New York, Raven Press, 1983, pp 47–60.

159. Zimmerman HJ: Anesthetic agents, in Zimmerman HJ (ed): *Hepatotoxicity: Adverse Effects of Drugs and Other Chemicals on the Liver.* New York, Appleton-Century-Crofts, 1978, pp 370–394.

160. Farell GC: Postoperative hepatic dysfunction, in Zakim D, Boyer TD (eds): *Hepatology. A Text Book of Liver Disease,* 2nd ed. Philadelphia, Saunders, 1990, pp 869–890.

161. Trowell J, et al: Controlled trial of repeated halothane anaesthetics in patients with carcinoma of the uterine cervix treated with radium. *Lancet* 1975; 1:821–824.

162. Van Dyke RA, et al: Studies on irreversible binding of radioactivity from [14C] halothane to rat hepatic microsomal lipids and proteins. *Drug Metab Dispos Biol Fate Chem* 1974; 2: 469–476.

163. Muller R, et al: Modification of liver microsomal lipids by halothane metabolites: A multi-nuclear NMR spectroscopic study. *Naunyn Schmiedebergs Arch Pharmacol* 1982; 321:234–237.

164. Satoh H, et al: Human anti-endoplasmic reticulum antibodies in sera of patients with halothane-induced hepatitis are directed against a trifluoroacetylated carboxylesterase. *Proc Natl Acad Sci U S A* 1989; 86:322–326.

165. Trudell JR, et al: The effect of alcohol and anesthetic metabolites on cell membranes. A possible direct immune mechanism. *Ann N Y Acad Sci* 1992; 625:806–817.

166. Christen U, et al: Halothane metabolism: Kupffer cells carry and partially process trifluoroacetylated protein adducts. *Biochem Biophys Res Commun* 1991; 175:256–262.

167. Lewis JH, et al: Enflurane hepatotoxicity. A clinicopathological study of 24 cases. *Ann Intern Med* 1983; 98:984–992.

168. Eger EI, et al: Is enflurane hepatotoxic? *Anesth Analg* 1986; 65:21–30.

169. Fisher NA, et al: Hepatic necrosis associated with herpes virus after isoflurane anesthesia. *Anesth Analg* 1985; 64:1131–1133.

170. Gregoire S, et al: Acute hepatitis in a patient with mild factor IX deficiency after anesthesia with isoflurane. *Can Med Assoc J* 1986; 135:645–646.

171. Carrigan TW, et al: A report of hepatic necrosis and death following isoflurane anesthesia. *Anesthesiology* 1987; 67:581–583.

172. Brunt EM, et al: Fulminant hepatic failure after repeated exposure to isoflurane anesthesia. A case report. *Hepatology* 1991; 13:1017–1021.

173. Stoelting RK, et al: Hepatic dysfunction after isoflurane anesthesia. *Anesth Analg* 1987; 66:147–153.

174. Jones RM, et al: A prospective study of liver function in infants and children exposed to daily isoflurane for several weeks. *Anaesthesia* 1991; 46:686–688.

175. Wallin RF, et al: Sevoflurane: A new inhalational anesthetic agent. *Anesth Analg* 1975; 54:758–766.

176. Lind RC, et al: Sevoflurane biotransformation and hepatotoxicity in the guinea pig (abstract). *Anesthesiology* 1989; 71:A310.

177. Ghantous HN, et al: Sevoflurane is biotransformed by guinea pig liver slices but causes minimal cytotoxicity. *Anesth Analg* 1992; 75:436–440.

178. Holaday DA, et al: Clinical characteristics and biotransformation of sevoflurane in healthy human volunteers. *Anesthesiology* 1981; 54:100–106.

179. Kikuchi H, et al: Clinical evaluation and metabolism of sevoflurane in patients. *Hiroshima J Med Sci* 1987; 36:93–97.

180. Eger II EI, et al: Studies of the toxicity of I-653, halothane, and isoflurane in enzyme-induced, hypoxic rats. *Anesth Analg* 1987; 66:1227–1229.

181. Jones RM, et al: Biotransformation and hepato-renal function in volunteers after exposure to desflurane (I-653). *Br J Anaesth* 1990; 64:482–487.

182. Weiskopf RB, et al: Desflurane does not produce hepatic or renal injury in human volunteers. *Anesth Analg* 1992; 74:570–574.

183. Keating MA, et al: Flutamide in the treatment of advanced prostate cancer (abstract). *J Urol* 1986; 135:203A.

184. Johansson JE, et al: Clinical evaluation of flutamide and estramustine as initial treatment of metastatic carcinoma of prostate. *Urology* 1987; 29:55–59.

185. Lund F, et al: Flutamide versus stilboestrol in the management of advanced prostatic cancer. A controlled prospective trial. *Br J Urol* 1988; 61:140–142.

186. Gomez JL, et al: Incidence of liver toxicity associated with the use of flutamide in prostate cancer patients. *Am J Med* 1992; 92:465–470.

187. Hart W, et al: Flutamide and hepatitis (letter). *Ann Intern Med* 1989; 110:943–944.

188. Corkery JC, et al: Flutamide-related fulminant hepatic failure. *J Clin Gastroenterol* 1991; 13:364–365.

189. Gomez JL, et al: Simultaneous liver and lung toxicity related to the nonsteroidal antiandrogen nilutamide (Anandron): A case report. *Am J Med* 1992; 92:563–566.

190. Lundgren R: Flutamide as primary treatment for metastatic prostate cancer. *Br J Urol* 1987; 59:156–158.

191. Friis H, et al: Drug-induced hepatic injury: An analysis of 1100 case reports to the Danish Committee on Adverse Drug Reactions between 1978–1987. *J Intern Med* 1992; 232:133–138.

192. Hautekeete ML, et al: Hypersensitivity with hepatotoxicity to melsalazine after hypersensitivity to sulfasalazine. *Gastroenterology* 1992; 103:1925–1927.

193. Mulder H, et al: Azodisalicylate (Dipentum)-induced hepatitis? *J Clin Gastroenterol* 1989; 11:708–711.

194. Kowdley KV, et al: Prolonged cholestasis due to trimethoprim sulfamethoxazole. *Gastroenterology* 1992; 102:2148–150.

195. Tanner AR: Hepatic cholestasis induced by trimethoprim. *BMJ* 1986; 293:1072–1073.

196. Mitchell MC, et al: Granulomatous hepatitis associated with carbamazepine treatment. *Am J Med* 1981; 71:733–735.

197. Williams SJ, et al: Carbamazepine hepatitis: The clinicopathological spectrum. *J Gastroenterol Hepatol* 1986; 1:159–168.

198. Horowitz S, et al: Hepatotoxic reactions associated with carbamazepine therapy. *Epilepsia* 1988; 29:149–154.

199. Larrey D, et al: Carbamazepine-induced acute cholangitis. *Dig Dis Sci* 1987; 32:554–557.

200. Forbes GM, et al: Carbamazepine hepatotoxicity: Another cause of the vanishing bile duct syndrome. *Gastroenterology* 1992; 102:1385–1388.

201. Zimmerman HJ: Hepatotoxic effects of oncotherapeutic agents. *Prog Liver Dis* 1986; 8:621–642.

202. Horsmans Y, et al: Reversible cholestasis with bile duct injury following azathioprine therapy. A case report. *Liver* 1991; 11:89–93.

203. Mion F, et al: Azathioprine induced liver disease: Nodular regenerative hyperplasia of the liver and perivenous fibrosis in a patient treated for multiple sclerosis. *Gut* 1991; 32:715–717.

204. Jaskiewicz K, et al: Hepatic sinusoidal fibrosis associated with the use of cytotoxic drugs. *S Afr Med J* 1992; 81:626–627.

205. Geller RB, et al: Allogenic bone marrow transplantation after high-dose busulphan and cyclophosphamide in patients with acute non-lymphocytic leukemia. *Blood* 1989; 73:2209–2218.

206. Morgan M, et al: The toxicity of busulphan and cyclophosphamide as the preparative regimen for bone marrow transplantation. *Br J Haematol* 1991; 77:529–534.

207. Kasai M, et al: Toxicity of high-dose busulphan and cyclophosphamide as a preparative regimen for bone marrow transplantation. *Transplant Proc* 1992; 24:1529–1530.

208. Tutschka PJ, et al: Bone marrow transplantation for leukemia following a new busulphan and cyclophosphamide preparative regimen. *Blood* 1987; 70:1382.

209. Brodsky R, et al: Frequency of veno-occlusive disease of the liver in bone marrow transplantation with a modified busulphan/cyclophosphamide preparative regimen. *Am J Clin Oncol* 1990; 13:221.

210. Essell JH, et al: Marked increase in veno-occlusive disease of the liver associated with methotrexate use for graft-versus-host disease prophylaxis in patients receiving busulphan/cyclophosphamide. *Blood* 1992; 79:2784–2788.

211. Adachi N, et al: Veno-occlusive disease of the liver after combined adjuvant chemotherapy for a 1-year old boy with rhabdomyosarcoma: Potential usefulness of the Gabexate Mesylate (FOY). *J Pediatr Gastrolentero Nutr* 1992; 14:314–318.

212. D'Angio GJ: Unexpected toxicity encountered in the National Wilms' Tumour Study. *Cancer Treat Rep* 1987; 71:993.

213. Nybonde T, et al: Wilms' tumour complicated by veno-occlusive disease of the liver (VOD): Current concepts and a case report. *Pediatr Hematol Oncol* 1988; 5:53–60.

214. Devergie A, et al: Changes in endothelial and coagulation parameters after allogenic bone marrow transplant (BMT) as a means of prediction of veno-occlusive disease (VOD). *Exp Hematol* 1986; 14:430.

215. Shulman HM, et al: Hepatic veno-occlusive disease after bone marrow transplantation. Immunohistochemical identification of the material within occluded central venules. *Am J Pathol* 1987; 127:549–558.

216. Gluckman E, et al: Use of prostaglandin E1 for prevention of liver veno-occlusive disease in leukaemic patients treated by allogenic bone marrow transplantation. *Br J Haematol* 1989; 74:277–281.

217. Shepherd PCA, et al: Thioguanine used in maintenance therapy of chronic myeloid leukemia causes non-cirrhotic portal hypertension. *Br J Haematol* 1991; 79:185–192.

218. Kemney N, et al: New syndrome: Ascites, hyperbilirubinemia, and hypoalbuminemia after biochemical modulation of fluorouracil with N-phosphonaacetyl-L-aspartate (PALA). *Ann Intern Med* 1991; 115:947–951.

219. Erlichman C: An overview of the clinical pharmacology of N-phosphonacetyl-L-aspartate (PALA), a new antimetabolite. *Recent Results Cancer Res* 1980; 74:65–71.

220. Kufe DW, et al: Enhancement of 5-fluorouracil incorporation into human lymphoblast ribonucleic acid. *Biochem Pharmacol* 1981; 30:129–133.

221. Peters GJ, et al: Do antimetabolites interfere with the glycosylation of cellular glycoconjugates? *Eur J Cancer* 1990; 26:516–523.

222. Feinberg B, et al: Phase 1 trial of intravenously-administered recombinant tumor necrosis factor-alpha in cancer patients. *J Clin Oncol* 1988; 6:1328–1334.

223. Schilling PJ, et al: Novel tumor necrosis factor toxic effects. *Cancer* 1992; 69:256–260.

224. Khoruts A, et al: Circulating tumor necrosis factor, interleukin-1 and interleukin-6 concentrations in chronic alcoholic patients. *Hepatology* 1991; 13:267–276.

225. Colletti LM, et al: Role of tumor necrosis factor-α in the pathophysiologic alterations after hepatic ischemia/reperfusion injury in the rat. *J Clin Invest* 1990; 85:1936–1943.

226. Adamson GM, et al: Tumor necrosis factor induced oxidative stress in isolated mouse hepatocytes. *Arch Biochem Biophys* 1992; 294:223–229.

227. Mion F, et al: Hepatite aigue medicamenteuse: Un cas de cytolyse aigue appres prise de Fipexide. *Gastroenterol Clin Biol* 1990; 14:513–514.

228. Durand F, et al: Fipexide-induced fulminant hepatitis. Report of three cases with emergency transplantation. *J Hepatol* 1992; 15:144–146.

229. Lauritsen K, et al: Effect of omeprazole and cimetidine on duodenal ulcer. *N Engl J Med* 1985; 312:958–961.

230. Jochem V, et al: Fulminant hepatic failure related to omeprazole. *Am J Gastroenterol* 1992; 87:523–525.

231. Zimmerman HJ: Update of hepatotoxicity due to classes of drugs in common clinical use: Nonsteroidal anti-inflammatory drugs, antibiotics, antihypertensives, and cardiac and psychotropic agents. *Semin Liver Dis* 1990; 10:322–338.

232. Kromann-Andersen H, et al: Reported adverse reactions to and consumption of nonsteroidal anti-inflammatory drugs in Denmark over a 17-year period. *Dan Med Bull* 1988; 35:187–192.

233. García Rodríguez LA, et al: The role of non-steroidal anti-inflammatory drugs in acute liver injury. *BMJ* 1992; 305:865–868.

234. Carson JL, et al: The feasibility of studying drug-induced acute hepatitis with use of Medicaid data. *Clin Pharmacol Ther* 1992; 52:214–219.

235. Friis H, et al: Drug-induced hepatic injury: An analysis of 1100 cases reported to The Danish Committee on Adverse Drug Reactions between 1978 and 1987. *J Intern Med* 1992; 232:133–138.

236. Tarazi EM, et al: Sulindac-associated hepatic injury: Analysis of 91 cases reported to the Food and Drug Administration. *Gastroenterology* 1993; 104:569–574.

237. Nuki G: Non-steroidal analgesic and anti-inflammatory agents. *BMJ* 1983; 287:39–43.

238. Hepps KS, et al: Severe cholestatic jaundice associated with piroxicam. *Gastroenterology* 1991; 101:1737–1740.

239. Sherman KE, et al: Hepatotoxicity associated with piroxicam (letter). *Gastroenterology* 1992; 103:354–355.

240. Paterson D, et al: Piroxicam induced submassive necrosis of the liver. *Gut* 1992; 33:1436–1438.

241. Lee SM, et al: Subacute hepatic necrosis induced by piroxicam. *BMJ* 1986; 293:540–541.

242. Planas R, et al: Fatal submassive necrosis of the liver associated with piroxicam. *Am J Gastroenterol* 1990; 85:468–470.

243. Bismuth H, et al: Emergency liver transplantation for fulminant hepatitis. *Ann Intern Med* 1987; 107:337–341.

244. Armen R, et al: Phencyclidine-induced malignant hyperthermia causing submassive liver necrosis. *Am J Med* 1984; 77:167–172.

245. Kew M, et al: Liver damage in heat-stroke. *Am J Med* 1970; 49:192–202.

246. Randall T: Ecstasy-fueled 'rave' parties become dances of death for English youths. *JAMA* 1992; 268:1505–1506.

247. Hopkins PM, et al: Evidence for related myopathies in exertional heat stroke and malignant hyperthermia. *Lancet* 1991; 338:1491–1492.

248. Larner AJ: Complications of "ecstasy" misuse (letter). *Lancet* 1992; 340:726.

249. Henry JA, et al: Toxicity and deaths from 3,4-methylenedioxymethamphetamine ("ecstasy"). *Lancet* 1992; 340:384–387.

250. Bourdi M, et al: Anti-liver microsomes autoantibodies and dihydralazine-induced hepatitis: Specificity of autoantibodies and inductive capacity of the drug. *Mol Pharmacol* 1992; 42:280–285.

251. Leeder JS, et al: Human anti-cytochrome P450 antibodies in aromatic anticonvulsant-induced hypersensitivity reactions. *J Pharmacol Exp Ther* 1992; 263:360–367.

252. Babany G, et al: Severe monochlorobenzene-induced liver cell necrosis. *Gastroenterology* 1991; 101:1734–1736.

253. Cam C, et al: Acquired toxic porphyria cutanea tarda due to hexachlorobenzene. Report of 348 cases caused by this fungicide. *JAMA* 1963; 183:88–91.

254. Brodie BB, et al: Possible mechanism of liver necrosis caused by aromatic organic compounds. *Proc Natl Acad Sci U S A* 1971; 68:160–164.

255. Johansson I, et al: Benzene metabolism by ethanol-, acetone-, and benzene-inducible cytochrome P450 (IIE1) in rat and rabbit liver microsomes. *Cancer Res* 1988; 48:5387–5390.

256. Hetu C, et al: Effect of chronic ethanol administration on bromobenzene liver toxicity in the rat. *Toxicol Appl Pharmacol* 1983; 67:166–177.

257. Lau SS, et al: Hepatic microsomal epoxidation of bromobenzene to phenols and its toxicological implication. *Toxicol Appl Pharmacol* 1979; 50:309–318.

258. Lau SS, et al: Metabolic activation and detoxification of bromobenzene leading to cytotoxicity. *J Pharmacol Exp Ther* 1980; 214:703–708.

259. Zampaglione N, et al: Role of detoxifying enzymes in bromobenzene-induced liver necrosis. *J Pharmacol Exp Ther* 1973; 187:218–227.

260. Lauterburg BH, et al: Glutathione deficiency in alcoholics: Risk factor for paracetamol hepatotoxicity. *Gut* 1988; 29:1153–1157.

261. MacGregor FB, et al: Hepatotoxicity of herbal remedies. *BMJ* 1989; 299:1156–1157.

262. Harvey J, et al: Mistletoe hepatitis. *BMJ* 1981; 282:186–187.

263. Katz M, et al: Herbal hepatitis: Subacute hepatic necrosis secondary to chaparral leaf. *J Clin Gastroenterol* 1990; 12:203–206.

264. Beuers S, et al: Hepatitis after chronic abuse of senna. *Lancet* 1991; 337:372–373.

265. Davies EG, et al: Chinese herbs for eczema (letter). *Lancet* 1991; 336:177.

266. Carlsson C: Herbs and hepatitis (letter). *Lancet* 1990; 2:1068.

267. Larrey D, et al: Hepatitis after Germander *(Teucrium chamaedrys)* administration: Another instance of herbal medicine hepatotoxicity. *Ann Intern Med* 1992; 117:129–132.

268. Hodgson MJ, et al: Liver disease associated with exposure to 1,1,1-trichloroethane. *Arch Intern Med* 1989; 149:1793–1798.

269. Hodgson MJ, et al: 1,1,1-Trichloroethane and the liver. *Arch Intern Med* 1991; 151:2322–2326.

270. Guzelian PS: 1,1,1-Trichloroethane and the liver. *Arch Intern Med* 1991; 151:2321–2322.

271. Hodgson M, et al: Obesity and hepatotoxins as risk factors for fatty liver disease. *Br J Ind Med* 1991; 48:690–695.

272. Chen JD, et al: Exposure to mixtures of solvents among paint workers and biochemical alterations of liver function. *Br J Ind Med* 1991; 48:696–701.

273. Jie L, et al: Persistent ethanol drinking increases liver injury induced by trinitrotoluene exposure: An in plant case-control study. *Hum Exp Toxicol* 1991; 10:405–409.

274. Froment O, et al: Immunoquantitation of von Willebrand factor (factor VIII-related antigen) in vinyl chloride exposed workers. *Cancer Lett* 1991; 61:201–206.

275. Kessel D, et al: Thorium dioxide forgotten but not gone. *Br J Radiol* 1991; 64:1067–1069.

276. Mattocks AR: Toxicity of pyrrolizidine alkaloids. *Nature* 1968; 217:723–728.

277. Glowaz SL, et al: Detection of a reactive pyrrole in the hepatic metabolism of the pyrrolizidine alkaloid, monocrotaline. *Toxicol Appl Pharmacol* 1992; 115:168–173.

278. Mattocks AR, et al: Trapping and measurement of short-lived alkylating agents in a recirculating flow system. *Chem Biol Interact* 1990; 76:19–30.

279. Fleming LE, et al: Liver injury in workers exposed to dimethylformamide. *Scand J Work Environ Health* 1990; 16:289–292.

280. Mithöfer K, et al: Mitochondrial poisons cause depletion of reduced glutathione in isolated hepatocytes. *Arch Biochem Biophys* 1992; 295:132–136.

281. Gasbarrini A, et al: Fructose protects rat hepatocytes from anoxic injury. Effect on intracellular ATP, Ca^{2+}_i, Na^+_i, and pH_i. *J Biol Chem* 1992; 267:7545–7552.

282. Weis M, et al: N-Acetyl-p-benzoquinone imine induces Ca^{2+} release from mitochondria by stimulating pyridine nucleotide hydrolysis. *J Biol Chem* 1992; 267:804–809.

283. Richter C, et al: Cyclosporine A inhibits mitochondrial pyridine nucleotide hydrolysis and calcium release. *Biochem Pharmacol* 1990; 40:779–782.

284. Broekemeier KM, et al: Cyclosporin A protects hepatocytes subjected to high Ca^{2+} and oxidative stress. *FEBS Lett* 1992; 304:194–194.

285. Gunter TE, et al: Mechanisms by which mitochondria transport calcium. *Am J Physiol* 1990; 259:C755–C786.

286. Kass GEN, et al: Cyclosporin A protects hepatocytes against prooxidant-induced killing of isolated rat hepatocytes: A study on the role of mitochondrial Ca^{2+} cycling in cytotoxicity. *Biochem Pharmacol* 1992; 44:1995–2003.

287. Corcoran GB, et al: The role of the nucleus and other compartments in toxic cell death produced by alkylating hepatotoxicants. *Toxicol Appl Pharmacol* 1992; 113:167–183.

288. Bellomo G, et al: Demonstration of nuclear compartmentalization of glutathione in hepatocytes. *Proc Natl Acad Sci U S A* 1992; 89:4412–4416.

CHAPTER 5

Alcoholic Liver Disease

Rowen K. Zetterman, M.D.

Professor, Department of Internal Medicine, University of Nebraska Medical Center, and Liver Study Unit, Veteran Affairs Medical Center, Omaha, Nebraska

Substance abuse remains a common problem in the United States, with abuse of at least one illegal substance admitted to by 14.5 million Americans. Ethanol consumption is also frequent, with an average of 45 million Americans consuming at least one alcoholic beverage weekly.[1] Thus it should be no surprise that ethanol and substance abuse by physicians is also likely. In a position paper from the American College of Physicians (ACP), the magnitude of the problem and its assessment and recommendations for training programs are discussed.[2] Table 1 outlines these recommendations. The ACP considers it imperative that each training program establish a formal program of identification and treatment, and the reader is referred to the position paper for further details.

The biological markers of alcoholism and of alcohol-related liver injury continue to be pursued. In a study of 157 Spanish patients with alcoholic cirrhosis, α_1-antitrypsin, transferrin, orosomucoid, plasminogen, haptoglobin, group-specific component, phosphoglucomutase, acid phosphatase, esterase, adenylate kinase, and 6-phosphogluconate dehydrogenase markers were determined.[3] Although strong associations with the α_1-antitrypsin Pi*Z allelle, the haptoglobin HP*1 allelle, and the acid phosphatase ACP AC phenotype were observed, their biological significance and predictive value were less clear. Furthermore, they should also do additional studies of alcoholics in whom only minimal or no liver injury develops. In earlier studies, HLA subtypes were not useful in identifying those at risk, although country-specific differences have been observed. In yet another study of 41

TABLE 1.

Recommendations for Training Programs to
Address Problems of Ethanol and Other Substance
Abuse Among Physicians-in-Training*

1. A formal, organized process should be present
   to address the problem of substance abuse
   among residents in training programs.
2. All housestaff and attending faculty should
   know of the policies of the medical center
   regarding substance abuse and impairment.
3. Information should be provided to orient
   residents and their families to the problem of
   substance abuse among physicians.
4. A clearly defined process should exist for
   referral (and self-referral) of residents who are
   abusing alcohol and other drugs or both.
5. Residents and staff physicians should be aware
   of how to seek help for a resident who is
   suspected of substance abuse.

*From National Institute on Drug Abuse: *National House-
hold Survey on Drug Abuse, Population Estimates, 1988.*
Rockville, Md, US Department of Health and Human Services, 1989, DHHS Publication No ADM 89–1636.

mixed-race, alcoholic cirrhosis patients of the French West Indies, it initially appeared that there was an increase in HLA-A2 and a decrease in HLA-B2 frequency
when compared with 51 healthy controls and 41 heavy drinkers with no liver disease.[4] However, these differences did not persist with additional comparisons, and
this again shows that HLA subtypes will not segregate alcoholics with various forms
of liver disease.

That the quantity of ethanol consumed is a risk factor for the development of
cirrhosis was again confirmed in a study of 33 men and 36 women with newly
diagnosed alcoholic cirrhosis as compared with age- and gender-matched controls.[5]
When ethanol consumption exceeded the equivalent of 40 g/day or more, there
was a significantly increased risk of cirrhosis with a greater proportional increase
for risk in women than men as ethanol intake increased above this limit. This is a
lower level of intake in men than has been implicated in past studies and should be
a worry to some because it approximates only four beers or three mixed drinks
daily. It again reiterates the greater risk of women for alcohol-induced cirrhosis
with increasing ethanol consumption. Alcohol consumption also increases the risk
of hepatocellular carcinoma (HCC) developing in both men and women even in
the absence of coexisting cirrhosis.[6] In this study, when alcoholism resulted in cirrhosis, the risk for HCC was similar to that of chronic hepatitis B virus (HBV)
disease in Western countries. Excessive alcohol consumption does not seem to affect the outcome of acute viral hepatitis B, however.[7]

To assess the demographics of ethanol abuse in a large patient population using

Department of Veterans Affairs (VA) facilities, 62,829 inpatients hospitalized for either alcoholism treatment (43.9%), detoxification (14.8%), or other medical disorders but with a secondary diagnosis of alcoholism (41.3%) were compared with all 602,881 male patients who used VA inpatient care in 1987.[8] Male alcoholics tended to be younger, less likely to be married, and of similar ethnicity as nonalcoholic patients. There also tended to be more non-Caucasians among younger alcoholics, and younger alcoholics were less likely to be married than older drinkers. Hispanic and African-American alcoholics of all ages were more likely to be hospitalized for non–alcohol-related diagnoses and, if enrolled, less likely to complete alcohol treatment than were Native American or Caucasian alcoholics. Although underreporting of alcoholism in all groups may have been present, it does indicate the need to look for alcoholism in all groups of inpatients and to offer appropriate alcohol treatment when identified.

Although many recent studies have evaluated the relationship between modest ethanol consumption and cardiovascular mortality, few have explored the relationship of age, gender, and ethnicity with the quantity of alcohol use and overall mortality. Patients enrolled in the Kaiser Permanente Medical Care Program completed an additional questionaire regarding ethanol consumption during their routine health evaluation.[9] Between 1978 and 1985, 128,934 persons (78.8% of all patients) were identified with usable data regarding alcohol use, personal demographics, and clinical outcome. During this interval, there was 1,031,630 person-years of follow-up. They defined nondrinkers as no alcohol use in the past year and exdrinkers as no use in the past year with ethanol consumption before that time. Drinkers were current consumers of alcohol-containing beverages. Overall mortality was significantly increased in exdrinkers and heavier drinkers when compared with lifelong nondrinkers. In those who consumed ethanol, the lowest risk of death was in those who drank more than one alcohol-containing beverage per month but less than one per day. The higher risk of death in these groups was from noncardiovascular causes, especially cirrhosis, unnatural causes, and tobacco-related cancers. The lower mortality in the minimal ethanol intake group was due to a reduction in cardiovascular causes. Although there were no significant racial differences in mortality, gender did seem to play a role inasmuch as women tended to have a greater mortality than men at higher levels of ethanol consumption, largely because of an increase in death from unnatural causes and from a relatively higher risk of cancer and respiratory and cardiovascular disease. Although there was no difference in overall mortality due to various types of alcoholic beverages, there did tend to be fewer cardiovascular deaths among wine drinkers, especially female wine drinkers. Curiously, when smoking subsets were evaluated, the greatest risk of mortality in heavy drinkers was in nonsmokers and in those patients with light alcohol consumption; only exsmokers and smokers had a reduction in mortality. This study adds further evidence to the presumption that minimal alcohol consumption is associated with a reduction in mortality, especially of cardiovascular disease, even suggesting that wine consumption could be especially beneficial. However, this study also indicates that the "safe" limit of alcohol consumption is smaller than suggested by some earlier studies and that women especially may not benefit from current recommendations for daily ethanol consumption. Obviously, each patient must be counseled in view of other factors and family history.

Alcohol consumption may also affect the response to operations with increased postoperative morbidity.[10] Fifteen symptom-free drinkers who consumed more than 60 g equivalent of ethanol daily were compared for outcome following colorectal surgery with diagnosis-, weight-, gender-, nutritional status–, cardiopulmonary status–, age-, anesthesia-, and operation-matched controls who consumed less than 25 g of ethanol daily. During preoperative assessment, drinkers were more likely to have impairment of left ventricular function and delayed-type hypersensitivity and, when compared intraoperatively, to have longer bleeding times and greater surgical stress (higher serum catecholamine levels). Drinkers also had more post-operative complications (67% vs. 20%) and longer hospital stays (20 vs. 12 days) than nondrinkers. Thus, alcohol consumption can have a significant effect on operative outcome and should be carefully assessed during preoperative evaluation. Although older studies had indicated a greater operative risk for patients with alcoholic hepatitis, this study suggests that some of this risk is with ethanol alone regardless of the severity of underlying liver injury. How long one needs to wait before proceeding with operative intervention after stopping alcohol consumption is unclear from this study.

Despite their frequent concurrence in alcoholics, tobacco use does not seem to be an additive factor for the development of cirrhosis, although it is associated with a greater risk of development of chronic pancreatitis.[11] The age of onset of pancreatitis in smoking alcoholics was also less than for alcoholic nonsmokers. If the abdominal habitus of patients is classified by ultrasonography, it will be discovered that patients in whom alcoholic cirrhosis develops are of a different morphotype than those in whom alcoholic pancreatitis develops.[12] This is an interesting finding although it may also reflect differences in dietary intake between the groups over time and the effects of ethanol on fat storage. Ethanol will increase energy expenditure while decreasing lipid oxidation and result in increased fat storage.[13]

ETHANOL METABOLISM

The controversy about the role of the stomach in the metabolism of ethanol may have been put to rest. Alcohol dehydrogenase (ADH) activity does exist in the stomach, and the reduction in gastric ADH activity in women has been suggested to increase the delivery of ethanol to the liver, with the consequent greater exposure of hepatocytes to acetaldehyde (because all of the ethanol would be metabolized in the liver cell) resulting in greater liver injury. Ethnic differences in gastric ADH have also been noted.[14] Furthermore, the inhibiting effect of certain histamine 2 receptor antagonists (H$_2$RA) on gastric ADH activity has been implied to increase blood alcohol levels above legal driving limits in otherwise moderate drinkers.[15]

Omeprazole seems to be without such effect.[16] Studies in rats did show that several medications will affect gastric ADH activity in vitro.[17] However, the effect was minimal in vivo and, for cimetidine, not demonstrable when ethanol was administered in the fed state. This was subsequently confirmed when ethanol was consumed after breakfast in 20 healthy males who were receiving ranitidine, 150 mg twice daily.[18] Via a double-blind, crossover technique, the peak plasma ethanol level was the same whether subjects were receiving ranitidine or not. Finally, another recent randomized crossover study of 25 healthy males that used all commercially available H_2RAs (cimetidine, ranitidine, famotidine, and nizatidine) as compared with placebo showed that there was no difference in any group whether peak blood ethanol levels were measured or the area under the curve of the blood alcohol levels following ethanol consumption in the fed state (Fig 1).[19] Thus, the potential effect of H_2RA on blood ethanol levels need not be considered when they are prescribed. In a companion editorial to this study, Dr. Levitt called into question those prior studies that suggested that stomach ADH of the rat was capable of metabolizing approximately 50% of ingested ethanol since only 20% of ingested ethanol is normally absorbed from the stomach.[20] These recent studies should dispel any continuing concern over the choice of H_2RA in a patient who consumes alcoholic beverages and remove this as an argument for why an automobile driver's blood alcohol level was too high when tested.

Polymorphism of ADH enzymes and the alteration of ADH and aldehyde dehydrogenase (AlDH) activities continue to be studied in alcoholic patients in an at-

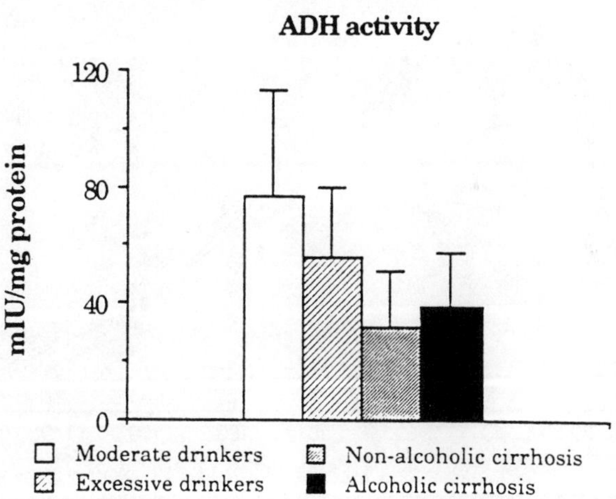

FIG 1.

Effect of H_2 blocker treatment on the serum ethanol concentration. Serum ethynol concentrations in 23 men following postprandial ingestion of 0.3 g of ethanol per kilogram of body weight after 7 days of cimetidine, famotidine, nizatidine, ranitidine, or no treatment were determined at the times indicated. Ethanol was measured by head-space gas chomatography. *Bars* represent the largest standard error of the mean of the five values at each time point. (From Raufman J-P, Notar-Francesco V, Raffaniello D, et al: *Ann Intern Med* 1993; 118:488–494. Used by permission.)

tempt to identify risk factors for the development of alcoholic liver disease. Prior studies have suggested that acetaldehyde, the highly reactive intermediate of ethanol, may have a role in the development of liver injury. Thus anything that could increase the intracellular acetaldehyde concentration (e.g., enhanced ADH or reduced AlDH activities) could be central to the pathogenesis of liver injury with ethanol consumption. In yet another study,[21] the relative importance of altered ADH and AlDH enzyme activity seems limited. Liver biopsy samples from 31 patients with alcoholic cirrhosis were compared with those of 25 patients with cirrhosis of other causes and with those of 62 patients with excessive ethanol consumption and 43 patients with moderate alcohol intake who lacked liver injury. No differences in ADH polymorphism were observed between groups. Furthermore, the reduction in ADH (Fig 2) and AlDH activity observed in alcoholic cirrhotics could also be observed in cirrhosis of other causes, thus suggesting that reduced ADH activity is a consequence and not a cause of liver disease. There are, however, regional (intra-acinar) differences in the distribution of ADH and AlDH activities within the liver between men and women that might play a role.[22] Alcohol-related hepatocyte injury is greatest in the perivenular (centrilobular) portion of the liver lobule. If there was a reason for higher acetaldehyde levels in these cells, this might explain the preponderance of injury at that site. Indeed,

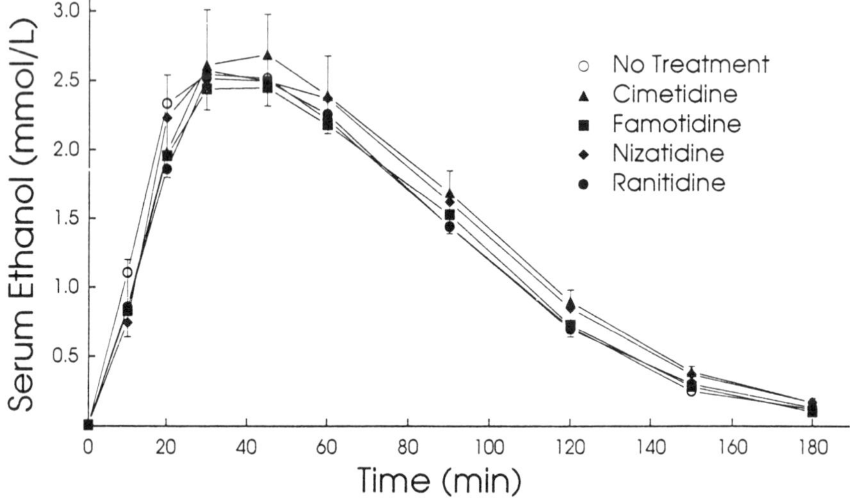

FIG 2.

Hepatic alcohol dehydrogenase (ADH) activity. In cirrhotic patients ADH activities (expressed as milli-international units per milligram protein) were significantly lower than in excessive drinkers and moderate drinkers ($P < .05$ and $P < .001$). Alcohol dehydrogenase activity was not different between the two groups of cirrhotic patients (alcoholic cirrhosis and nonalcoholic cirrhosis). Mean ADH activity was significantly lower in the excessive drinkers than in the moderate drinkers ($P < .001$). *Error bars* indicate standard deviations. (From Poupon RE, Nalpas B, Coutelle C, et al: *Hepatology* 1992; 15:1017–1022.)

younger women (less than 53 years of age) tend to have greater ADH activity in perivenular hepatocytes, whereas in younger males it is distributed in intermediate (midacinar) hepatocytes. With an increase in age, greater ADH activity in perivenular hepatocytes develops in men, and the distribution becomes the same in men as in women. No lobular differences in distribution of AlDH activity were observed. This interesting study seems to give a rationale for the greater risk of alcoholic liver injury in younger women with a subsequent peak of liver injury in older men. However, many more studies will be required to cement this concept. There are many other gender differences to consider in the development of alcoholic liver disease as well. We await further studies.

RELATIONSHIPS OF ALCOHOLIC LIVER DISEASE WITH HEPATITIS C VIRUS

Prior studies have indicated that serum antibodies to hepatitis C virus (HCV) are frequently identified in patients with alcoholic liver disease and have raised the question of whether HCV coinfection of alcoholics could explain why liver cirrhosis develops in a few whereas it does not in the majority of alcoholics. Although this hypothesis remains to be proved, it is becoming more clear that HCV may account for some of the histologic abnormalities previously attributed to ethanol. When liver biopsy specimens of 27 chronic alcoholics were compared, the 11 who only had features of alcoholic hepatitis were found to be serum HCV-associated RNA (HCV-RNA) negative whereas the 16 who had histologic features of both alcoholic and chronic hepatitis were all HCV-RNA positive.[23] In the latter group, the inflammation was principally portal in location with mononuclear cell preponderance, and the cells were mostly suppressor/cytotoxic thymus dependent (T8 cells) in type. In addition, in those positive for HCV, class I HLA antigens were displayed on hepatocytes in areas of hepatocellular necrosis but not in those with alcohol-related changes only. Although this study supports prior studies that indicate that the chronic hepatitis observed in patients with chronic alcoholism may be due to HCV, it does not address the effect of the virus on the development of "alcoholic cirrhosis." When 164 patients with alcoholic cirrhosis were assessed for antibodies to HCV by the first-generation enzyme-linked immunosorbent assay (ELISA-1) method, 29 (18%) were positive.[24] All anti-HCV–positive patients had more mononuclear inflammation and a less typical alcoholic hepatitis appearance with a similar degree of fat, fibrosis, and necrosis as anti-HCV–negative subjects. Twenty-four patient sera were also tested by recombinant immunoblot assay (RIBA) and found to be positive in 11. The RIBA-positive group had more hepatocellular necrosis and the RIBA-negative group more perisinusoidal and perinodular fibrosis. However, one cannot automatically assume that the the lack of chronic hepatitis features means that HCV is not present. In an evaluation of 62 chronic alcoholics, of 36 found to be anti-HCV positive, 22 were also RIBA positive, and of these, 18 were serum HCV-RNA positive.[25] Twelve HCV-RNA–positive patients had liver biopsy findings with typical alcohol-related features in 7 and mixed alcohol-viral lesions in 5. Thus, although HCV may be associated with histologic chronic hepatitis, it is not a universal finding and simultaneous HCV infection cannot be excluded on this basis alone.

IMMUNOLOGIC FACTORS IN ALCOHOLIC LIVER DISEASE

No review would be complete without a litany of the latest immune studies in alcoholic liver disease inasmuch as there are many past studies that have implicated a role for immune mechanisms in human alcohol-related liver injury. This year's collection of studies amplifies but does little to extend this hypothesis.

Previous studies have identified serum elevations of interleukin-6 (IL-6) in patients with alcoholic hepatitis. In a study of 30 patients with moderate to severe alcoholic hepatitis, serial IL-6 levels were determined and correlated with clinical parameters and outcome.[26] Interleukin-6 levels were elevated at the outset, correlated with the severity of liver disease as indicated by the Maddrey discriminant function score, and fell in a pattern similar to that of bilirubin or other acute-phase reactants such as C-reactive protein. Although IL-6 seems to be a marker for the severity of alcoholic hepatitis and may regulate or augment its acute-phase response, its role in the pathogenesis of the disease is less clear. It is possible that it is even more important for repair than for liver cell injury.

When identified in the liver by indirect immunofluorescence using a monoclonal anti–IL-6 antibody, IL-6 is principally distributed along endothelial cells and not with infiltrating mononuclear cells.[27] It has also been observed that immunoglobulin A (IgA) is deposited along the sinusoids of patients with alcoholic liver disease. The interrelation of IL-6 and IgA was explored in 12 alcoholic cirrhotics with a Child classification of B as compared with 12 controls.[28] The spontaneous secretion of IgA and IgG by peripheral blood mononuclear cells (PBMCs) in vitro was correlated with lipopolysaccharide-induced secretion of IL-6 in vitro. The addition of polymeric IgA to PBMCs caused an increase in mRNA for IL-6 and enhanced IL-6 secretion. Thus it appears that IgA can enhance secretion of IL-6, which will further enhance IgA production. Such amplification of immunoglobulin secretion could explain the hypergammaglobulinemia that occurs in alcoholic liver disease.

Alcoholic hepatitis is characterized histologically by the centrilobular accumulation of polymorphonuclear leukocytes (PMNs). What draws these cells to the liver is unclear. One study indicates that the chemotactic stimulus for these cells may arise from hepatocytes.[29] The supernatant from cultures of hepatocytes isolated from rats fed ethanol long-term was chemotactic for PMNs, and the production of these chemotactic factors was impaired by inhibitors of protein synthesis. These factors might be metabolites of leukotriene B_4 (LTB_4) since two novel metabolites of LTB_4 chemotactic for PMNs were only formed by hepatocytes in the presence of ethanol.[30] Such factors may, at least in part, explain the accumulation of PMNs within the liver in patients with alcoholic hepatitis. However, if it was simply due to altered LTB_4 metabolism, PMN accumulation would occur in all patients with alcohol consumption and not only those with advanced alcohol-related liver disease.

Only a little progress has been made in the role of acetaldehyde-protein adducts in the pathogenesis of liver injury from ethanol. An additional study has found circulating serum acetaldehyde adducts in some heavy consumers of alcohol.[31] With chromatographic techniques they identified two site-specific acetaldehyde-hemoglobin adducts that appear to be acetaldehyde-modified α and β N-termini of hemoglobin. Although the identification of these adducts could be markers of alcohol consumption, they are also indicators of the potential for adduct formation by acetaldehyde. It seems reasonable to assume that adducts are also formed with integral hepatocyte proteins and could even be the immunologic trigger for an immune pathogenesis of alcoholic liver injury. Circulating IgA antibody to a 200-kd hepatocyte cytosolic protein-acetaldehyde adduct has also been identified.[32] When various populations of patients with alcoholic liver disease were studied, those with alcoholic hepatitis were most likely to have circulating antibody present (Table 2). Thus, another stimulus for the production of IgA has been identified. However, what this adduct's role is in the development of alcoholic liver disease remains to be clarified. Since it is found in patients with mild alcoholic liver injury and in other types of liver disease, little role for it in the pathogenesis of liver injury from ethanol can be implied. However, additional adducts have also been observed and need further study. I suspect, however, that if there is a role for acetaldehyde adducts in alcoholic liver disease pathogenesis, it will be with the cellular immune and not the humoral immune component.

LIVER IMAGING

There have been several attempts to use various imaging techniques to establish liver disease diagnoses by looking at liver texture. This has not proved very

TABLE 2.

Prevalence of Circulating IgA Antibodies to a 200-kd Acetaldehyde-Protein Adduct*

Patient Group	Percent Positive	P Value
Alcoholic hepatitis ± cirrhosis ($n = 23$)	70	—
Inactive alcoholic cirrhosis ($n = 10$)	30	<.05
Alcoholics with no overt liver disease ($n = 10$)	20	<.02
Nonalcoholic liver disease ($n = 17$)	35	<.05
Control, social drinkers ($n = 20$)	25	<.005

*Adapted from Koskinas J, Kenna JG, Bird JL, et al: *Gastroenterology* 1992; 103:1860–1867.

useful. One interesting study looked at other ultrasound findings in patients with chronic liver diseases to see whether there were other features that permitted a diagnosis of alcoholic liver disease.[33] When hepatic and splenic vessels were evaluated in patients with alcoholic liver cirrhosis, larger hepatic arteries, smaller splenic arteries, and smaller spleens were observed more frequently in patients with alcoholic cirrhosis than in those with cryptogenic cirrhosis, chronic hepatitis B cirrhosis, or primary biliary cirrhosis. When they calculated the hepatic-to-splenic artery size ratio, it was greater than 0.9 in 25 of 26 patients with alcoholic cirrhosis and less than 0.9 in 55 of 62 of the patients with other liver diseases. The sensitivity and specificity of this ratio for alcoholic cirrhosis was 96% and 88%, respectively. The difference was a consequence of finding both larger hepatic arteries in the alcoholics and larger splenic arteries in those with other liver diseases. Perhaps reticuloendothelial hyperplasia is greater in these other diseases and accounts for the larger spleens and arteries. Despite this interesting observation, the role of ultrasound may still be limited since it is likely that the history was also sensitive to the diagnosis of underlying alcoholism and thus of alcoholic liver disease.

Computed tomography (CT) might also assist in the differentiation of alcoholic cirrhosis from other types of liver disease. With the injection of ionic contrast, the time to peak contrast enhancement of the liver (in Housfield units) can be compared with the time to peak enhancement of the aorta.[34] It is no surprise that this interval is longer in those with cirrhosis than in patients with normal livers. Interestingly, however, the time is even longer in patients with alcoholic cirrhosis as compared with posthepatitic cirrhosis. The difference in the cirrhotic must be a consequence of the vascular derangement where the distribution of contrast would be slower than in normal individuals because of intrahepatic shunting and nodule formation. Perhaps the difference in patients with alcoholic cirrhosis reflects even greater intrahepatic shunting than in nonalcoholics or differences due to micronodular cirrhosis. It would also be important to evaluate this finding in patients with active alcoholic cirrhosis where inflammation and necrosis may continue to limit vascular inflow and compared them with those with inactive cirrhosis or those with macronodular transformation.

The newest entry into the attempt to diagnose diffuse liver disease by imaging techniques is quantitative tomoscintigraphy (single-photon emission computed tomography [SPECT]). In a study of conventional liver scanning (planar scintigraphy [PS]) vs. SPECT, 114 patients with alcoholic liver disease including 24 with fatty liver, 18 with alcoholic hepatitis, and 72 with cirrhosis were compared with 70 nonalcoholic controls referred for possible metastatic disease of the liver.[35] Patients were studied by multiple techniques including PS and SPECT, hepatic ultrasound, and CT. Calculated liver volume, spleen volume, spleen-to-liver volume and uptake ratio, nonhomogeneity, marrow-to-liver uptake ratio, left lobe-to-right uptake ratio, and a calculated score were the criteria assessed by SPECT. These criteria for SPECT in identifying liver disease were 79% sensitive for fatty liver and 97% for alcoholic cirrhosis. In comparison to other imaging modalities, SPECT

Moving?

I'd like to receive my **Current Hepatology** without interruption.
Please note the following change of address, effective:

Name: ____

New Address: ______________________________________

____

City: _________________________ State: _______ Zip: _______

Old Address: ______________________________________

____

City: _________________________ State: _______ Zip: _______

Reservation Card

Yes, I would like my own copy of **Current Hepatology**. Please begin my subscription with the current edition according to the terms described below.* I understand that I will have 30 days to examine each annual edition. If satisfied, I will pay just $79.95 plus sales tax, postage and handling (price subject to change without notice).

Name: ____

Address: ____

City: _________________________ State: _______ Zip: _______

Method of Payment
○ Visa ○ Mastercard ○ AmEx ○ Bill me ○ Check (in US dollars, payable to Mosby, Inc.)

Card number: _____________________ Exp date: _____________

Signature: ____

LS-0909

*Your Current Service Guarantee:

When you subscribe to *Current*, we'll send you an advance notice of future volumes about two months before they publish. This automatic notice system is designed to take up as little of your time as possible. If you do not want *Current*, the advance notice makes it quick and easy for you to let us know your decision, and you will always have at least 20 days to decide. If we don't hear from you, we'll send you the new volume as soon as it's available. And, of course, *Current* is yours to examine free of charge for 30 days (postage, handling and applicable sales tax are added to each shipment.).

BUSINESS REPLY MAIL

FIRST CLASS MAIL   PERMIT No. 762   CHICAGO, IL

POSTAGE WILL BE PAID BY ADDRESSEE

Chris Hughes
Mosby-Year Book, Inc.
200 N. LaSalle Street
Suite 2600
Chicago, IL 60601-9981

BUSINESS REPLY MAIL

FIRST CLASS MAIL   PERMIT No. 762   CHICAGO, IL

POSTAGE WILL BE PAID BY ADDRESSEE

Chris Hughes
Mosby-Year Book, Inc.
200 N. LaSalle Street
Suite 2600
Chicago, IL 60601-9981

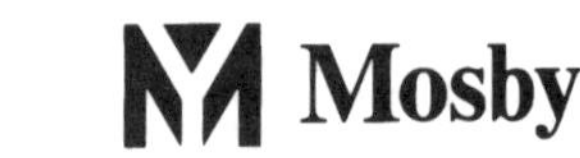

sensitivity was 89% to 66% for conventional liver scans, 88% to 53% for ultrasound, and 92% to 65% for CT.

Although these studies are all interesting, they continue to show us that a replacement for histologic diagnosis is yet to be discovered. However, for a patient too ill for liver biopsy or when the tissue sample is insufficient to establish the presence of cirrhosis, such techniques may be able to support the diagnosis of alcoholic cirrhosis.

HISTOLOGY

Previous studies have identified "giant mitochondria" by light microscopy in liver specimens obtained from patients with alcoholic liver diseases and suggested that their presence in alcoholic hepatitis is associated with a more benign clinical course. In a study of 103 liver specimens (53 with alcoholic liver disease and 50 with nonalcoholic disease), "giant mitochondria" were identified in 18 of 53 biopsy samples from alcoholic patients but in only 2 of 50 specimens from patients with other diseases.[36] Furthermore, giant mitochondria were even more likely in those with advanced liver disease. However, the investigators were unable to confirm the light microscopic observation of giant mitochondria by electron microscopy. Perhaps this is because what has been assumed to be large mitochondria at light microscopy is actually crystalloid bodies. In another study, examination of the liver specimen by both light and electron microscopy indicated that "giant mitochondria" were really crystalloid bodies with a latticelike structure whose formation may be related to degeneration of intracellular organelles.[37] Thus, although these bodies are more common in alcoholic liver disease, both their identification and significance may be less correct than prior studies would indicate.

COMPLICATIONS OF ALCOHOLIC CIRRHOSIS

Portal Hypertension

The continuing use of ethanol-containing beverages after variceal hemorrhage is thought to increase the risk of rebleeding and hasten mortality. However, a new study has challenged this concept. When 100 survivors of first-time variceal bleeding related to alcoholic cirrhosis were followed for up to 2 years, 15 did not redrink, 29 drank occasionally, and 56 continued to abuse alcohol.[38] Surprisingly, there was no difference in variceal rebleeding frequency or in mortality of the groups at 2 years. This study is contrary to previous studies of patients with cirrhosis where abstinence was reported as beneficial. For the patient who has bled from varices, what factors predict rebleeding? One study indicates that a hepatic venous pressure gradient (wedged hepatic venous pressure minus hepatic vein pressure) greater than 16 mm Hg, the presence of large esophageal varices at endoscopy, coexisting ascites, a high Pugh score, and prior variceal hemorrhage are all predictors of subsequent bleeding.[39] The presence of a pressure gradient over 16 mm Hg, prior bleeding, and an elevated Pugh score were also associated with a higher mortality. The implication of this study is that wedged hepatic venous pressure measurement may impart sufficient prognostic information to justify its routine use.

Portal hypertensive gastropathy (PHG) has been increasingly recognized in patients with cirrhosis. In 47 patients with cirrhosis, 20 of whom were alcoholic, 68% were found to have PHG.[40] No clinical features including esophageal variceal size, however, predicted its presence. When PHG was graded as severe, portal pressures were higher, sinusoidal resistance was greater, hepatic blood flow was less, and there was greater impairment of indocyanine green (ICG) clearance. Similarly, the factors that lead to PHG are also unclear. Although it is associated with portal hypertension, PHG is more frequently observed when the portal hypertension is due to cirrhotic than to noncirrhotic causes, when both esophageal and gastric varices are present, and when the severity of underlying liver disease is greater.[41] Since all of the patients in this study had bled from varices, many received sclerotherapy, and an even greater prevalence of PHG was seen after sclerotherapy.

Two studies have been reported this year that indicate a reduction in portal pressure upon the administration of clonidine.[42, 43] Clonidine did not affect hepatic blood flow or hepatic function as assessed by galactose elimination and ICG clearance[42] and decreased renal vascular resistance with an increase in the glomerular filtration rate.[43] Additional clinical trials of clonidine in the treatment of variceal hemorrhage due to cirrhosis are needed to assess its place in the management of patients with portal hypertension.

Ascites

Large-volume paracentesis has been shown to be effective in the management of patients with ascites due to liver cirrhosis. Although good-risk patients may not need plasma expansion with albumin following paracentesis, it is still widely used, especially in patients with poor hepatic function. Other plasma expanders may also be effective. Following 5-L paracentesis, patients were randomized to receive either intravenous albumin or dextran 70 (6 g/L of ascites removed).[44] There were no differences in subsequent liver or renal test results, electrolytes, plasma renin activity, clotting studies, or platelet count in either group, thus indicating that dextran can be used as an acceptable plasma expander in place of albumin following large-volume paracentesis. Although it is important to realize that these were all good-risk patients with no significant renal dysfunction, it does suggest that more cost-effective alternatives to albumin may be as efficacious in plasma volume expansion.

Infections

Spontaneous bacterial peritonitis (SBP) is a frequently recognized complication of ascites. Early studies indicated that in approximately 10% of ascitics SBP will eventually develop. This has been confirmed in the follow-up of 65 patients with cirrhosis and ascites (43/65 due to alcoholic cirrhosis) inasmuch as SBP developed in 7.7% during 21 months of follow-up.[45] One risk factor for SBP is gastrointestinal hemorrhage. When 119 patients with upper gastrointestinal bleeding were randomized to receive oral norfloxacin or placebo, bacterial infection developed in only 10% of treated patients as compared with 37% of controls.[46] Antibiotic treatment reduced the incidence of not only SBP but also bacteremia and urinary tract infection. This infection reduction was in gram-negative aerobic bacteria. However, despite this effect, the overall mortality of the two groups remained the same. This study also implies that the gastrointestinal tract is the likely source of bacterial infection in cirrhotics and that routine administration of oral antibiotics should be considered following upper gastrointestinal bleeding.

THERAPY

New reports of therapeutic trials have been limited but continue to indicate the importance of adequate nutrition for patients with advanced alcoholic liver disease and the role of corticosteroids in improvement of short-term survival of those with alcoholic hepatitis. In another large multicenter trial, insulin-glucagon infusions were of no benefit in the treatment of severe alcoholic hepatitis.[47] This study should put to rest any continuing question about their role.

Enteral Nutrition

Although no large studies of enteral or parenteral nutritional supplementation have conclusively shown benefit in mortality of patients with alcoholic hepatitis, another small study has indicated the importance of adequate nutrition in the treatment of advanced alcoholic liver injury as defined by a history of alcoholism, a bilirubin content greater than 51 μmol/L (3 mg/dL), and at least one of the following: prothrombin time over 4 seconds prolonged, serum albumin less than 3.0 g/dL, or the presence of ascites.[48] All patients were offered a "regular" diet (or a 2-g sodium diet in the presence of ascites or peripheral edema). Sixteen patients received 4 weeks of enteral supplementation with a casein-based formulation (Isocal HCN) sufficient to provide 167 kJ of energy and 1.5 g of protein per kilogram of ideal body weight, whereas 15 received the standard diet alone. The supplemented group achieved approximately twice the calorie and protein intake of the control group. The overall mortality, incidence of diarrhea, development of renal insufficiency, gastrointestinal bleeding or ascites, and anthropometric changes were similar in both groups. However, the enterally supplemented group had improvement in mean grade of encephalopathy during the first week of therapy (whereas encephalopathy in control patients deteriorated) and in serum bilirubin and antipyrine half-life. Since many patients with severe alcoholic liver disease are anorexic because of the severity of their illness and/or the mechanical effects of ascites, supplementation is an important consideration. This study also emphasizes the importance of adequate nutritional intake in the management of patients with alcoholic hepatitis and suggests that standard formulas can be used.[49]

Corticosteroids

In yet another trial of prednisolone, clinical benefit seems evident. Sixty-one patients with biopsy-proven (percutaneous in 7 and transvenous in 54) alcoholic hepatitis who had either a Maddrey discriminant function score of greater than 32 (57 patients) or spontaneous encephalopathy (4 patients) were randomized to receive prednisolone, 40 mg, as a single daily dose for 28 days or placebo.[50] If they were unable to take oral medications, prednisolone or a placebo infusion was administered parenterally. No patient was observed for longer than 1 month before initiating the therapy. Patients with acute gastroduodenal mucosal disease, persisting bacterial infection (more than 1 month before entry), neoplastic disease, simultaneous human immunodeficiency virus (HIV) or hepatitis B surface antigen (HBsAg) disease, and anticoagulant therapy were excluded from participation. All patients were offered a 3,000-kcal diet. There were significantly fewer deaths in the prednisolone-treated group (4/32) than in the placebo-treated group (16/29). When assessed by multivariate analysis, the factors significantly associated with improved outcome included receipt of prednisolone, serum bilirubin, and ascites. No gender differences in outcome or adverse side effects of corticosteroids were observed. This study again supports the role of corticosteroids in the management of patients who appear to have severe alcoholic hepatitis. All definitely had severe alcoholic hepatitis as proved by biopsy. Why corticosteroids should work is unclear. The study may support a role for immune mechanisms in pathogenesis. It would be interesting to see whether the effect of corticosteroids is due to improved dietary intake.

So whom do you treat and how? Although these recommendations may be controversial to some, it appears that all patients with severe alcoholic hepatitis should be treated with both short-term enteral supplementation and corticosteroids. Standard low-sodium enteral formulations appear adequate, and patients do not require the more expensive branched-chain amino acid formulations. For those with spontaneous hepatic encephalopathy or those with severe alcoholic liver disease, corticosteroids should be added. The Maddrey score[51] can be used to assist in the determination of whom to treat (those with scores greater than 32) as calculated by the formula. I suppose one question remains, and that is whether improved nutrition alone without steroids would be as adequate as the combination of both. However, it seems unlikely that this hypothesis will be tested soon.

Liver transplantation

The place of liver transplantation in the management of a patient with life-threatening complications of alcoholic liver disease is becoming more established. Although most liver transplant centers will at least consider liver transplantation for abstinent alcoholics, selection of candidates can still be difficult. In a study of 99 alcoholic candidates for liver transplantation, the group at the University of Michigan used a selection process that evaluated medical, surgical, and psychiatric factors.[52] Alcohol abuse or dependence was defined by *Diagnostic and Statistical Manual, Third Edition, Revised* (DMS-III-R) criteria. Acceptance of alcoholism, the prognosis for sobriety, and social stability were assessed by the University of Michigan alcoholism prognosis scale. Forty-five patients were suitable candidates and underwent liver transplantation with a 78% and 73% actuarial survival rate at 1 and 2 years, respectively. Of those who received transplants, 5 patients again consumed alcohol following transplantation, 2 with uncontrolled drinking. All patients who redrank were alive at the time of the report. Of the 54 who did not receive transplants, 17 were deemed too well to need transplantation with 93% and 59% 1- and 2-year survival rates, respectively, and 19 were considered too ill to undergo transplantation, with only a 35% survival rate at 3 months and a 0% survival rate at 1 year. Seventeen patients were refused liver transplantation because of the psychiatric assessment of poor prognosis for sobriety, and their corresponding survival rates were 65% and 43%, respectively, at 1 and 2 years. This study emphasizes several important features: (1) a defined period of abstinence is not a definite requirement for candidacy, (2) survival of patients with alcoholic liver disease following liver transplantation is similar to that of patients with other liver diseases, (3) those judged too well to need transplantation need continuing and careful follow-up to identify signs of deterioration that will require transplantation intervention, and (4) patients not selected for liver transplantation because of concerns about continuing sobriety have a poor survival. Several important questions raised by this study remain unanswered, however. How reliable is the history of recidivism?[53] What is the effect of continued alcohol ingestion following liver transplantation on patient outcome? Will recurrent alcoholic liver disease develop?

Is there an effect of alcohol on the incidence of rejection? Is there a "safe limit" of ethanol that can be consumed? What about those judged to be poor psychiatric candidates? What contributes to their high mortality? Were there also patients "too ill" for transplantation in this group who contributed to the mortality rate? Could any of them become adequate candidates later?

And what about ethanol intake in a nonalcoholic liver transplant patient? The University of Michigan group has also compared the drinking habits of alcohol-dependent and non–alcohol-dependent patients with chronic liver disease who were undergoing liver transplantation.[54] Of alcohol-dependent patients, 14% had some posttransplant ethanol consumption and 9% had symptomatic consumption, whereas 46% of patients who received transplants for other liver diseases had some degree of ethanol consumption. There were no differences in subjective appraisals of physical and psychological health between the groups at follow-up. Importantly, overall the alcohol-dependent group continued to have high rates of favorable prognostic factors for continued abstinence.

SUMMARY

Alcoholic liver disease continues to be an important cause of liver disease in the United States. Markers of alcoholism and of the potential for progression to cirrhosis have not been identified. Thus we must continue to carefully assess each patient we see for signs of alcoholism so that appropriate intervention can be undertaken. It may be that the quantity of ethanol required to result in liver cirrhosis (the equivalent of only 40+ g daily) is even lower than prior studies have indicated while causative mechanisms in alcoholic cirrhosis continue to elude investigators. Where HCV and immune mechanisms fit into pathogenesis will require continuing investigation. It does seem that we can put aside our worries about H_2 receptor antagonists and their effect on gastric ADH. In several recent studies they had no significant effect on blood alcohol levels. Last, the importance of supplemental nutrition and of short-term corticosteroids in treating patients with alcoholic hepatitis has again been emphasized.

REFERENCES

1. National Institute on Drug Abuse: *National Household Survey on Drug Abuse, Population Estimates, 1988.* Rockville, Md, US Department of Health and Human Services, 1989, DHHS Publication No. ADM 89–1636.

2. Aach RD, et al: Alcohol and other substance abuse and impairment among physicians in residency training. *Ann Intern Med* 1992; 116:245–254.

3. Lareu MV, et al: Genetic markers in alcoholic liver cirrhosis. *Hum Hered* 1992; 42:235–241.

4. Poupon RE, et al: HLA GM systems and susceptibility to alcoholic cirrhosis: A study of mixed-race subjects. *Alcohol Alcohol* 1991; 26:417–424.

5. Batey RG, et al: Alcohol consumption and the risk of cirrhosis. *Med J Aust* 1992; 156:413–416.

6. Adami H-O, et al: Alcoholism and liver cirrhosis in the etiology of primary liver cancer. *Int J Cancer* 1992; 51:898–902.

7. Laskus T, et al: Course and outcome of acute type b hepatitis in heavy alcohol abusers. *Digestion* 1991; 49:231–234.

8. Booth BM, et al: Age and ethnicity among hospitalized alcoholics: A nationwide study. *Alcohol Clin Exp Res* 1992; 6:1029–1034.

9. Klatsky AL, et al: Alcohol and mortality. *Ann Intern Med* 1992; 117:646–654.

10. Tonnesen H, et al: Postoperative morbidity among symptom-free alcohol misusers. *Lancet* 1992; 340:334–337.

11. Bourliere M, et al: Is tobacco a risk factor for chronic pancreatitis and alcoholic cirrhosis? *Gut* 1991; 32:1392–1395.

12. Pietri H, et al: Liver cirrhosis and chronic calcifying pancreatitis are associated with different morphotypes. *Digestion* 1991; 48:173–178.

13. Suter PM, et al: The effect of ethanol on fat storage in healthy subjects. *N Engl J Med* 1992; 15:983–987.

14. Baraona E, et al: Lack of alcohol dehydrogenase isoenzyme activities in the stomach of Japanese subjects. *Life Sci* 1991; 49:1929–1934.

15. Caballería J, et al: Effect of H_2-receptor antagonists on gastric alcohol dehydrogenase activity. *Dig Dis Sci* 1991; 36:1673–1679.

16. Roine R, et al: Effect of omeprazole on gastric first-pass metabolism of ethanol. *Dig Dis Sci* 1992; 37:891–896.

17. Palmer RH, et al: Effect of various concomitant medications on gastric alcohol dehydrogenase and the first-pass metabolism of ethanol. *Am J Gastroenterol* 1991; 86:1749–1755.

18. Fraser AG, et al: Ranitidine has no effect on postbreakfast ethanol absorption. *Am J Gastroenterol* 1993; 88:217–221.

19. Raufman J-P, et al: Histamine-2 receptor antagonists do not alter serum ethanol levels in fed, non-alcoholic men. *Ann Intern Med* 1993; 118:488–494.

20. Levitt MD: Do histamine-2 receptor antagonists influence the metabolism of ethanol? *Ann Intern Med* 1993; 118:564–565.

21. Poupon RE, et al: Polymorphism of alcohol dehydrogenase, alcohol and aldehyde dehydrogenase activities: Implication in alcoholic cirrhosis in white patients. *Hepatology* 1992; 15:1017–1022.

22. Maly IP, et al: Intraacinar profile of alcohol dehydrogenase and aldehyde dehydrogenase activities in human liver. *Gastroenterology* 1991; 101:1716–1723.

23. Freni MA, et al: HCV infection, hepatic HLA display and composition of the mononuclear cell inflammatory infiltrate in chronic alcoholic liver disease. *Eur J Clin Invest* 1991; 21:586–591.

24. Halimi C, et al: Pathogenesis of liver cirrhosis in alcoholic patients: Histological evidence for hepatitis C virus responsibility. *Liver* 1991; 11:329–333.

25. Nalpas B, et al: Hepatitis C viremia and anti-HCV antibodies in alcoholics. *J Hepatol* 1992; 14:381–384.

26. Hill DB, et al: Increased plasma interleukin-6 concentrations in alcoholic hepatitis. *J Lab Clin Med* 1992; 119:547–552.

27. Kakumu S, et al: Localisation of intrahepatic interleukin 6 in patients with acute and chronic liver disease. *J Clin Pathol* 1992; 45:408–411.

28. Deviere J, et al: Immunoglobulin A and interleukin 6 form a positive secretory feedback loop: A study of normal subjects and alcoholic cirrhotics. *Gastroenterology* 1992; 103:1296–1301.

29. Shiratori Y, et al: Generation of chemotactic factor by hepatocytes isolated from chronically ethanol-fed rats. *Dig Dis Sci* 1992; 37:650–658.

30. Shirley MA, et al: Chemotactic LTB_4 metabolites produced by hepatocytes in the presence of ethanol. *Biochem Biophys Res Commun* 1992; 185:604–610.

31. Gross MD, et al: The identification and partial characterization of acetaldehyde adducts of hemoglobin occurring in vivo: A possible marker of alcohol consumption. *Alcohol Clin Exp Res* 1992; 16:1093–1103.

32. Koskinas J, et al: Immunoglobulin A antibody to a 200-kilodalton cytosolic acetaldehyde adduct in alcoholic hepatitis. *Gastroenterology* 1992; 103:1860–1867.

33. Bolondi L, et al: Caliber of splenic and hepatic arteries and spleen size in cirrhosis of different etiology. *Liver* 1991; 11:198–205.

34. Sugano S, et al: Evaluation of hepatic density change by dynamic CT in healthy humans and in patients with chronic liver diseases. *Dig Dis Sci* 1992; 37:220–224.

35. Delcourt E, et al: Emission tomography for assessment of diffuse alcoholic liver disease. *J Nucl Med* 1992; 33:1337–1345.

36. Robertson NJ, et al: Liver giant mitochondria revisited. *J Clin Pathol* 1992; 45:412–415.

37. Inagaki T, et al: Ultrastructural identification of light microscopic giant mitochondria in alcoholic liver disease. *Hepatology* 1992; 15:46–53.

38. McCormick PA, et al: The effects of alcohol use on rebleeding and mortality in patients with alcoholic cirrhosis following variceal hemorrhage. *J Hepatol* 1992; 14:99–103.

39. Merkel C, et al: Prognostic usefulness of hepatic vein catheterization in patients with cirrhosis and esophageal varices. *Gastroenterology* 1992; 102:973–979.

40. Iwao T, et al: Portal hypertensive gastropathy in patients with cirrhosis. *Gastroenterology* 1992; 102:2060–2065.

41. Sarin SK, et al: Factors influencing development of portal hypertensive gastropathy in patients with portal hypertension. *Gastroenterology* 1992; 102:994–999.

42. Albillos A, et al: Oral administration of clonidine in patients with alcoholic cirrhosis. *Gastroenterology* 1992; 102:248–254.

43. Esler M, et al: Increased sympathetic nervous activity and the effects of its inhibition with clonidine in alcoholic cirrhosis. *Ann Intern Med* 1992; 116:446–455.

44. Fassio E, et al: Paracentesis with dextran 70 vs paracentesis with albumin in cirrhosis with tense ascites. *J Hepatol* 1992; 14:310–316.

45. Storgaard JS, et al: Incidence of spontaneous bacterial peritonitis in patients with ascites. Diagnostic value of white blood cell count and pH measurement in ascitic fluid. *Liver* 1991; 11:248–252.

46. Soriano G, et al: Norfloxacin prevents bacterial infection in cirrhotics with gastrointestinal hemorrhage. *Gastroenterology* 1992; 103:1267–1272.

47. Trinchet J-C, et al: Treatment of severe alcoholic hepatitis by infusion of insulin and glucagon: A multicenter sequential trial. *Hepatology* 1992; 15:76–81.

48. Kearns PJ, et al: Accelerated improvement of alcoholic liver disease with enteral nutrition. *Gastroenterology* 1992; 102:200–205.

49. Treatment of patients with alcoholic liver disease with casein-based enteral nutrition. *Nutr Rev* 1992; 50:204–206.

50. Ramond M-J, et al: A randomized trial of prednisolone in patients with severe alcoholic hepatitis. *N Engl J Med* 1992; 326:507–512.

51. Carithers RL, et al: Methylprednisolone therapy in patients with severe alcoholic hepatitis: A randomized multicenter trial. *Ann Intern Med* 1989; 110:685–690.

52. Lucey MR, et al: Selection for and outcome of liver transplantation in alcoholic liver disease. *Gastroenterology* 1992; 102:1736–1741.

53. Lucey MR, et al: Alcoholic liver disease: To transplant or not to transplant. *Alcohol Alcohol* 1992; 27:103–108.

54. Beresford TP, et al: The short-term psychological health of alcoholic and non-alcoholic liver transplant recipients. *Alcohol Clin Exp Res* 1992; 16:996–1000.

CHAPTER 6

Cirrhosis

Rudolf Preisig, M.D.

Professor of Medicine and Clinical Pharmacology, Department of Clinical Pharmacology, University of Berne, Inselspital, Berne, Switzerland

EXPERIMENTAL CIRRHOSIS

In recent years, much work has been devoted to elucidating the pathophysiology of chronic liver disease using experimentally induced cirrhosis in animals. For this purpose, two models in the rat now are well established, namely, chemically induced cirrhosis produced by a combination of phenobarbital and carbon tetrachloride (CCl_4-cirrhosis) and secondary biliary cirrhosis after bile duct ligation (BDL-cirrhosis) and excision.

When interpreting the results of such studies, it must be remembered that the two models of cirrhosis differ in important aspects of their structural distortion. Table 1 depicts two sets of morphometric analyses obtained in two different studies with CCl_4-cirrhosis and BDL-cirrhosis from the same laboratory[1, 2] BDL-cirrhosis is characterized by increased liver weight, and hepatocytes are replaced in part by bile ductular and connective tissue. In CCl_4-cirrhosis, the liver tends to be smaller, with connective tissue partially replacing hepatocytes. Results of biochemical liver tests also differ between the two models, with cholemia being the outstanding feature of BDL-cirrhosis.

TABLE 1.

Morphometric Analysis of Rat Liver Composition (Mean Values)*

Research Subjects	Liver Mass (g)	Hepatocyte Volume (%)	Connective Tissue Volume (%)	Bile Duct Volume (%)	Nonhepatic Parenchyma Volume (%)
Reference 1					
Controls (n = 5)	20.6	91.0	0.55	0.19	8.2
CCL$_4$-cirrhosis (n = 11)	17.4	73.9†	17.5†	2.92†	6.1†
Reference 2					
Controls (n = 5)	16.3	85.1	1.4	0.20	10.2
BDL-cirrhosis (n = 5)	32.5†	51.5†	15.2†	21.4†	7.8†

*Data from Gross JB, Reichen J, et al: *Hepatology* 1987; 7:457–463. Used by permission.
†P at least <.01.

Secondary Biliary Cirrhosis (Bile Duct Ligation–Cirrhosis)

BDL-induced secondary biliary cirrhosis in the rat is a progressive disease, exhibiting continuous deterioration of liver function despite relative maintenance of hepatocyte mass.[3] In one study, by 8 weeks after BDL, 8 of 14 animals had died with cirrhosis. Serial measurements of quantitative liver function (galactose, aminopyrine) predicted death with high accuracy. Thus, timing is a critical issue in studies using this model. Recent investigations have demonstrated that structural and functional changes induced by BDL are largely reversible after the establishment of a biliodigestive anastomosis.[4] Because it has been shown previously that secondary biliary cirrhosis has become established by 3 to 4 weeks after BDL,[5] this was the time chosen for the construction of a Roux-en-Y (RY) choledochojejunostomy in one group of animals. Recovery from BDL-cirrhosis after another 4 weeks then was compared with that of a group of rats undergoing BDL, in whom obstruction was maintained for 8 weeks, and also with appropriate, sham-operated controls. The essential findings were as follows: whereas biochemical parameters (serum bilirubin and liver enzyme levels) returned to normal within days after RY choledochojejunostomy, functional recovery (as assessed by the aminopyrine breath test) and reversal of portal hypertension occurred after 2 and 4 weeks, respectively. Stereologic analysis of the liver in the different treatment groups is provided in Table 2. Structural changes in the animals with RY anastomoses resolved almost completely, with the exception of some residual bile duct proliferation and fibrosis. This carefully evaluated model undoubtedly will serve as a useful basis for further studies of the pathophysiology of biliary obstruction and the effects of decompression.

The BDL-cirrhosis model appears attractive also for the investigation of circu-

TABLE 2.

Liver Weight and Stereologic Analysis of the Liver in the Different Treatment Groups*†

	BDL8	BDL4	RY4	SHAM
Liver weight (g/kg)	67.2 ± 17.2	61.0 ± 10.0	46.6 ± 2.1	37.5 ± 3.6
Parenchyma (g/kg)	30.8 ± 11.0	37.4 ± 10.0	39.3 ± 4.4	36.3 ± 3.4
Bile ducts (g/kg)	17.0 ± 5.7	16.0 ± 7.2	2.2 ± 0.9	0.1 ± 0.1
Vessels (g/kg)	1.2 ± 0.6	0.7 ± 0.2	0.8 ± 0.3	0.7 ± 0.2
Other structures	18.2 ± 9.1	6.8 ± 1.7	4.3 ± 1.5	0.3 ± 0.1

*From Zimmermann H, Reichen J, et al: *Gastroenterology* 1992; 103:579–589. Used by permission.

†Liver weight and stereologic analysis of the liver in rats with 8 and 4 weeks of obstruction (BDL), animals with 4 weeks of biliary drainage by a biliodigestive anastomosis (RY4), and sham-operated controls (SHAM). Mean ± 1SD are given. Differences were tested for statistical significance by the Kruskal-Wallis test; if this analysis of variance indicated a significant difference, the groups of interest were compared with the Mann-Whitney U test. Liver weight was increased significantly in both obstructed groups compared to RY4 (P <.02) and SHAM (P <.005). In contrast, the absolute volume of parenchyma did not differ statistically between the four groups; the same held true for vessels. Bile ducts did not differ between the two obstructed groups, but were significantly lower in RY4 (P <.005) and SHAM (P <.001); RY still had significantly more ductular structures than did SHAM (P <.005). A similar pattern was observed for other structures (mainly connective tissue), with the exceeption that this was increased significantly in BDL8 compared to BDL4 (P <.002).

latory derangements. On the basis of previous studies[6, 7] that demonstrated the existence of a hyperdynamic circulation, three recent investigations have taken advantage of this model. A French group examined systemic and splanchnic hemodynamics in BDL-cirrhotic rats (4 weeks postoperatively) after endotoxin infusion, platelet-activating factor (PAF) infusion, and the administration of PAF antagonists.[8] Endotoxin produced no significant hemodynamic effects (with the exception of an increased heart rate) in controls, but cirrhotic rats responded with a marked (P < .01) increase in peripheral resistance, a decrease in cardiac output, and a reduction in regional perfusion rates, particularly of the kidneys (by 50%). Similar effects on cardiac output and renal blood flow were observed after PAF administration, suggesting that PAF, which is released by endotoxin, may be an important mediator of the endotoxin effect. Because PAF antagonists partly prevented endotoxin-induced renal hypoperfusion, the authors suggest that this may represent a promising approach to the treatment of renal failure associated with infection in cirrhotic patients. The same authors also studied the effect of removing the sympathetic nervous system by pithing on the hyperdynamic circulation in rats undergoing BDL and, for comparison, in animals with portal vein stenosis.[9] Although pithing reduced portal pressure in both models, cardiac output and portal flow remained increased in the cirrhotic rats, suggesting that humoral factors may be involved. Such a factor may be adenosine, an ubiquitous vasodilator, as pointed out by a Canadian study.[10] Using a selective adenosine antagonist (8-phenyltheophylline [8-PT]), cirrhotic rats responded with a greater than 40% reduction in intestinal blood flow; cardiac output, arterial pressure, and other regional blood flows were not affected. Unfortunately, these results are at variance with those of a previous study, in which no significant effects of 8-PT were observed.[11] Further investigations will be necessary before adenosine is accepted as a humoral factor involved in the circulatory changes of cirrhosis. Similarly, the speculation that increased synthesis and release of nitric oxide may play a role[12] has not been substantiated in the BDL model[13]; nevertheless, it has found some support in rats with portal hypertension resulting from partial portal vein ligation.[14]

Experimental cirrhosis is a "sine qua non" for gaining insight into adaptive responses of subcellular structures. Although information is available on structural changes after BDL,[15–17] the functional consequences are ill-defined. In experiments carried out in the perfused cirrhotic liver and in homogenates from these livers, mitochondrial function was measured and related to stereologically assessed structures.[18] The following picture emerged.

Whereas mitochondrial volume fraction increased per hepatocyte (by 28%), activities of most enzymes were unchanged. Conversely, oxygen consumption and glucose production were decreased (by 49% and 90%, respectively). Despite the "adaptive strategy" of increasing mitochondrial volume fraction, presumably for the maintenance of hepatic energy metabolism, BDL-cirrhosis clearly resulted in the impairment of mitochondrial metabolic function.

Chemically Induced Cirrhosis (CCl₄-Cirrhosis)

CCl_4-cirrhosis in rats, which is thought to mimic more closely the alcoholic or posthepatitic type of cirrhosis in man, usually is produced using a technique designed by McLean and coworkers.[19] Chronic exposure to phenobarbital (in the drinking water) and CCl_4 vapors results within 10 to 12 weeks in a type of cirrhosis that has been well characterized by both conventional histology and morphometric methods[1, 20] (see Table 1).

Similar to BDL-cirrhosis, CCl_4-cirrhosis has been used extensively for hemodynamic studies. Using sophisticated methodology that had been well established in previous studies,[21–23] Swedish investigators confirmed the hyperdynamic circulation in nonanesthetized rats with CCl_4-cirrhosis, as demonstrated by higher cardiac output and expanded blood volume in the face of normal mean arterial pressures.[24] With a balloon-equipped catheter placed in the right atrium, it was possible to block venous return and produce a brief circulatory arrest, allowing researchers to measure mean circulatory filling pressure (an index of total blood volume and vascular compliance). Because vascular compliance in cirrhotic rats was comparable to that of controls, the authors argue that venodilatation with augmented venous capacity could be the essential change leading to a hyperdynamic circulation.

Pharmacologic manipulation also has been used to gain insight into the basic mechanisms of hemodynamic derangement. In one study,[25] a competitive inhibitor of nitric oxide (NO) biosynthesis (Nw-nitro-L-arginine [NNA]) was used because it had been established previously that NO release accounts for (or may be identical with) the potent vasodilating effect of endothelium-derived relaxing factor.[26–28]

In conscious, cirrhotic rats with ascites, NNA administration caused a dose-dependent increase in the mean arterial pressure that was significantly greater than that in control animals (Fig 1). Using a dose range of NNA between 25 and 250 µg/kg/min, the glomerular filtration rate and urinary sodium excretion were enhanced without any change in renal plasma flow in cirrhotic animals, renal vasoconstriction was observed in controls. These results were interpreted to argue in favor of a role for NO, at least in the arterial segment of the circulation, in influencing the hyperdynamic state. Another study by the same investigators defined the effects of endothelin administration.[29] Endothelin represents a family of peptides with powerful vasoconstrictive action[30–32]; it also is involved in the synthesis and release of endogenous vasoactive substances, such as atrial natriuretic factor, renin, aldosterone, and vasopressin.[31] Unexpectedly, bolus injection of synthetic porcine endothelin produced markedly increased urinary sodium excretion in cirrhotic rats with ascites, presumably as a result of the inhibition of tubular sodium reabsorption. Because this natriuretic effect was demonstrable despite diminished renal plasma flow and glomerular filtration rate, and because it was associated with an increase in endogenous atrial natriuretic factor, the authors speculate that endothelin somehow may have increased renal sensitivity to atrial natriuretic factor.

The CCl$_4$-cirrhosis model clearly has a place in the search for compounds with a potentially favorable effect in preventing or ameliorating cirrhosis. For this pur-

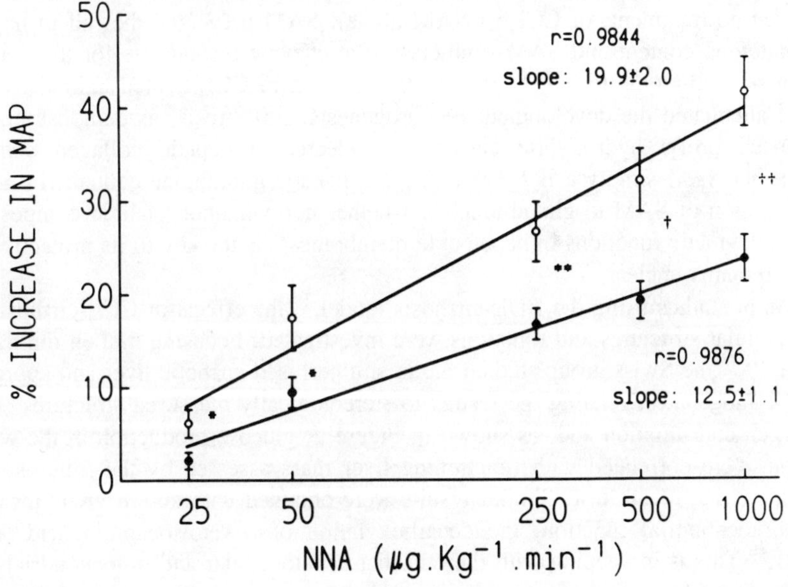

FIG 1.
Percentage increase in mean arterial pressure *(MAP)* induced by Nw-nitro-L-arginine *(NNA)* with respect to baseline values in cirrhotic *(open circles)* and control *(closed circles)* rats. *P <.05, **P <.01, †P <.005, ‡P <.001 between cirrhotic and control rats. (From Clària J, Jiménez W, Ros J, et al: *Hepatology* 1992; 15:343–349. Used by permission.)

pose, an antioxidant, such as vitamin E, is a logical choice, because the toxic effect of CCl_4 results from the formation of a trichloromethylperoxy radical, which initiates cell damage by covalent binding and lipid peroxidation.[33, 34]

An Italian group with extensive experience in this field[35–37] has presented a detailed study of the effects of dietary vitamin E supplementation on the development of CCl_4-cirrhosis.[38] Comparing rats pretreated over a period of 3 weeks with a vitamin E–supplemented diet (250 mg/kg) with animals receiving a normal diet (vitamin E content: 50 mg/kg) in whom CCl_4-cirrhosis subsequently was induced (intraperitoneal injection of CCl_4 over 5 weeks), the following was shown: (1) Vitamin E stores in the livers of control and cirrhotic animals were increased threefold by dietary supplementation. (2) Although vitamin E did not interfere with radical formation from CCl_4, it provided significant (but incomplete) protection against the development of cirrhosis. (3) Vitamin E was ineffective in preventing fatty liver. The authors assume, therefore, that vitamin E interferes with as yet ill-defined processes that lead to cell necrosis and fibrosis.

Another promising agent, S-adenosylmethionine (SAM), which reached the stage of clinical investigation, albeit with controversial results,[39, 40] was investigated in the CCl_4-cirrhosis model.[41] Protective effects of SAM previously had been shown in acute acetaminophen-induced liver injury.[42] In the present study, animals simultaneously receiving CCl_4 (intraperitoneally) and SAM (intramuscularly, 3 mg/kg/day) over 9 weeks were compared with appropriate control animals (which received no treatment, or CCl_4 or SAM alone). SAM prevented the fall in hepatic glutathione content and SAM-synthetase (the enzyme responsible for the conversion of methionine to SAM) activity that is seen in CCl_4-treated animals. SAM also attenuated the development of fibrogenesis and fibrosis, as demonstrated by reduced prolyl hydroxylase activity and decreased hepatic collagen content. Whether SAM simply acts by restoring the hepatic glutathione content (by transsulfuration of SAM to glutathione) or whether normalization of lipid composition and enzymatic functions in hepatocyte membranes[43] is the key to its protective effect remains unclear.

As in studies using the BDL-cirrhosis model,[18] the effects of CCl_4-cirrhosis on subcellular structures and functions were investigated. Focusing first on mitochondria,[44, 45] the Swiss group studied the in situ perfused cirrhotic liver and appropriate homogenates, relating the results to stereologically measured structures. Both oxygen consumption and, as shown in Figure 2, glucose production in the whole organ were correlated with functioning liver mass assessed by the (microsomal) aminopyrine breath test. Similar results were obtained with an "in vivo" measure of mitochondrial function, the decarboxylation of α-ketoisocaproic acid (Kica test).[46] This is in keeping with the fact that hepatocellular and mitochondrial volumes in cirrhotic livers were reduced to the same extent (by 39% and 40%, respectively). Both inner and outer mitochondrial membranes also were diminished, but key enzyme activities (adenosine triphosphatase, cytochrome oxidase) were increased in the inner membrane, suggesting a compensatory mechanism for the relative maintenance of mitochondrial function in cirrhosis. Another paper by the same

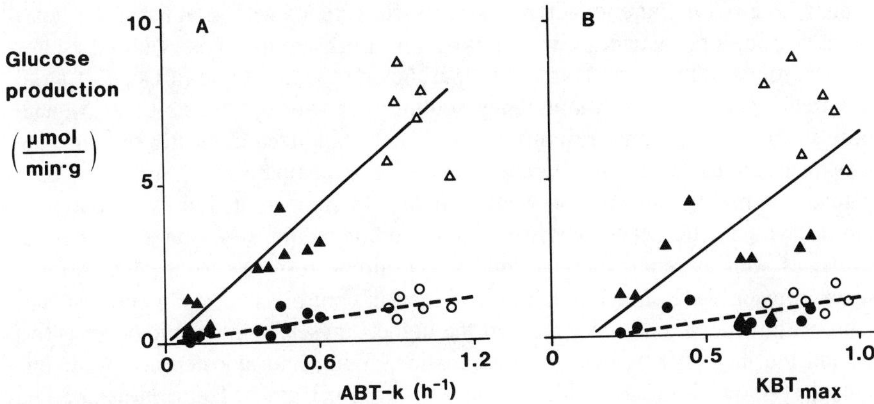

FIG 2.
Relationship between liver function test results in vivo and glucose production by the perfused liver. Liver function was measured with the microsomal aminopyrine breath test *(ABT-k)* and the mitochondrial KICA breath test *(KBT$_{max}$)*. Basal glucose production is indicated by *circles* and L-alanine/glucagon–stimulated glucose production by *triangles;* cirrhotic and control animals are represented by *closed* and *open* symbols, respectively. (From Krähenbühl S, Reichen J, Zimmermann A, et al: *Hepatology* 1990; 12:526–532. Used by permission.)

group was devoted to lysosomal function and transcellular vesicular transport,[47] again in search of structural-functional relationships. Lysosomal enzyme activity (such as that of β-hexosaminidase) was found to be increased in relation to the severity of cirrhosis, as assessed by the aminopyrine breath test. Stereologic analysis revealed an increase in pericanalicular lysosomes. From studies in the perfused cirrhotic liver, it became apparent that, despite maintenance of bile flow, biliary elimination by transcytotic vesicular transport (measured with markers such as horseradish peroxidase and epidermal growth factor) was reduced markedly. Thus, the increased number of lysosomes in cirrhosis may be interpreted as a consequence of accumulation rather than as an adaptive response.

CIRRHOSIS AND THE SYMPATHETIC NERVOUS SYSTEM

As pointed out in an excellent review by Henriksen and colleagues,[48] since 1981, an average of more than 10 papers per year have been devoted to elucidating the role of catecholamines and sympathetic nervous system activity in the circulatory derangement of cirrhosis. Consequently, we presented some of the key papers in last year's volume of *Current Hepatology*. Meanwhile, interest in this topic continues. As a follow-up to their landmark paper using microneurographic recordings of muscle sympathetic nerve activity,[49] the Toronto group has expanded their studies in search of a relationship of sympathetic nerve activity with renal responsiveness to atrial natriuretic factor.[50] Twenty-six patients with established cirrhosis (19 alcoholic, 7 postnecrotic) were divided into three groups: those without ascites (by ultrasonography; n = 9), those with ascites responding to an infusion of atrial natriuretic factor after a 20-mmol/day sodium diet with natriuresis (n = 5), and those without a natriuretic response (n = 12) characterized clinically by tense ascites resistant to high-dose diuretic therapy. For comparison, 7 age- and sex-matched normal volunteers also were included. In compensated cirrhotic patients, muscle sympathetic nerve activity, plasma noradrenaline, renin, and aldosterone levels, as well as renal function and the natriuretic response to atrial natriuretic factor infusion were comparable to those seen in control subjects. In contrast, patients with refractory ascites exhibited the highest muscle sympathetic nerve activity and the largest increases in noradrenaline, renin, and aldosterone; by definition, they showed no natriuretic response to atrial natriuretic factor infusion. The group with "early ascites" had only moderately increased sympathetic nerve activity associated with normal noradrenaline, renin, and aldosterone levels. Renal clearance of lithium, which was reduced significantly in all patients with cirrhosis and ascites, remained unchanged after the infusion of atrial natriuretic factor. Based on these results, the authors suggest that, in patients with cirrhosis, the early phase of sodium retention is associated with increased sympathetic nerve activity, thus contributing to ascites formation; they speculate that the effects of highly activated sympathetic nerve activity on renal function (in particular, the lack of effect of atrial natriuretic factor) may explain the development of refractory ascites.

Previous studies already have suggested that blocking the increased sympathetic nerve activity may be beneficial in the hyperdynamic circulation that is associated with portal hypertension.[51, 52] An extension of those reports is the subject of two recent papers[53, 54] in which the effects of clonidine, a centrally acting α_2-agonist, were examined. The Australian group[53] studied the acute (intravenous clonidine) inhibitory effects of the drug on increased noradrenaline release into the circulation and the subsequent hemodynamic changes in patients with stable alcoholic cirrhosis (Child-Pugh score: 9A, 21B, 14C). As a first and important result, the authors demonstrated that noradrenaline spillover, which was highest in patients in class C, was blocked effectively by clonidine from the body as a whole, as well as from the kidneys and the splanchnic circulation (Fig 3). This effect was dose-dependent, and was particularly pronounced in the splanchnic circulation; it was associated with significant reductions in portal pressure (median, 25%), whereas hepatic blood flow remained unchanged. A complementary study by Spanish investigators[54] demonstrated that these potentially beneficial effects are maintained after long-term (2 months) oral administration of clonidine. In addition to the decrease in the hepatic venous pressure gradient (Fig 4), these authors also showed that, in the 15 cirrhotic patients studied, hepatic blood flow and hepatic function (measured with galactose and indocyanine green) remained unaltered. The major side effect encountered was dry mouth.

Is clonidine a new alternative to β-blockers in the pharmacotherapy of portal hypertension? I have considerable doubts, for the following reasons:

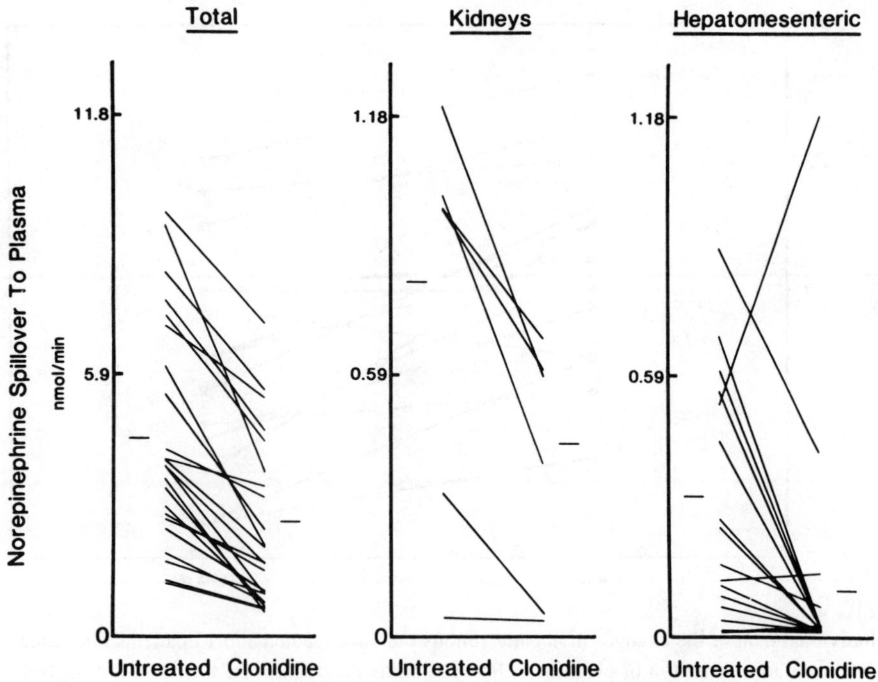

FIG 3.

Effect of clonidine, 2.5 μg/kg of body weight intravenously, on norepinephrine spillover to plasma from the body as a whole (total; $P <.001$), from the kidneys ($P <.018$), and from the hepatomesenteric area ($P <.009$). Mean values are indicated by the *horizontal lines*. (From Esler M, Dudley F, Jennings G, et al: *Ann Intern Med* 1992; 116:446–455. Used by permission.)

1. The number of patients studied, duration of treatment, and drug effects achieved are as yet insufficient to warrant conclusions applicable to clinical practice.
2. So far, it has not been shown that the aim of this therapy, namely, the prevention of variceal bleeding, can be achieved.
3. The arterial hypotensive (and possibly the sedative) actions of clonidine may place serious constraints on effective dosing of the drug for the reduction of portal pressure.

METABOLIC ABNORMALITIES IN CIRRHOSIS

Increased blood levels of methionine are a well-established phenomenon in cirrhosis.[55, 56] This is thought to be the result of blockage of the transsulfuration pathway (i.e., the conversion of methionine to cystine and taurine).[57] This concept has

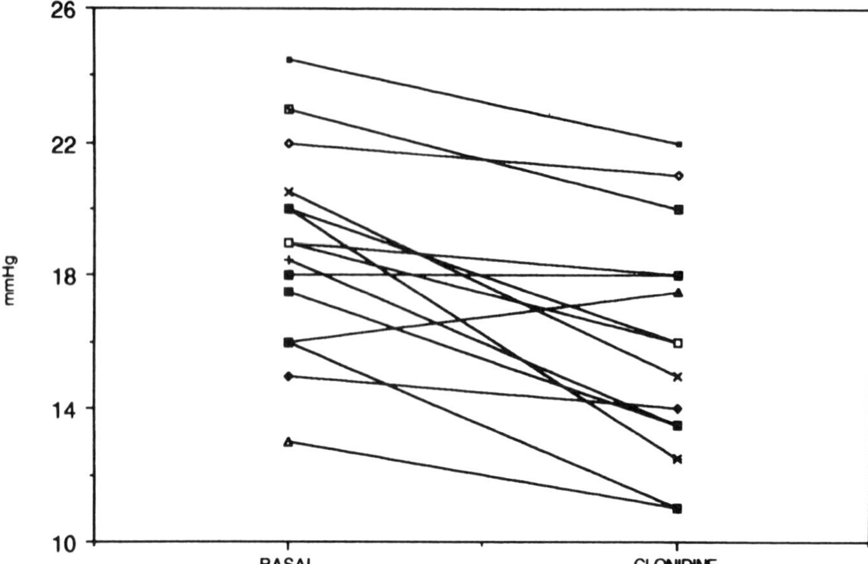

FIG 4.

Individual data of the changes in hepatic venous pressure gradients in 15 patients after long-term oral administration of clonidine. (From Albillos A, Banares R, Barrios C, et al: *Gastroenterology* 1992; 102:248–254. Used by permission.)

not been proven, however, and the relationship of impaired methionine metabolism to severity of liver disease is not known. Italian investigators presented the results of a study in which methionine plasma clearance was measured under steady-state conditions (intravenous infusion of methionine) in 12 patients with cirrhosis and 6 healthy research subjects.[58] They confirmed that fasting methionine plasma levels in cirrhotic patients on average were almost doubled compared to those of control subjects, and that they were correlated inversely ($r = -.84$) with methionine clearance. Methionine clearance was related to severity of functional impairment (galactose elimination capacity; Child-Pugh score; Fig 5). Degradation of methionine to urea was virtually absent in cirrhotic individuals and conversion to taurine was reduced markedly. Thus, increased methionine levels in chronic liver disease are caused by a metabolic defect in methionine disposition. Whether this defect is located in the transmethylation or transsulfuration pathway remains to be established.

Two studies have reexamined some aspects of carbohydrate metabolism in cirrhosis with the use of sophisticated techniques. The aim of the first investigation was to shed light on the hyperinsulinism and impaired glucose tolerance that are encountered frequently in patients with cirrhosis.[59] Twenty-six patients with cirrhosis of various causes (alcoholic, primary biliary cirrhosis [PBC], postnecrotic) and differing disease severity (Child-Pugh score: 12A, 14B) were subjected to glucose clamp protocols together with indirect calorimetry. Maximum cellular glucose disposal was reduced to 60% of the values obtained in a group of 10 control subjects. Insulin-induced increases in glucose oxidation and lipogenesis were un-

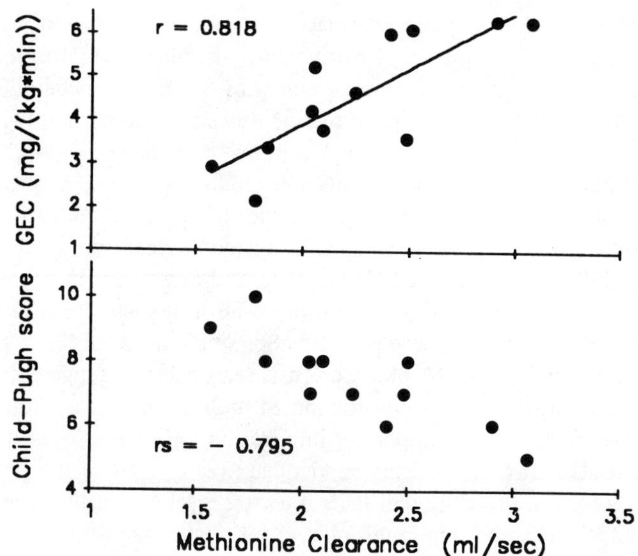

FIG 5.

Correlation between methionine clearance and galactose elimination capacity *(GEC; upper panel)* or Child-Pugh score *(lower panel)* in cirrhotic patients. *rs* = Spearman rank correlation. (From Marchesini G, Bugianesi E, Bianchi G, et al: *Hepatology* 1992; 16:149–155. Used by permission.)

changed, but the plasma lactate level—when matched for normal glucose disposal—was increased markedly. Thus, impairment of insulin-induced glucose metabolism and resistance to insulin is a feature of cirrhosis, independent of its etiology, because of reduced glucose storage. Extrahepatic mechanisms, such as defective muscle storage, are important contributing factors. The second investigation examined hepatic fructose metabolism assessed by dynamic [31]phosphorus magnetic resonance spectroscopy (^{31}P-MRS), a method that allows noninvasive measurement of intermediary metabolic steps (such as phosphorylation).[60] Comparing nine patients with nonalcoholic cirrhosis with six normal volunteers, metabolic abnormalities in cirrhotic patients after an intravenous fructose load (250 mg/kg) consisted of significantly decreased formation of monophosphate esters ($P < .01$) and diminished use of inorganic phosphate ($P < .005$). These changes were correlated with severity of functional impairment as measured by galactose elimination capacity. Although the number of clinical studies using dynamic ^{31}P-MRS still is limited, little doubt exists that this elegant approach is destined to provide new insights into metabolic events in health and disease.

DRUG DISPOSITION IN CIRRHOSIS

Despite the fact that spironolactone (SP) has been in use for more than 30 years, and despite extended experience with this drug in cirrhotic patients, little information is available concerning the pharmacokinetics and metabolism of SP in this population. Recently, however, sensitive and specific high-performance liquid chromatography methods for the measurement of SP and its metabolites were designed to fill the gap.[61] As a first surprise, it was shown in normal volunteers that 7α-thiomethylspironolactone (7-A) and not, as previously believed, canrenone (Can) is the major metabolite of SP; this was confirmed in a subsequent investigation.[3] A second surprise came with the results of a recent study, in which nine decompensated cirrhotic patients were investigated[62]; mean serum half-lives of SP (9 hours) and its two major metabolites (24 to 58 hours) were increased some sixfold to eightfold compared to those of normal control subjects. Because the changes in renal sodium clearance in these patients after single doses of SP were correlated best with the clearances of 7-A plus Can, it is reasonable to suggest that these two metabolites are largely responsible for the SP-induced diuresis. From a practical point of view, there are two important implications: (1) a single daily dose of SP in decompensated cirrhotic patients is adequate; (2) in view of the long half-lives of the metabolites, it probably will take at least 2 weeks to reach steady-state conditions. This, then, is the minimum interval for dosage adjustment.

Resistance to diuretic therapy in cirrhotic patients with ascites is explained in part by overactivation of the renin-angiotensin-aldosterone system.[63, 64] Consequently, the use of angiotensin converting enzyme (ACE) inhibitors appears to be a logical choice. A recent study from Holland[65] suggests that the addition of low-dose captopril may lead to a striking improvement in the diuretic efficacy of a combination of SP and furosemide in at least half of all patients with ascites and edema. In this and previous investigations,[66, 67] patient response to ACE inhibitors was quite variable and the dosage used appeared to be critical to maintaining good kidney function. Thus, the question arose again whether changes in pharmacokinetics may be responsible for this heterogeneity of effect, because ACE inhibitors are prodrugs that require deesterification by hepatic microsomal esterases to become active metabolites. Using perindopril, a nonsulfhydryl ACE inhibitor, as a model compound, French investigators studied its disposition in 10 alcoholic patients with cirrhosis of different severity (Child-Pugh score 5 to 11) after a single oral dose.[68] The results were similar to those of a previous study using enalapril[69]: although partial metabolic clearance of the parent drug to its active metabolites was reduced to about half (consistent with impaired hepatic deesterification), maximum inhibition of plasma ACE activity was comparable to that in control subjects. The authors conclude that dosage adjustment of perindopril in patients with cirrhosis is not required; nevertheless, the lack of differences in pharmacodynamic effects between patients with cirrhosis and control subjects remains unexplained. Thus, there is as yet no answer concerning the heterogeneous response of cirrhotic patients to ACE inhibitors during blunted diuresis.

It is becoming more and more evident that the presence of chronic liver disease may have quite different effects on the various pathways of hepatic drug metabolism. Until recently, it was thought that the glucuronidation of xenobiotics was well maintained in cirrhosis.[70] Since 1983, however, different groups have established clear-cut exceptions to this "rule." The elimination of compounds such as zomepirac,[71] naproxen,[72] and zidovudine,[73] all of which are glucuronidated extensively in normal man, was shown to be impaired significantly in cirrhotic patients. To this list now can be added diflunisal, a salicylic acid derivative.[74] Investigation of the hepatic handling of this compound was of particular interest because, in healthy volunteers, about half a given dose is recovered as acyl glucuronide, one third as phenolic glucuronide, and the rest as sulfate.[75] Comparing the results in five (presumably compensated) cirrhotic patients with those in five age- and sex-matched control subjects after a single oral dose of 250 mg of diflunisal, plasma clearance of total diflunisal was comparable in both groups, whereas that of unbound diflunisal was impaired significantly in patients with cirrhosis. The unbound partial clearances of both the phenolic and the acyl glucuronides were reduced in parallel; clearance of the sulfate conjugate, on the other hand, was maintained.

A timely and interesting study has been published concerning the disposition of dapsone in cirrhosis.[76] It is timely because this classic "orphan drug," used for many years in the treatment of leprosy, is of renewed interest in the treatment of complications associated with the acquired immunodeficiency syndrome.[77] It is interesting because dapsone is metabolized by two different pathways, acetylation and N-hydroxylation. The essential findings may be summarized as follows: in the 14 cirrhotic patients investigated (who were compared with 70 control subjects), the acetylation of dapsone was reduced significantly; however, this was not correlated with oral dapsone clearance. In contrast, despite considerable overlap in the urinary dapsone recovery ratio (which is calculated from the N-hydroxylamine metabolite divided by the sum of the metabolite and the parent compound; Fig 6), the reduction in oral clearance of dapsone in the cirrhotic subjects (by 22%) resulted almost exclusively from impairment of the hydroxylation pathway. The authors' general recommendation that "dosage modification is not required" in the presence of cirrhosis, unfortunately, is not supported by their results. Thus, only half their cirrhotic patients are characterized sufficiently to allow assessment of disease severity; these 7 patients had a Child-Pugh score of 5 to 7 (mild to moderate disease). In decompensated cirrhosis, further reduction in the oral clearance of dapsone could be anticipated. Patients with Child-Pugh stage C disease, therefore, may require dosage reduction.

PRIMARY BILIARY CIRRHOSIS AND PRIMARY SCLEROSING CHOLANGITIS

The interest of hepatologists seems to have shifted away somewhat from PBC and primary sclerosing cholangitis (PSC), because surprisingly few papers were published during this review period concerning these entities. Nevertheless, some important new findings are available. A combined effort between laboratories in the United States and Australia resulted in the synthesis of a recombinant protein

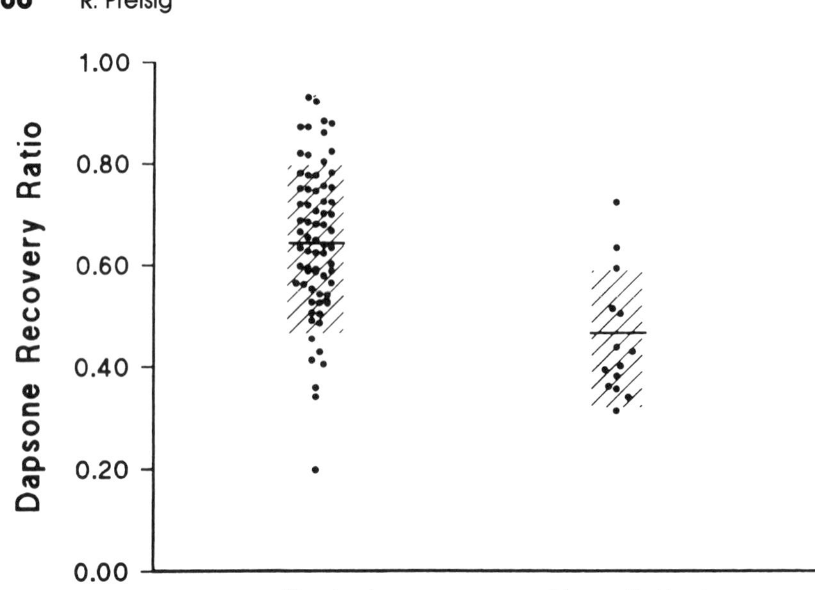

FIG 6.
Comparison of the 8-hour urinary dapsone recovery ratio in 70 normal research subjects and 14 patients with cirrhosis. The *cross-hatched area* is 1 S.D. around the mean; $P <$ .001. (From May DG, Arns PA, Richards WO, et al: *Clin Pharmacol Ther* 1992; 51:689–700. Used by permission.)

specially tailored to the immunodiagnosis of PBC.[78] After cloning of the E2 subunits of the pyruvate dehydrogenase and the branched chain 2-oxo-acid dehydrogenase complexes,[79–83] more than 90% of patients with PBC were demonstrated to react with one or both these enzymes. The remainder, however, recognize only E2 subunits of 2-oxo-acid dehydrogenase. To overcome this problem, these investigators used recombinant technology to design a molecule that expresses the dominant epitopes of both pyruvate dehydrogenase and 2-oxo-acid dehydrogenase. This hybrid molecule then was used in an enzyme-linked immunosorbent assay for the diagnosis of PBC. As expected, 78 of 84 sera from patients with PBC who reacted to both fragments also reacted to the hybrid molecule; in contrast, no immunoreaction was seen to sera from patients with chronic active hepatitis, those with PSC, or normal volunteers. This work undoubtedly will be the basis for the development of a relatively simple, standardized enzyme-linked immunosorbent assay for measuring antimitochondrial antibodies, which should be available soon for general use.

Over the years, there have been some indications that a "genetic disposition" may be involved in the pathogenesis of PBC. Thus, immunologic abnormalities were described in healthy relatives of patients with PBC,[84, 85] and "familial PBC" was reported in rare instances.[86–91] A Japanese group reported its findings in 18 healthy first-degree relatives from two families (7 from one family and 11 from the other). In both families, two members (cases A1, A2, B1, and B2) had established PBC.[92] As shown in Figure 7, in the two families, different antibodies were found in 5 relatives (mean age, 32 years), most frequently of the antithyroid type. Only 1 family member had low titers of antimitochondrial and antinuclear antibodies, but no evidence of disease. Concanavalin A–induced lymphocyte transformation was reduced significantly ($P < .001$) in 7 family members, who tended to be older (mean age, 42 years) compared to the other relatives (mean age, 32 years); this impairment was not associated with HLA haplotypes. Immunoglobulin levels, on the other hand, were normal in all family members. The authors propose that impairment of concanavalin A–inducible lymphocytes (which are mainly suppres-

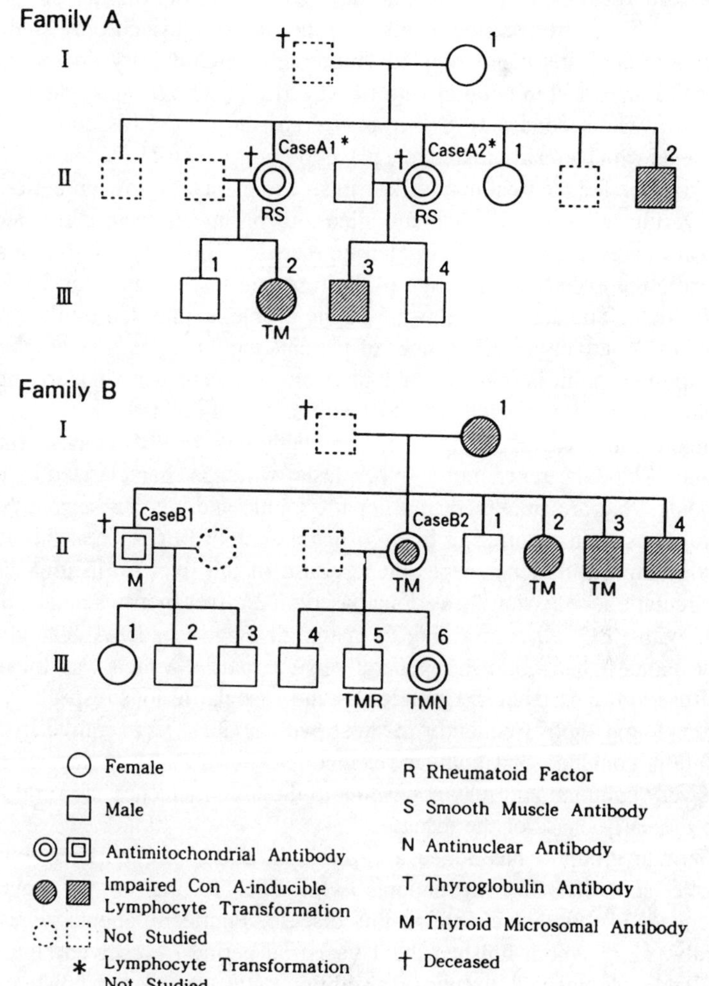

FIG 7.
Family trees of the two families studied. (From Tsuji H, Murai K, Akagi K, et al: *Dig Dis Sci* 1992; 37:353–360. Used by permission.)

sor T cells) may represent a (genetically determined?) contributing factor in the development of PBC.

The original description of PBC by Addison and Gull in 1851 was a disease characterized by jaundice, vitiligo, and planar as well as tuberous xanthomas.[93] It took a century to link the xanthomatosis with hyperlipidemia, as first was established by Ahrens.[94] Although it was shown that elevations in low-density and high-density lipoprotein levels progress in parallel with the severity of PBC,[95] little attention was paid to the potentially increased risk of arteriosclerosis in patients with PBC. A Mayo Clinic study now has focused on this problem.[96] An initial group of 50 consecutive patients with PBC had detailed serum lipid profiles performed. As shown in Table 3, triglyceride levels were normal or elevated only slightly, contrasting with cholesterol, low-density lipoprotein, high-density lipoprotein levels, which were increased in parallel with the severity of disease, reaching peak values in stage III. The second part of the study consisted of a retrospective analysis of 312 patients who had participated in a placebo-controlled trial. About half had taken cholestyramine for the treatment of pruritus. The median follow-up period was 7.4 years. During this time, 128 patients died. According to death certificate data, 7 deaths were attributable to arteriosclerotic disease. This was not significantly different from the expected death rate (4.2) from arteriosclerosis using United States mortality data. The authors are aware of the problems imposed by their study design and the relatively small number of patients included. As they emphasize, the most important point is that the pathophysiologic mechanisms underlying the hypercholesterolemia associated with PBC are as yet ill-defined.

An interesting contribution to the hepatic pathology of PBC comes from an Italian group.[97] Nodular regenerative hyperplasia, which is characterized by regenerative nodules that are smaller than a hepatic lobule and without surrounding fibrosis, rarely has been reported in livers of patients with PBC.[98–100] This lesion has been considered a rather nonspecific response of the liver to disturbances in the microcirculation.[101] A study was done based on 35 liver biopsies obtained from 30 patients with PBC, all conforming to histologic stage I or II. Amazingly, almost half the patients had nodular regenerative hyperplasia, which was focal in 80% and diffuse in the remainder. Granulomas and vascular lesions (especially of arteries) were found more frequently in those with nodular regenerative hyperplasia. The authors conclude that nodular regenerative hyperplasia in stages I and II of PBC is very common and may contribute to the high incidence of portal hypertension in the early phase of the disease.[102]

A German group[103] has added a 1-year, placebo-controlled trial with ursodeoxycholic acid (UDCA) in patients with PSC to the as yet very limited experience[104–106] with the drug in this disease. Fourteen patients were included originally, 12 of whom finished the 1-year trial period (5 received UDCA, 13 to 15 mg/kg/day; 7 received placebo). In addition to the usual serum biochemical tests (aspartate and alanine aminotransferase, bilirubin, and alkaline phosphatase levels, etc.), serum bile acids were measured and the aminopyrine breath test was performed. Liver biopsies were obtained before treatment began and after it ended.

TABLE 3.

Age, Stage, and Lipid Profile of 50 Patients With Primary Biliary Sclerosis*†

Stage	No. of Patients (%)	Age (mean ± S.D., yr)	Cholesterol (mg/dL)	Triglycerides (mg/dL)	HDL (mg/dL)	LDL (mg/dL)	A-I (mg/dL)
1	1 (2)	41	235 (188 ± 30.7)	126 (101 ± 63)	63 (56.2 ± 13.7)	152	168 (148.8 ± 20.7)
2	8 (16)	39.5 ± 6.8	256 ± 124.0 (178 ± 29.7)	98 ± 35.1 (104 ± 60)	81 ± 27.8 (50.4 ± 12.4)	159 ± 128.3	156 ± 36 (137.7 ± 16.9)
3	20 (40)	50.9 ± 9.1	300 ± 69.6 (210.7 ± 41.90)	159 ± 96.3 (144 ± 116)	80 ± 35.8 (50.5 ± 13.6)	195 ± 65.8	166 ± 26.8 (147.4 ± 21.9)
4	21 (42)	57.0 ± 9.2	291 ± 114.0 (210.7 ± 41.9)	128 ± 65.0 (144 ± 116)	66 ± 32.7 (50.5 ± 136.6)	203 ± 110.2	144 ± 32.7 (147.4 ± 21.9)

*From Crippin JS, Lindor KD, et al: *Hepatology* 1992; 15:858–862. Used by permission.
†Numbers in parentheses represent normal ranges for age. HDL = high-density lipoprotein; LDL = low-density lipoprotein; A-I = apoprotein A-I.

UDCA was tolerated well, but did not influence the clinical status; it had a favorable effect on serum enzyme levels, but not on serum bile acid levels or the aminopyrine breath test. Only 2 patients in the UDCA group had evidence of improvement in histologic score. Despite the careful execution of this study, it remains to be shown whether UDCA-induced changes in biochemical parameters are beneficial to the patient in influencing the natural history of PSC.

PALMAR ERYTHEMA

Local vascular changes seen through the skin (e.g., spider angiomas, palmar erythema) are considered hallmarks of liver disease. Some recent attempts have been made to understand the pathogenesis of spider angiomas[107] and their regional distribution[108]; however, strictly focal lesions, such as palmar erythema, have been "out of reach" of available techniques. New instruments, such as the laser-Doppler system,[109] now make it possible to overcome this difficulty. An exciting report by Italian investigators describes the use of this technique for the measurement of local cutaneous blood flow comparing the dorsum and palm of the hand in 34 cirrhotic patients (Child-Pugh score: 12A, 13B, 9C) and 24 healthy research subjects.[110]

In 11 cases of cirrhosis, palmar erythema was present. Measurements of cutaneous focal blood flow were obtained before and after venous occlusion (which was created with a blood pressure cuff inflated to 40 mm Hg) as a means of assessing the venoarterial vasoconstrictor reflex. The cutaneous vascular resistance index was calculated from the ratio of mean arterial pressure and focal blood flow. The findings in the group with cirrhosis on the palmar side of the hand are depicted in Figure 8. Evidently, focal blood flow in the resting state was higher and the vascular resistance index was lower in cirrhosis, a difference noted exclusively in patients with palmar erythema; these individuals also showed little adaptation to venous occlusion. On the dorsum of the hand, the only significant difference in patients with cirrhosis was a decrease in basal values of the vascular resistance index. All observed changes apparently were unrelated to the Child-Pugh score. Once again, these results attest to the well-known vasodilation in cirrhosis, which was evident on both the dorsum and the palm of the hand. Because the venoarterial reflex was depressed only in the palm of patients with cirrhosis, and because this defect also was evident in the absence of palmar erythema, the authors propose that impairment of autonomic nervous function may be responsible for malfunctioning of arteriovenous anastomoses, which normally are present in great numbers in the palm.

SUMMARY

Two models of experimental cirrhosis in rats are used widely: a type induced by BDL (BDL-cirrhosis) that leads to secondary biliary cirrhosis, and another type

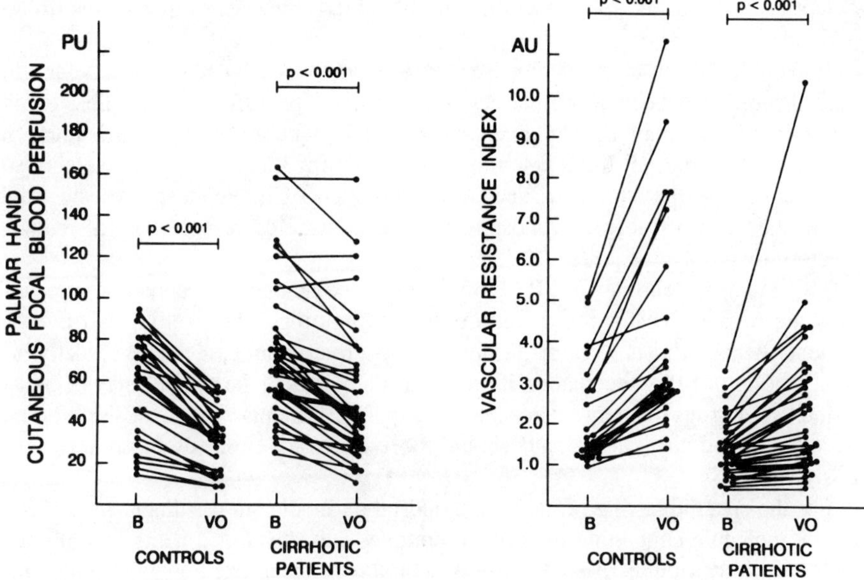

FIG 8.
Palmar side of the hand: behavior of the absolute values of focal blood perfusion *(left panel)* and of the vascular resistance index *(right panel)*. *B* = basic condition; *BD* = venous occlusion. (From Leonardo G, Arpaia MR, del Guercio R, et al: *Scand J Gastroenterol* 1992; 27:326–332. Used by permission.)

induced by carbon tetrachloride administration (CCI_4-cirrhosis). BDL-cirrhosis is largely reversible, provided biliary drainage is reestablished with a functioning RY choledochojejunostomy. On the other hand, dietary supplementation with vitamin E or parenteral injection of SAM attenuates the development of CCI_4-cirrhosis. Both models of cirrhosis exhibit a hyperkinetic circulatory state. Humoral factors potentially involved in its pathogenesis (such as PAF, adenosine, and NO) and blockage by selective antagonists have been studied extensively. The sequence of events may be viewed as follows: Increased resistance to portal inflow (e.g., resulting from cirrhosis) leads to portal hypertension. The development of collaterals may reduce portal pressure; however, this is counteracted by splanchnic vasodilatation, which is part of the hyperdynamic circulatory state. The factors responsible for this latter aspect remain unclear. Finally, structural-functional relationships of subcellular components (mitochondria, lysosomes) were investigated in the two models showing differing adaptive responses.

Much evidence points to a key role of the sympathetic nervous system in the pathogenesis of portal hypertension and ascites in cirrhotic patients. Possibly, sympathetic hyperactivity diminishes the action of atrial natriuretic factor on the kidney, resulting in the development of refractory ascites. The α_2-agonist clonidine blocks increased spillover of noradrenaline, especially in the splanchnic circulation, with a resultant decrease in the hepatic venous pressure gradient; its potential role in the pharmacotherapy of portal hypertension remains to be defined.

Impaired, insulin-induced glucose metabolism caused by reduced cellular glucose disposal has been confirmed again in cirrhosis of different etiologies. Resistance to insulin may be explained by reduced glucose storage, particularly in muscles. Dynamic ^{31}P-MRS is a noninvasive tool for studying hepatic metabolism in vivo. Using this approach, decreased formation of monophosphate esters and diminished use of inorganic phosphates were considered responsible for reduced fructose disposal.

Two major metabolites of SP (thiomethylspironolactone and canrenone) presumably are responsible for the diuretic effect of the drug. Their serum half-lives in patients with cirrhosis (24 and 58 hours, respectively) suggest that once-daily administration of SP is adequate. Diflunisal, a salicylic acid derivative, may be added to the list of drugs that require dosage adjustment in patients with cirrhosis. Whether decompensated cirrhotic patients should receive reduced doses of dapsone remains unsettled.

For the specific testing of antimitochondrial antibodies in the diagnosis of PBC, a new molecule containing the critical epitopes was developed using recombinant technology. It should permit the use of a simple, standardized enzyme-linked immunosorbent assay. Familial occurrence of PBC again has been described; impairment of lymphocyte transformation was found in 7 of 18 healthy first-degree relatives. Increases in cholesterol and low-density and high-density lipoprotein levels related to the severity of disease are the essential derangements of lipid metabolism in PBC. A retrospective study suggests that, despite these changes, the risk of arteriosclerotic disease is not increased.

The vascular defect leading to palmar erythema was investigated with a laser-Doppler technique. In cirrhosis, evidence of vasodilation was obtained on both the dorsum and the palm of the hand. The venoarterial reflex was depressed only in the palm, however, independent of the presence or absence of erythema. This defect may be attributable to deranged autonomic nervous function.

Acknowledgments

The author is extremely grateful for the careful preparation of the manuscript by Mrs. M. Sommer, and for the artwork by Mrs. M. Kappeler.

REFERENCES

1. Knuchel J, et al: Effect of secretin on bile formation in rats with cirrhosis in the liver: Structure-function relationship. *Gastroenterology* 1989; 97:950–957.

2. Gross JB, et al: The evolution of changes in quantitative liver function tests in a rat model of biliary cirrhosis: Correlation with morphometric measurement of hepatocyte mass. *Hepatology* 1987; 7:457–463.

3. Gardiner P, et al: Spironolactone metabolism: Steady-state serum levels of the sulfur-containing metabolites. *J Clin Pharmacol* 1989; 29:342–347.

4. Zimmermann H, et al: Reversibility of secondary biliary fibrosis by biliodigestive anastomosis in the rat. *Gastroenterology* 1992; 103:579–589.

5. Kontouras J, et al: Prolonged bile duct obstruction: A new experimental model for cirrhosis in the rat. *Br J Exp Pathol* 1984; 65:305–311.

6. Lee SS, et al: Hemodynamic characterization of chronic bile duct-ligated rats: Effect of pentobarbital sodium. *Am J Physiol* 1986; 251:G175–180.

7. Vorobioff J, et al: Hyperdynamic circulation in portal-hypertensive rat model: A primary factor for maintenance of chronic portal hypertension. *Am J Physiol* 1983; 244:G52–G57.

8. Kleber G, et al: Hemodynamic effects of endotoxin and platelet activating factor in cirrhotic rats. *Gastroenterology* 1992; 103:282–288.

9. Abergel A, et al: Persistence of a hyperdynamic circulation in cirrhotic rats following removal of the sympathetic nervous system. *Gastroenterology* 1992; 102:656–660.

10. Lee SS, et al: Adenosine receptor blockade reduces splanchnic hyperemia in cirrhotic rats. *Hepatology* 1992; 15:1107–1111.

11. Champigneulle B, et al: Adenosine and hemodynamic alterations in cirrhotic rats. *Am J Physiol* 1991; 260:G543–G547.

12. Vallance P, et al: Hyperdynamic circulation in cirrhosis: A role for nitric oxide? *Lancet* 1991; 237:776–778.

13. Sogni PH, et al: Evidence for normal nitric oxide-mediated vasodilator tone in conscious rats with cirrhosis. *Hepatology* 1992; 16:980–983.

14. Fa-Yauh L, et al: The role of nitric oxide in the vascular hyporesponsiveness to methoxamine in portal hypertensive rats. *Hepatology* 1992; 16:1043–1048.

15. Carruthers JS, et al: Experimental extrahepatic biliary obstruction: Fine structural changes of liver cell mitochondria. *Gastroenterology* 1962; 42:419–430.

16. Yamauchi H, et al: Morphometric studies on the rat liver in biliary obstruction. *Tohoku J Exp Med* 1976; 119:9–25.

17. Gall JAM, et al: A quantitative analysis of the liver following ligation of the common bile duct. *Liver* 1990; 10:116–125.

18. Krähenbühl S, et al: Stereological and functional analysis of liver mitochondria from rats with secondary biliary cirrhosis: Impaired mitochondrial metabolism and increased mitochondrial content per hepatocyte. *Hepatology* 1992; 15:1167–1172.

19. McLean EK, et al: Instant cirrhosis. An improved method for producing cirrhosis of the liver in rats by simultaneous administration of carbon tetrachloride and phenobarbitone. *Br J Exp Pathol* 1969; 50:502–506.

20. Reichen J, et al: Aminopyrine N-demethylation by rats with liver cirrhosis: Evidence for the intact cell hypothesis. A morphometric-functional study. *Gastroenterology* 1987; 93:719–726.

21. Carbonell LF, et al: Hemodynamic alterations in chronically conscious diabetic rats. *Am J Physiol* 1987; 252:H900–905.

22. Salom MG, et al: Effects of converting-enzyme inhibitor on hemodynamic actions of ANP in renal hypertensive rats. *Am J Physiol* 1989; 257:R365–369.

23. Inglés AC, et al: Limited cardiac preload reserve in conscious rats. *Am J Physiol* 1991; 260:H1912–1917.

24. Inglés AC, et al: Increased total vascular capacity in conscious cirrhotic rats. *Gastroenterology* 1992; 103:275–281.

25. Clària J, et al: Pathogenesis of arterial hypotension in cirrhotic rats with ascites: Role of endogenous nitric oxide. *Hepatology* 1992; 15:343–349.

26. Palmer RMJ, et al: Nitric oxide release accounts for the biological activity of endothelium-derived relaxing factor. *Nature* 1987; 327:524–526.

27. Palmer RMJ, et al: Vascular endothelial cells synthesize nitric oxide from L-arginine. *Nature* 1988; 333:664–666.

28. Ress DD, et al: Role of endothelium-derived nitric oxide in the regulation of blood pressure. *Proc Natl Acad Sci U S A* 1989; 86:3375–3378.

29. Clàra J, et al: Doses of endothelin have natriuretic effects in conscious rats with cirrhosis and ascites. *Kidney Int* 1991; 40:182–187.

30. Goetz KL, et al: Cardiovascular, renal and endocrine responses to intravenous endothelin in conscious dogs. *Am J Physiol* 1988; 255:1064–1068.

31. Miller WL, et al: Integrated cardiac, renal and endocrine actions of endothelin. *J Clin Invest* 1989; 83:317–320.

32. King AJ, et al: Systemic hemodynamic effects of endothelin in rats. *Am J Physiol* 1990; 258:H787–H792.

33. Slater TF: Free radical mechanisms in tissue injury. *Biochem J* 1984; 222:1–15.

34. Dianzani MU, et al: Lipid peroxidation and haloalkylation in CCl_4-induced liver injury, in Poli G, Cheeseman KH, Dianzani MU, et al (eds): *Free Radicals in Liver Injury.* Oxford, IRL Press, 1985, pp 149–158.

35. Poli G, et al: The role of lipid peroxidation in liver damage. *Chem Phys Lipids* 1987; 45:117–142.

36. Poli G, et al: Lipid peroxidation and covalent binding in the early functional impairment of liver Golgi apparatus by carbon tetrachloride. *Cell Biochem Funct* 1990; 8:1–10.

37. Biasi F, et al: In vivo and in vitro evidence concerning the role of lipid peroxidation in the mechanism of hepatocyte death due to carbon tetrachloride. *Cell Biochem Funct* 1991; 9:111–118.

38. Parola M, et al: Vitamin E dietary supplementation protects against carbon tetrachloride-induced chronic liver damage and cirrhosis. *Hepatology* 1992; 16:1014–1021.

39. Frezza M, et al: Oral S-adenosylmethionine in the symptomatic treatment of intrahepatic cholestasis: A double-blind, placebo-controlled study. *Gastroenterology* 1990; 99:211–215.

40. Ribalta J, et al: S-adenosyl-L-methionine in the treatment of patients with intrahepatic cholestasis of pregnancy: A randomized, double-blind, placebo-controlled study with negative results. *Hepatology* 1991; 13:1084–1089.

41. Corrales F, et al: S-adenosylmethionine treatment prevents carbon tetrachloride-induced S-adenosylmethionine synthetase inactivation and attenuates liver injury. *Hepatology* 1992; 16:1022–1027.

42. Bray GP, et al: S-adenosylmethionine and N-acetylcysteine in paracetamol hepatotoxicity, in Rodés J, Arroyo J (eds): *Therapy in Liver Diseases.* Barcelona, Ediciones Doyma, 1991, pp 343–347.

43. Muriel P, et al: Characterization of membrane fraction lipid composition and function of cirrhotic rat liver. *J Hepatol* 1992; 14:16–21.

44. Krähenbühl S, et al: Mitochondrial function in carbon tetrachloride-induced cirrhosis in the rat. *Biochem Pharmacol* 1989; 38:1583–1588.

45. Krähenbühl S, et al: Mitochondrial structure and function in CCl_4-induced cirrhosis in the rat. *Hepatology* 1990; 12:526–532.

46. Michaeltz PA, et al: Assessment of mitochondrial function in vivo with a breath test utilizing α-ket-isocaproic acid. *Hepatology* 1989; 10:829–832.

47. Dufour J-F, et al: Hepatic accumulation of lysosomes and defective transcytotic vesicular pathways in cirrhotic rat liver. *Hepatology* 1992; 16:997–1006.

48. Henriksen JH, et al: Aspects of sympathetic nervous system regulation in patients with cirrhosis: A 10-year experience. *Clin Physiol* 1991; 11:293–306.

49. Floras JS, et al: Direct evidence from intra-neural recordings for increased sympathetic outflow in patients with cirrhosis and ascites. *Ann Intern Med* 1991; 114:373–380.

50. Gilles A, et al: Muscle sympathetic nerve activity and renal responsiveness to atrial natriuretic factor during the development of hepatic ascites. *Am J Med* 1991; 91:383–392.

51. Mastai R, et al: Effects of alpha-adrenergic stimulation and beta-adrenergic blockade on azygos blood flow and splanchnic haemodynamics in patients with cirrhosis. *J Hepatol* 1987; 4:71–79.

52. Willett IR, et al: Sympathetic tone modulates portal venous pressure in alcoholic cirrhosis. *Lancet* 1986; 2:939–943.

53. Esler M, et al: Increased sympathetic nervous activity and the effects of its inhibition with clonidine in alcoholic cirrhosis. *Ann Intern Med* 1992; 116:446–455.

54. Banares AAR, et al: Oral administration of clonidine in patients with alcoholic cirrhosis. *Gastroenterology* 1992; 102:248–254.

55. Kinsell LT, et al: Rate of disappearance from plasma of intravenously administered methionine in patients with liver damage. *Science* 1947; 106:589–590.

56. Horowith JH, et al: Evidence for impairment of transsulfuration pathway in cirrhosis. *Gastroenterology* 1981; 81:668–675.

57. Stipanuk MH: Metabolism of sulfur-containing amino acids. *Annu Rev Nutr* 1986; 6:179–209.

58. Marchesini G, et al: Defective methionine metabolism in cirrhosis: Relation to severity of liver disease. *Hepatology* 1992; 16:149–155.

59. Müller MJ, et al: Mechanism of insulin resistance associated with liver cirrhosis. *Gastroenterology* 1992; 102:2033–2041.

60. Dufour J-F, et al: Alterations in hepatic fructose metabolism in cirrhotic patients demonstrated by dynamic ^{31}phosphorus spectroscopy. *Hepatology* 1992; 15:835–842.

61. Overdiek HWPM, et al: New insights into the pharmacokinetics of spironolactone. *Clin Pharmacol Ther* 1985; 38:469–474.

62. Sungaila I, et al: Spironolactone pharmacokinetics and pharmacodynamics in patients with cirrhotic ascites. *Gastroenterology* 1992; 102:1680–1685.

63. Arroyo V, et al: Renin, aldosterone and renal haemodynamics in cirrhosis with ascites. *Eur J Clin Invest* 1979; 9:69–73.

64. Wilkinson SP, Williams R: Renin-angiotensin-aldosterone system in cirrhosis. *Gut* 1980; 21:545–554.

65. Vliet AA, et al: Efficacy of low-dose captopril in addition to furosemide and spironolactone in patients with decompensated liver disease during blunted diuresis. *J Hepatol* 1992; 15:40–47.

66. Pariente EA, et al: Acute effects of captopril on systemic and renal hemodynamics in cirrhotic patients with ascites. *Gastroenterology* 1985; 88:1255–1259.

67. Daskalopoulos G, et al: Effects of captopril on renal function in patients with cirrhosis and ascites. *J Hepatol* 1987; 4:330–336.

68. Thiollet M, et al: The pharmacokinetics of perindopril in patients with liver cirrhosis. *Br J Clin Pharmacol* 1992; 33:326–328.

69. Ohnishi A, et al: Kinetics and dynamics of enalapril in patients with liver cirrhosis. *Clin Pharmacol Ther* 1989; 45:657–665.

70. Howden CW, et al: Drug metabolism in liver disease. *Pharmacol Ther* 1988; 40:439–474.

71. Witassek F, et al: Abnormal glucuronidation of zomepirac in patients with cirrhosis of the liver. *Hepatology* 1983; 11:415–422.

72. Williams RL, et al: Naproxen disposition in patients with alcoholic cirrhosis. *Eur J Clin Pharmacol* 1984; 27:291–296.

73. Taburet A-M, et al: Pharmacokinetics of zidovudine in patients with liver disease. *Clin Pharmacol Ther* 1990; 47:731–739.

74. Macdonald JI, et al: Both phenolic and acyl glucuronidation pathways of diflunisal are impaired in liver cirrhosis. *Eur J Clin Pharmacol* 1992; 42:471–474.

75. Loewen GR, et al: Effect of dose on the glucuronidation and sulphation kinetics of diflunisal in man: Single dose studies. *Br J Clin Pharmacol* 1988; 26:31–39.

76. May DG, et al: The disposition of dapsone in cirrhosis. *Clin Pharmacol Ther* 1992; 51:689–700.

77. Lee BL, et al: Dapsone, trimethoprim, and sulfamethoxazole plasma levels during treatment of Pneumocystis pneumonia in patients with the acquired immunodeficiency syndrome (AIDS). *Ann Intern Med* 1989; 110:606–611.

78. Leung PSC, et al: Use of designer recombinant mitochondrial antigens in the diagnosis of primary biliary cirrhosis. *Hepatology* 1992; 15:367–372.

79. Coppel RL: Primary structure of the human M2 mitochondrial autoantigen of primary biliary cirrhosis: Dihydrolipoamide acetyltransferase. *Proc Natl Acad Sci U S A* 1988; 85:7317–7321.

80. Fussey SP, et al: Identification and analysis of the major M2 autoantigens in primary biliary cirrhosis. *Proc Natl Acad Sci U S A* 1988; 85:8654–8658.

81. Fussey SP, et al: The E1 alpha and beta subunits of the pyruvate dehydrogenase complex are M2'd' and M2'e' autoantigens in primary biliary cirrhosis. *Clin Sci* 1989; 77:365–368.

82. Surh CD, et al: Antimitochondrial autoantibodies in primary biliary cirrhosis recognize cross-reactive epitope(s) on protein X and dihydrolipoamide acetyltransferase of pyruvate dehydrogenase complex. *Hepatology* 1989; 10:127–133.

83. Fregeau DR, et al: Primary biliary cirrhosis: Inhibition of pyruvate dehydrogenase complex activity by autoantibodies specific for E1 alpha, a non-lipoic acid containing mitochondrial enzyme. *J Immunol* 1990; 144:1671–1676.

84. Galbraith RM, et al: High prevalence of seroimmunologic abnormalities in relatives of patients with active chronic hepatitis or primary biliary cirrhosis. *N Engl J Med* 1974; 290:63–70.

85. Feizi T, et al: Mitochondrial and other tissue antibodies in relatives of patients with primary biliary cirrhosis. *Clin Exp Immunol* 1972; 10:609–622.

86. Walker JG, et al: Chronic liver disease and mitochondrial antibodies: A family study. *BMJ* 1972; 1:146–148.

87. Klatskin G, et al: Mitochondrial antibody in primary biliary cirrhosis and other diseases. *Ann Intern Med* 1972; 77:533–541.

88. Chohan MR: Primary biliary cirrhosis in twin sisters. *Gut* 1973; 14:213–214.

89. Tong MJ, et al: Immunological studies in familial primary biliary cirrhosis. *Gastroenterology* 1976; 71:305–307.

90. Jaup BH, et al: Familial occurrence of primary biliary cirrhosis associated with hypergammaglobulinemia in descendants: A family study. *Gastroenterology* 1980; 78:549–555.

91. Kato Y, et al: Familial primary biliary cirrhosis. *Am J Gastroenterol* 1981; 75:188–191.

92. Tsuji H, et al: Familial primary biliary cirrhosis associated with impaired concanavalin A-induced lymphocyte transformation in relatives. *Dig Dis Sci* 1992; 37:353–360.

93. Addison T, et al: On a certain affection of the skin—vitiligoidea-a. plana b. tuberosa. *Guys Hosp Rep* 1851; 7:265–277.

94. Ahrens EH, et al: Primary biliary cirrhosis. *Medicine (Baltimore)* 1950; 29:299–364.

95. Jahn CE, et al: Lipoprotein abnormalities in primary biliary cirrhosis; association with hepatic lipase inhibition as well as altered cholesterol esterification. *Gastroenterology* 1985; 89:1266–1278.

96. Crippin JS, et al: Hypercholesterolemia and atherosclerosis in primary biliary cirrhosis: What is the risk? *Hepatology* 1992; 15:858–862.

97. Colina F, et al: Nodular regenerative hyperplasia of the liver in early histological stages of primary biliary cirrhosis. *Gastroenterology* 1992; 102:1319–1324.

98. Mac Sween RNM: Primary biliary cirrhosis, in Mac Sween RNM, et al (eds): *Pathology of the Liver*. New York, Churchill Livingstone, 1979, pp 306–314.

99. McMahon RFT, et al: Nodular regenerative hyperplasia of the liver, CREST syndrome and primary biliary cirrhosis: An overlap syndrome? *Gut* 1989; 30:1430–1433.

100. Nakanuma Y, et al: Nodular hyperplasia of the liver in primary biliary cirrhosis of early histological stages. *Am J Gastroenterol* 1987; 82:8–10.

101. Wanless IR: Micronodular transformation (nodular regenerative hyperplasia) of the liver. A report of 64 cases among 2,500 autopsies and a new classification of benign hepatocellular nodules. *Hepatology* 1990; 11:787–797.

102. Navasa M, et al: Portal hypertension in primary biliary cirrhosis. Relationship with histological features. *J Hepatol* 1987; 5:292–298.

103. Beuers U, et al: Ursodeoxycholic acid for treatment of primary sclerosing cholangitis: A placebo-controlled trial. *Hepatology* 1992; 16:707–714.

104. Chazouillères O, et al: Ursodeoxycholic acid for primary sclerosing cholangitis. *J Hepatol* 1990; 11:120–123.

105. O'Brien CB, et al: Ursodeoxycholic acid for the treatment of primary sclerosing cholangitis: A 36-month open pilot trial. *Hepatology* 1991; 14:838–847.

106. Stiehl L, et al: Effect of ursodeoxycholic acid in patients with primary sclerosing cholangitis, in Paumgartner G, et al (eds): *Bile Acids as Therapeutic Agents*. Dordrecht, The Netherlands, Kluwer Academic Publishers, 1991, pp 305–307.

107. Pirovino M, et al: Cutaneous spider nevi in liver cirrhosis: Capillary microscopical and hormonal investigations. *Klin Wochenschr* 1988; 66:298–302.

108. Okumura H, et al: Regional differences in peripheral circulation between upper and lower extremity in patients with cirrhosis. *Scand J Gastroenterol* 1990; 25:883–889.

109. Nilsson GE, et al: A new instrument for continuous measurement of tissue blood flow by light beating spectroscopy. *IEEE Trans Biomed Eng* 1980; 22:12–19.

110. Leonardo G, et al: Local deterioration of the cutaneous venoarterial reflex of the hand in cirrhosis. *Scand J Gastroenterol* 1992; 27:326–332.

CHAPTER 7

Liver Metastasis of Colorectal Carcinoma: Diagnosis, Treatment, and Prognosis of Resectable Lesions*

Yeu-Tsu Margaret Lee, M.D.

Colonel, Medical Corps, United States Army; Chief, Surgical Oncology Section, Department of Surgery, Tripler Army Medical Center; Associate Clinical Professor in Surgery, John A. Burns School of Medicine, University of Hawaii, Honolulu, Hawaii; Clinical Associate Professor of Surgery, F. Edward Hebert School of Medicine, Uniformed Services University of the Health Sciences, Bethesda, Maryland

The liver is a frequent site of metastasis for many types of cancer. More than 150,000 Americans have colorectal (CR) carcinoma diagnosed each year[1] and about half eventually die, most of liver metastasis. Hepatic metastasis has been shown to have an overriding influence on the natural course of CR cancer, despite concurrent pulmonary, peritoneal, or lymph node involvement.[2] Therefore, aggressive treatment of secondary cancer of the liver is warranted.

Although patients with liver metastasis of CR carcinoma survive longer than do those with liver metastasis from other primary tumors, only patients who undergo

*The opinions and assertions contained herein are the private views of the author and are not to be construed as official or as reflecting the views of the Department of the Army or the Department of Defense.

liver resection have a reasonable chance of long-term survival. Before 1985, only 11 patients were known to have survived for more than 5 years with histologically proven hepatic metastasis of CR carcinoma.[3]

The only currently available curative treatment of CR carcinoma metastatic to the liver is hepatic resection. Controversy does exist in the surgical literature, however, regarding the role of liver resection. Silen[4] in particular states that hepatic resection for metastasis of CR carcinoma is of dubious value. What is the basis for this assertion? What factors and data are necessary for proper analysis of this issue?

As is the case with many other surgical approaches, appropriate patient selection is essential to decrease operative risks and improve long-term outcome. How often does CR carcinoma metastasize only to the liver? What diagnostic tests are useful in determining the resectability of liver metastases before and during surgery? In volume 10 of *Current Hepatology,* operative complications and survival rates from 1983 to 1988 were reviewed.[3] In this chapter, treatment guidelines and surgical results for resectable liver metastasis of CR carcinoma are discussed.

HOW OFTEN DOES LIVER METASTASIS OCCUR IN PATIENTS WITH COLORECTAL CARCINOMA?

The overall cure rate and incidence of liver metastasis of CR cancer have remained relatively constant for the past several decades.[5] About 10% to 30% of patients have liver metastasis at the time of initial laparotomy for resection of the primary CR tumor (synchronous metastasis).[6, 7] The proportion of liver-only metastases that are solitary or few is difficult to discern from the literature, but may be about 25%.[5] Thus, 3% to 8% of patients may have resectable synchronous liver metastasis. In a series of 2,411 patients with CR cancer, 3% with Dukes A or B lesions and 6% with Dukes C lesions underwent curative resection of liver metastasis.[8]

After surgical resection of primary CR cancer, liver metastasis will develop in 8% to 25% of patients (metachronous metastasis).[9, 10] In a study of adjuvant therapy for patients with high-risk colon cancer (Dukes stage B2 or C) who were followed up for a median of 5.5 years, 27% had recurrent tumor in the liver.[11] Among patients with high-risk rectal cancer, 17% had liver involvement (about 9% liver only).[12]

These percentages increased when patients with tumor recurrence were used as the denominators. Willet and colleagues[13] noted that liver metastases were seen in 54% of all recurrent colonic disease and that 19% of all recurrences occurred in the liver only. Welch and Donaldson[14] observed that 71% of all patients with recurrent CR cancer after curative resection had liver metastasis, and that 20% of all recurrent disease was confined to the liver. In an autopsy series, Pestana and associates[15] reported liver involvement in 70% of those patients who died of disseminated CR cancer.

Liver metastasis is being diagnosed more accurately in randomized protocols now because of the use of biopsy confirmation.[11] Accordingly, the prognosis of patients with CR cancer has improved significantly even without the use of adjuvant therapy (5-year survival of Dukes B2 and C lesions is 77% and 47%,[11] respectively, now compared to 45% and 22% before 1982).[16]

HOW USEFUL ARE LABORATORY TESTS IN THE DIAGNOSIS OF LIVER METASTASES?

Liver metastases may be completely silent. Among 107 patients who underwent exploration for presumed resectable liver metastases, only 20% had any abdominal symptoms preoperatively.[17] Lefor and coworkers[17] reported that 67% of the patients had elevated lactic dehydrogenase (LDH) levels and that 85% had abnormal carcinoembryonic antigen (CEA) levels.

Kemeny and associates[18] described 100 patients who underwent exploration for known liver metastasis. Preoperative transaminase levels, bilirubin levels, and prothrombin times were elevated in less than 10% of the patients. The CEA level was increased (>2.5 ng/mL) in 86%, and the LDH and alkaline phosphatase (AP) levels were high in 61% to 63% of the patients. A correlation was noted between the extent of liver involvement and the absolute levels of CEA, LDH, and AP: CEA, LDH, and AP levels were elevated in 73%, 30%, and 40%, respectively, of patients with resectable lesions and in 93%, 78%, and 73%, respectively, of those with unresectable lesions. Parker and colleagues[19] noted biopsy-proven liver metastasis in 12 of 121 patients with newly diagnosed CR cancer. All 12 patients had LDH, AP, or CEA levels greater than 100 ng/mL.

Although CEA levels greater than 10 ng/mL usually indicate metastatic disease in patients with cancer, 26% of patients without metastatic spread may have abnormal CEA levels.[20] Tartter and coworkers[21] observed that the accuracy with which liver metastases are diagnosed could be improved by using both CEA (>10 ng/mL) and AP levels (>135 IU/L). The accuracy rate was 88% when the results of both tests were abnormal, compared to 73% and 62%, respectively, for each individual test.

WHAT PREOPERATIVE STAGING STUDIES SHOULD PATIENTS UNDERGO?

Patients who are operative candidates with presumed resectable liver metastasis should undergo studies to exclude both lesions outside the abdomen and extrahepatic intra-abdominal disease. In addition to routine physical examination, liver function tests, and determination of the CEA level, the following staging procedures have been recommended by various authors[17, 22-24]:

1. Colonoscopy to rule out new or recurrent colonic lesions.
2. Computed tomography (CT) of the chest, abdomen, and pelvis.
3. Optional external ultrasound (US) study of the liver and magnetic resonance imaging (MRI) of the abdomen in selected patients.
4. Hepatic angiography to define the arterial anatomy of the liver and to detect additional hepatic metastases.
5. Radioisotopic bone scanning or upper gastrointestinal studies for symptoms.

These preoperative staging studies can eliminate 38%[22] to 40%[25] of patients referred for resection of liver metastasis because obvious extrahepatic metastases were discovered.

Isotopic scanning of the liver (rarely used today), CT, and US all are useful for detecting liver metastasis, but each technique does have limitations.[26] CT and US have an overall median accuracy rate of 88% (range, 85% to 96%), a sensitivity rate of 80% (range, 65% to 91%), and a specificity rate of 93% (range, 65% to 91%). These figures result in a median false-negative rate of 20% and a false-positive rate of 7%.

The combination of any two tests improves the sensitivity rate, but lowers the specificity rate. Thus, accuracy is not improved by performing more tests. CT scanning and US are comparable and complementary, however, and MRI is particularly useful in demonstrating the relationship of tumors to hepatic and portal veins. The latter technique should be reserved for patients with equivocal or conflicting findings on CT and US, and in whom strong suspicion of a liver neoplasm exists.

HOW ACCURATE ARE RADIOLOGIC STUDIES IN DEFINING THE EXTENT OF METASTATIC LESIONS OF THE LIVER?

A major limitation in evaluating patients with liver metastasis from CR cancer is the inadequacy of available preoperative diagnostic imaging techniques. Mittal and colleagues[27] studied 41 patients with total or partial liver resection and showed that CT missed 31% of the metastases that ranged in size from 0.1 to 1.6 cm. About one of five missed lesions was larger than 1 cm.

Kemeny and associates[18] found CT scans to reveal accurately the extent of liver metastasis when more than 80% of the liver parenchyma was infiltrated with the tumor. Among 60 patients with discrete lesions at laparatomy, CT accurately identified the location and number of metastases in 26 patients (43%). In another 40%, CT showed a lower number of lesions, and in 13%, it indicated more lesions. Lesion site was identified incorrectly in 4% of patients.

In a recent prospective study of patients who had undergone exploration for liver metastasis, preoperative CT failed to show any disease in 7% (10 of 139 patients).[28] Five of the patients had bilobar disease. Overall, CT underestimates the number of lobes involved in 33% of patients, and overestimates this number in 12%. Extrahepatic disease was found in 12% of patients with negative results on preoperative CT scanning. Angiography helped in identifying lesions that were not visible on CT or liver scanning in 11% of patients.

Reinig and coworkers[29] compared CT with MRI in 16 patients with 155 liver metastases. Regular CT detected 50% of the lesions, whereas the sensitivity of T1 MRI images was 95% and that of T2 images was 51%. Sitzmann and associates[30] compared three imaging techniques in 100 patients with suspected resectable liver metastasis (52 had CR cancer). A total of 227 lesions were identified at operation. The sensitivity for tumor detection was 66% for standard CT, 70% for MRI, and 94% for arteriographically enhanced CT (AECT). The advantage of AECT was most marked for lesions less than 1 cm in diameter (82% vs. 20% for MRI and 5% for CT). AECT also was sensitive in assessing tumor margins, whereas MRI was most useful in detecting vascular involvement. They concluded that the combination of AECT and MRI was the best predictor of liver metastasis (86%), but that no imaging technique was sensitive for extrahepatic involvement.

At operation, a mass palpated in the liver can be benign 5% to 8% of the time. Hughes and Sugarbaker[31] noted that a liver thought to be free of metastasis at palpation by the surgeon actually could harbor metastasis in 5% of cases. Among 150 patients explored for resection of liver metastasis, 2% were free of liver disease at the time of laparotomy.[28]

Intraoperative US and palpation have shown CT to detect about half of all liver metastases smaller than 1 cm, and preoperative US and angiography to detect about one third of all lesions 1 to 2 cm in size.[32] The routine use of intraoperative US can reveal lesions of 3 to 5 mm, even in the left lobe or deep in the liver parenchyma.[23] Among 167 lesions detected by intraoperative US, 76% were visible on preoperative US, 61% on CT, and 52% on angiography.

AT EXPLORATORY LAPAROTOMY, HOW OFTEN ARE PATIENTS EXCLUDED FROM HEPATIC RESECTION?

Among 247 consecutive patients with CR cancer metastases to the liver, Fortner and colleagues[33] reported in 1984 that 30% underwent resection. Among 100 patients who underwent exploratory laparotomy for liver metastasis between 1985 and 1988, Sitzmann and coworkers[30] reported that 57% had hepatic resection, 17% had insertion of a hepatic arterial catheter, and 14% had diagnostic laparotomy only. About 12% of patients expected to undergo resection after preoperative CT, AECT, and MRI studies had unresectable lesions.

Steele and associates[23] reported that one third of their patients undergoing surgery for liver resection were found intraoperatively to have previously undiagnosed

TABLE 1.

Outcome of Patients With Colorectal Liver Metastases Who Were Referred to Surgeons for Resection

	Number of Patients (%)			
Reference (Period)	Referred for Surgery	Underwent Exploration	Underwent Liver Resection	Explored but No Resection
August et al., 1985[22] (1976–1983)	81(100)	50(62)	37(46)	13(26)
Lefor et al., 1988[17] (1978–1986)	145(100)	107(74)	66(46)	41(38)
Kemeny et al., 1986[18] (1982–1985)	100(100)	75(75)	30(30)	45(60)
Steele et al., 1991[28] (1984–1988)	N/A	150	87	63(42)

liver or extrahepatic lesions that obviated resection. This is similar to the 25% to 42% of patients who could not undergo resection in other studies (Table 1). Table 2 summarizes the various reasons that liver metastasis cannot be resected at the time of exploration.

Among 150 patients who underwent exploration for liver metastasis of CR cancer, Steele and coworkers[28] reported that 87 (58%) had resection and 63 (42%) did not. Of those patients who underwent resection, 46% had curative resection and 12% had noncurative resection. Of those patients who did not undergo liver resection, 43 (68%) had anatomically unresectable lesions and 20 (32%) had extrahepatic disease.

Lefor and associates[17] found that 28 of 107 patients (26%) undergoing surgical exploration had extrahepatic spread. The presence of extrahepatic disease correlated with the presence of symptoms, Dukes C primary tumors, and greater than 25% hepatic replacement by tumor. None of these factors was predictive, however. Occasionally, extrahepatic tumor deposits were misdiagnosed as intrahepatic metastases.[34]

Kemeny and colleagues[18] reported that CT accurately detected the presence and

TABLE 2.

Reasons for Inability to Resect Liver Metastases at Exploration

	Number of Patients (%)						
Reference (Period)	Unresectable	Extensive Liver Metastases	Celiac Lymph Node	Portal Lymph Node	Peritoneal Spread	Omental Spread	Other Sites
August et al., 1983[22] (1976–1983)	13	6	1	5	1	—	—
Lefor et al., 1988[17] (1978–1986)	41	13	9	6	7	2	4
Kemeny et al., 1986[18] (1982–1985)	45	10	8	14	9	1	3
Lefor et al. and Kemeny et al.[17, 18]	86(100)	23(27)	17(20)	20(23)	16(19)	3(4)	7(8)

absence of extrahepatic disease in 68% of cases. None of 14 patients with a positive portal node, however, had this finding noted on CT scanning. Thus, even with the combination of late-generation CT scanning and biochemical testing, the accurate measurement and localization of hepatic metastases and extrahepatic disease still requires surgical assessment.

WHAT TYPE OF LIVER RESECTION WAS PERFORMED AND WHAT WERE THE OPERATIVE MORTALITY AND MORBIDITY RATES?

The types of liver resection used include trisegmentectomy, right or left lobectomy, left lateral segmentectomy, and wedge resection. Usually, the size, number, and location of the metastatic lesions determine the extent of resection. In recent years, the use of trisegmentectomy is decreasing and that of wedge resection is increasing (Table 3).

Hughes and Sugarbaker[31] showed a resection margin of greater than 1 cm to be associated with improved survival. Most surgeons define negative margins as being 1 cm or more in width and having no microscopic involvement.

Surgical complication rates also vary with the size, number, and location of liver metastases, and with the extent of hepatic resection. In 1983, Niederhuber and Ensinger[49a] reviewed several large series and found the overall mortality of wedge and some extended liver resections to be less than 10%. Lee[3] reviewed 22 reports published from 1983 to 1988 of the resection of CR cancer metastasis to the liver (involving a total of 1,028 patients) and found the operative mortality to be acceptable (median, 4%; range, 0% to 14%). Table 4 presents the surgical mortality and morbidity rates of liver resection for metastasis of CR cancer.

Butler and associates[42] reported an operative mortality for liver resections of 29% from 1950 to 1967; this decreased to 2% from 1968 to 1981. The complication rate remained stasble at 26%. Savage and Malt[48] reviewed 300 patients who underwent liver resection between 1962 and 1988. For the 252 patients with liver metastases of CR cancer, the operative mortality rate decreased from 13.6% before 1980 to 4.8% after 1980. Multiple factors were studied and the authors found that thoracoabdominal exposure of the liver was associated with a mortality rate of 20% vs. 8.6% for abdominal exposure. Segmental and wedge resection had 5.3% mortality vs. 14.7% for major hepatic resection.

In 1984, Fortner and coworkers[33] reported an operative mortality rate of 7% for 75 patients who underwent resection of CR cancer liver metastases from 1971 to 1982. The median age of their patients was 58 years (range, 24 to 75 years). Their operative mortality rate decreased to 4% from 1980 to 1982. In 1990, Fortner and Lincer[50] reported an operative mortality rate of 3.3% for 90 patients older than 64 years who underwent liver resection between 1970 and 1988 (66 had CR cancer). The rate was 4.4% for those with major hepatic resection and 1.4% for those with segmental resection. The mortality rate increased with age: it was 0.7% for pa-

TABLE 3.

Type of Liver Resection for Hepatic Metastases of Colorectal Cancer

| Reference | Year | Period | Number of Patients | Lobectomy | | Trisegmentectomy (%) | LLS* (%) | Wedge (%) | Others (%) |
				Right	Left				
Rajpal et al.[35]	1982	1972–81	34	18	1	4	3	8	—
Thompson et al.[36]	1983	1955–80	22	7	3	4	5	2	1
Iwatsuki et al.[37]	1983	1964–82	24	8	3	1	6	1	—
Fortner et al.[33]	1984	1971–82	75	27	10	14	9	10	5
Tomas-dela Vega et al.[38]	1984	1972–82	42	9	3	6	—	24	—
Kortz et al.[39]	1984	1974–82	16	10	2	1	—	3	—
Cady and McDermott[40]	1985	1966–84	23	15	5	—	—	3	—
Gennari et al.[41]	1986	1948–80	48	18	1	3	6	20	—
Butler et al.[42]	1986	1950–81	62	11	9	2	6	34	—
Nordlinger et al.[43]	1987	1970–85	80	28	4	11	12	25	—
Bozzetti et al.[44]	1987	1980–84	45	17	1	3	6	18	—
Patt et al.[45]	1987	N/A	23	3	3	6	10	1	—
Iwatsuki et al.[46]	1988	1964–87	90	30	14	28	9	3	6
Holm et al.[47]	1989	1971–86	35	9	3	2	7	12	2
Summary of above 14 studies	—	1950–87	619	210	62	85	69	173	15
			(100%)	(34%)	(10%)	(14%)	(11%)	(28%)	(2%)
Savage and Malt[48]	1991	1962–79	84	33%	21%	17%	19%	8%	1%
	1991	1980–88	216	34%	16%	22%	14%	10%	—
Younes et al.[49]	1991	1987–89	116	41%	9%	6%	24%	21%	—
Steele et al.[28]	1991	1984–88	87	30%	10%	7%	11%	37%	4%

*LLS = left lateral segmentectomy.

TABLE 4.

Operative Mortality and Morbidity for Liver Resection of Colorectal Metastases

References	Year	Period	Number of Patients	Mortality (%)	Morbidity (%)	Comment
Lee[3] (review of 22 papers)	1990	1955–87	1,028	0	13	Minimum
				14	43	Maximum
				4	27	Median
Holm et al.[47]	1989	1971–86	35	0	46	—
Fortner and Lincer[50]	1990	1970–88	66	3.3	N/A	>65 yr
Savage and Malt[48]	1991	1962–88	126	6.3	37	—
Hodgson et al.[51]	1992	1981–88	33	0	18	22 pts. had colorectal cancer

tients younger than 55 years, 3.6% for those between 55 and 64 years, and 11.1% for those older than 64 years. Sixty percent of the operative deaths in this series resulted from hepatic insufficiency. These investigators commented that extended right hepatic lobectomy should be performed only in selected cases.

Among 22 studies reported in the literature from 1983 to 1988, the surgical complication rate was moderate. As presented in Table 4, the median morbidity rate was 27% (range, 13% to 43%). Thompson and coworkers[36] reported major complications after hepatic resection to be intra-abdominal sepsis (17%), biliary leakage (11%), hepatic failure (8%), and hemorrhage (6%).

Holm and associates[47] reported postoperative complications in 46% of their 35 patients: 52% of those undergoing major resection and 33% of those undergoing wedge resection. Excluding bile leakage in 6% of patients, the most common complications were atelectasis (14%) and prolonged jaundice (9%). These authors did not report any cases of hemorrhage, sepsis, or hepatic failure. They found intraoperative blood loss of more than 3,500 mL to correlate significantly with postoperative complications (71% vs. 29%).

Hodgson and colleagues[51] found the use of an ultrasonic dissector to simplify major liver resection and decrease mean blood loss to only 1,020 mL. Among 33 patients undergoing liver resection, the authors reported no operative deaths and a low postoperative complication rate of 18% (4 of 6 patients had hepatorenal failure).

For 263 patients who survived liver resection for various indications, Savage and Malt[48] reported an overall complication rate of 37%. Definite reductions were noted in the rates of local, pulmonary, and wound complications after 1980. A thoracoabdominal exposure was used in 57% of procedures performed before 1980 and in 19% of those performed after 1980. Thoracoabdominal incision was associated with a morbidity rate of 45%, compared to 29% for abdominal incision. The rate of pulmonary complications was 21% with the thoracoabdominal approach vs. 10% for the abdominal approach. Similarly, the rate of subphrenic sepsis was 17% for thoracic vs. 4% for abdominal procedures.

Recently, Terblanche and colleagues[52] initiated a standard protocol using routine vascular inflow occlusion and fibrin sealant to reduce blood loss during hepatic resection. No deaths have occurred among ten consecutive patients and the postoperative course has been remarkably smooth.

WHAT ARE THE THERAPEUTIC RESULTS OF RESECTION OF COLORECTAL CANCER METASTASIS TO THE LIVER?

Historically, Cattell was the first surgeon to perform hepatic wedge resection for metastatic disease in 1940. The first formal lobectomy was done by Wangensteen in 1949 for a metastatic carcinoma from the stomach.[5] In 1976, Wilson and Adson[53] of the Mayo Clinic described 60 patients who had resection of CR cancer hepatic metastases from 1949 to 1972. The 5-year survival rate was 28% and the 10-year survival rate was 19%. Attiyeh and associates[54] also reported 5- and 10-year survival rates of 40% and 28%, respectively.

A 1978 survey[55] of 345 patients who underwent resection of liver metastases at different hospitals showed a 5-year survival rate of 30% for those with CR cancer. In 1990, Lee[3] reviewed 22 reports of 1,028 patients who underwent resection of CR cancer metastases to the liver from 1955 to 1986. The median 5-year survival rate was 34% (range, 15% to 49%). The median survival time was 31 months (median range, 21 to 59 months). Two recent reports showed similar results (5-year survival, 35%[51] and 40%[50]).

In a registry of hepatic metastases,[56] which recorded 859 patients who underwent liver resection of CR carcinoma metastases at 24 institutions between 1948 and 1985, there were 798 patients who had curative removal of isolated hepatic metastases. These individuals had a 5-year actuarial survival rate of 33% and a 5-year actuarial disease-free survival rate of 22%. Many clinicopathologic factors influence the 5-year survival rate. These are discussed in detail in the next section.

Jaffee and coworkers[2] reviewed 390 patients with various untreated liver metastases seen from 1940 to 1966. Their median length of survival was 75 days from diagnosis. Patients with metastases of CR cancer had the longest survival: a median of 146 days (20% lived for more than 1 year). Wagner and associates[57] described 252 patients with biopsy-proven, untreated, solitary and multiple unilobar metastatic lesions. Median survival times were 21 and 15 months, respectively. More than 20% of patients who had solitary liver lesions that were not resected lived for 3 years or more. Almost all died by 5 years, however.

In a review of the world literature done by Hughes and colleagues[31] in 1988, only 14 patients could be found who survived liver metastases for longer than 5 years without undergoing resection. Eleven patients were reported before 1985.[3] Thus, Adson commented that survival for 2 to 3 years is determined more by the natural course of malignant hepatic disease than by the removal of such lesions. Long survival of 5 or more years, however, is determined more often by removing the tumor than by slowing its growth.

Because there is no curative radiotherapy or chemotherapy for metastatic CR cancer, the only potentially curative treatment of metastatic liver tumors is hepatic resection. Silen[4] argued that hepatic resection for metastases of CR carcinoma is of dubious value. He based his view on the data that only 8% to 27% of all patients with hepatic metastases from CR cancer are candidates for hepatic resection. Because the 5-year survival rate after resection is about 25%, only 2% to 7% of all patients with hepatic metastases will benefit. Adson[58] is less pessimistic and has emphasized the fact that some patients with hepatic metastases live much longer if their liver lesions are removed. His own personal data and many other reports in the literature show that patients with no evidence of residual primary, regional, or other metastatic disease at the time of hepatic resection have a 30% to 50% chance of surviving for 5 or more years.

This debate cannot be resolved by anything less than a formal prospective trial in which surgically staged patients are randomized either to undergo resection of their liver metastases for cure or not to undergo resection. Such a trial, however, although intellectually appealing, never will be acceptable to either surgeons or patients.[28]

In the absence of a randomized trial, comparative data from the University of Erlangen in West Germany were reported by Hughes and associates[8] in 1989. There were 2,411 patients with Dukes A to C CR cancers, 125 of whom underwent potentially curative resection of their primary tumor and liver metastases from 1960 to 1986. No patient was lost to follow-up, and the survival data were compiled as of January 1, 1988. Patients who had Dukes A to C primary colon cancer without liver metastasis at the time of initial diagnosis and those with similar primary and curative resection of their liver metastasis had similar survival curves up to 7 years, stage for stage. This finding suggested that lymph node status was the determinate variable in patients with large-bowel cancers and that, when hepatic metastases were resected completely, they had little or no impact on prognosis.

WHAT FACTORS INFLUENCE THE PROGNOSIS OF PATIENTS WHO HAVE RESECTION OF THEIR LIVER METASTASES?

As discussed previously, about one third of the patients who undergo resection of their liver metastases survive for 5 or more years. Several clinicopathologic characteristics of the tumor and host, however, can increase or decrease survival.

It is well documented that only curative resection of metastatic lesions will improve patients' chance of survival. Metastases treated with palliative resection and regional chemotherapy currently have the same survival rates as do untreated metastases.[8] When hepatic metastases are resected for cure, several factors have been found to have no effect on long-term survival; these are listed in Table 5. These factors occasionally are reported to have some influence, but it usually is only minor.

TABLE 5.

Factors That Had no Significant Effect on Long-term Survival After Resection of Hepatic Metastases

Factor	Reference Number	Comments
Age	5,56	Subgroups <40, 40–70, >70 yrs.
Sex	5	
Location of primary cancer	5	Colon vs. rectum
Synchronous or metachronous	5,8	
Location of metastases in liver	5,8	Right vs. left vs. both lobes
Size of solitary metastasis	5,8,56	Cutoff by 5 or 8 cm
Satellite nodule adjacent to main mass	5,59	Satellite usually 1 cm or less
Extent of multiple metastases	8,49	Unilobar or bilobar
Type of resection	56,49	Wedge or anatomic, major or minor
Amount of hepatic tissue resected	5	
Tumor DNA content	5	

The extent of liver resection and the number of metastases that can be resected have been the subject of much debate. Cobourn and colleagues[59] and Stehlin and associates[60] reported 5-year survival rates of 33% to 48% for patients who undergo resection of solitary metastases vs. 0% to 6% for those who undergo resection of multiple lesions. Cady and McDermott[40] noted that more than 80% of patients with four metastases died with further liver metastases, compared to only 17% of those with fewer lesions.

In recent years, segmental or wedge hepatic resection has been used whenever possible to allow economical but radical resection of multiple metastases and to decrease operative mortality.[8, 24] Hughes and coworkers[8] noted that 13 patients who had resection of four or more metastases had survival rates similar to those of 112 patients who had resection of 1 to 3 metastases. Minton and colleagues[24] used a "Swiss cheese" procedure in 98 consecutive patients to excise 1 to 13 liver metastases. Six of 9 patients who were followed for more than 5 years survived.

Table 6 outlines the factors that do have significant influence on patient prognosis after hepatic resection. Extensive extrahepatic disease, even when it can be resected, indicates a poor prognosis. Adson and coworkers[61] reported a 3-year survival rate of 11% for patients who underwent resection of liver and extrahepatic metastases. None lived for 5 years. By comparison, among patients without extrahepatic metastases, 63% survived for 3 years and 46% survived for 5 years.

Hughes and Sugarbaker[31] reported that patients with positive hepatic or celiac nodes died by 3 years, despite removal of the nodes at the time of liver resection. In a multi-institutional study,[8] only 1 of 25 patients survived for 5 years after the resection of hepatic or celiac nodes. Among 37 patients who underwent resection of noncontiguous extrahepatic metastases (i.e., lung, peritoneum, adrenal gland, etc.), the 5-year survival rate was only 4%.

Several authors have shown that resection of liver metastases of Dukes B primary cancers is associated with better 5-year survival than is resection of Dukes C primary lesions (range, 33% to 55% vs. 15% to 23%).[3] For patients who undergo

TABLE 6.

Factors That Had Significant Effect on the Prognosis After Resection of Hepatic Metastases of Colorectal Cancers

Factor	Reference Number	Comments
Extrahepatic metastases	8,31,61	Poor survival even if all resected
Extent of liver involved (number of metastases)	5,8,49,62,65	5-yr survival: 37% vs. 18% for 1 vs. 3 or more lesions
Dukes' stage of primary cancer	3,8,56	5-yr survival: 32%–55% vs. 15%–23% for Dukes B vs. Dukes C cancers
Disease-free interval between primary cancer and liver metastases	5,8,31	5-yr survival: 24% vs. 42%; >1-yr vs. <1-yr 5-yr survival: 7% vs. 70%; 1-yr vs. 4-yr
Carcinoembryonic antigen level (ng/mL)	8,49,56	5-yr survival: 47% vs. 29%; <5 vs. >5 5-yr survival: 42% vs. 14%; 5 vs. 30
Symptoms of liver metastases (performance status)	56	5-yr survival: 45% vs. 32%; negative vs. positive for symptoms
Resection margin	56,65	5-yr survival: 23% vs. 47%; 1 cm vs. more than 1 cm
Intraoperative hypotensive episode and duration (min.)	49	Significance $P = .0006$
Perioperative blood transfusions	62,63	Median disease-free survival: 26 vs. 12 months for 3–5 units transfused vs. 6 or more units transfused

resection of isolated liver metastases, the 5-year survival rate is 47% vs. 23% $(P = .001)$.[56]

Although the resection of synchronous and metachronous metastases had similar survival rates, patients with longer disease-free intervals did much better than did those with shorter disease-free intervals.[5, 18] Patients who had 1 to 2 metastases fared better than did those who had 3 or more lesions.[56] Resection margins of 1 cm or more indicate adequate removal.[56] Elevated CEA levels and the presence of systemic symptoms both suggest more advanced liver involvement.[56]

In the multi-institutional study,[56] multivariate analysis identified five independent prognostic factors: (1) stage of the primary tumor, (2) number of metastases, (3) presence of a lesion greater than 8 cm, (4) length of disease-free interval before hepatic resection, and (5) age older than 70 years. All these factors, except age, were highly significant in the multivariate analysis $(P < .01)$. Age was of borderline significance $(P < .05)$.

Stephenson and colleagues[62] studied 55 patients who had resection of CR liver metastases (the 5-year overall survival rate was 30%). Multivariate analysis showed that the number of units of blood transfused intraoperatively and during the first 2 postoperative weeks, the size of the metastatic tumor, and the number of metastatic nodules were independent prognostic factors that jointly predicted overall survival. The difference in survival rate between those who received 3 to 10 and those who received more than 10 units of blood was especially significant for patients who had resection of metastases less than 3 cm or those who had only 1 to 2 nodules (P = .02 and .002, respectively). Blumberg and coworkers[63] studied the association between perioperative blood transfusion and later recurrence of solid tumors (120 of their 216 patients had CR cancer). Patients who received three or fewer units of red cell concentrates had no greater risk of recurrence than did those who received no transfusions. Their findings suggested that the transfusion of stored blood plasma caused earlier tumor recurrence in some instances. Fernandez and coworkers[64] showed that even 2.5 units of packed red cells caused an exaggerated decrease in T-helper lymphocytes at 5 to 10 days after operation and failure to demonstrate rebound of a proliferative immunologic response 45 to 90 days later.

Younes and colleagues[49] studied 116 patients who had complete hepatic resection of CR metastases between 1987 and 1989. With a median follow-up period of 13.2 months, about 21% of the patients were free of disease at 2 years. By univariate analysis, the number of units of whole blood transfused was one of the nine factors found to affect the recurrence rate after resection. By multivariate analysis, however, only four factors remained significant: the site of the primary tumor (right colon, left colon, sigmoid, rectum), preoperative CEA levels, the number of metastases, and the number of hypotensive episodes that occurred during the operation.

After curative removal of isolated hepatic metastases, patients with symptoms of metachronous metastases appeared to have a small but statistically significant reduction in survival when compared with patients without symptoms.[56] Individuals who were asymptomatic at presentation and who had fewer than three metastases had a median survival of 24 months without resection of their liver metastases, which is considerably longer than the 4- to 6-month survival periods reported in unselected populations of patients.[65]

The poor prognosis of patients with Dukes C cancer reflects the greater chance of extrahepatic disease recurrence when mesocolic lymph nodes are involved by tumor.[8] Among the 859 patients registered in the multi-institutional study, no patient with Dukes C disease and three or more liver metastases survived for 5 years after resection.[56] Patients with Dukes C lesions who were older than 70 years or who had a lesion greater than 8 cm also had a low survival rate (less than 15%).

The patients most likely to benefit from the resection of hepatic metastases appear to be those with Dukes B primary CR cancer who have a solitary, isolated metastasis resected with a clear margin after a long disease-free interval; their 5-year survival rate exceeds 50%.[5] Despite these general conclusions, Hughes and colleagues[56] found that, among 140 patients who survived for 5 years after hepatic resection, some had had poor prognostic factors. Thus, Hughes and colleagues[8] emphasized that our current level of knowledge does not allow us to identify a group of patients that should be excluded from hepatic surgery. Saenz and associates[5] believe that patients with suitable biologic metastatic disease should be sought, evaluated diagnostically, and urged to undergo potentially curative hepatic resection with the expectation of a substantial chance of long-term survival.

SUMMARY

About 10% to 30% of patients with CR cancer will have liver metastases at the time of diagnosis, and similar numbers will have liver metastases after resection of their primary tumor. Among all patients with recurrent CR lesions, 50% to 70% have liver metastases (half appear to have recurrence only in the liver).

Among patients with liver metastases, only 20% have any abdominal symptoms. Of the many tests available, only the measurement of LDH, AP, and CEA levels appears to have diagnostic value. These three levels are elevated in 60% to 85% of patients with liver metastases. CT and US have an overall median accuracy rate of 88%. Either test may miss 20% of the hepatic lesions, however, and diagnose tumors inaccurately 7% of the time. The use of arteriography, enhanced CT, and MRI may improve the detection and delineation of metastatic lesions in the liver. No imaging technique, however, is very sensitive in the diagnosis of extrahepatic involvement.

Preoperative staging using colonoscopy, CT scanning, US, and other tests can remove from consideration 25% to 40% of patients referred for resection of liver metastases. Among patients who have exploratory laparotomy, about 30% to 50% do not undergo liver resection, for three primary reasons: (1) the liver metastases are too extensive, (2) there is extrahepatic lymph node involvement, or (3) there is peritoneal spread of metastasis to other sites.

Surgery offers the only hope of cure for patients with liver metastases. Whenever possible, the metastatic lesions should be resected with at least a 1-cm margin. In the last 2 to 3 decades, operative mortality has decreased to 0% to 5% with a lesser extent of resection and improved operative and postoperative care. The surgical complication rate, however, remains at 20% to 40%.

Overall, about one third of patients who undergo resection of liver metastases of CR cancer will survive for 5 or more years (5-year actuarial disease-free survival rate, 20% to 25%). This is much better than the natural history of patients with unresected liver metastases, almost all of whom die by 3 years after diagnosis.

Data from a German hospital demonstrated the therapeutic effectiveness of resecting liver metastases. Patients with Dukes A to C primary CR cancer without liver metastases and those with Dukes D lesions but with similar primary and curative resection of their liver metastases had similar survival curves for as long as 7 years, stage for stage.

Many clinicopathologic factors have a significant effect on patient prognosis after the resection of liver metastases, including the presence or absence of extrahepatic involvement, the extent of liver metastases, Dukes' stage of primary CR cancer, the length of the disease-free interval, the CEA level, resection margins, the number of intraoperative hypotensive episodes, and the amount of blood transfused perioperatively.

REFERENCES

1. Boring CC, et al: Cancer statistics, 1992. *CA Cancer J Clin* 1992; 42:19–38.

2. Jaffee BM, et al: Factors influencing survival in patients with untreated hepatic metastases. *Surg Gynecol Obstet* 1968; 127:1–11.

3. Lee YM: Metastatic colorectal cancer of the liver: Prognostic factors and results of surgical treatment, in Gitnick G (ed): *Current Hepatology*, vol 10. St Louis, Mosby-Year Book, 1990, pp 205–220.

4. Silen W: Hepatic resection for metastases from colorectal carcinoma is of dubious value. *Arch Surg* 1989; 124:1021–1022.

5. Saenz NC, et al: Experience with colorectal carcinoma metastatic to the liver. *Surg Clin North Am* 1989; 69:361–370.

6. Foster JH: Survival after liver resection for secondary tumors. *Am J Surg* 1978; 135:389–394.

7. Cady B, II, et al: Survival of patients after colonic resection for carcinoma with simultaneous liver metastasis. *Surg Gynecol Obstet* 1970; 131:697–700.

8. Hughes K, et al: Surgery for colorectal cancer metastatic to the liver: Optimizing the results of treatment. *Surg Clin North Am* 1989; 69:339–359.

9. Finlay IG, II, et al: Incidence and detection of occult hepatic metastases in colorectal carcinoma. *BMJ* 1982; 284:803–805.

10. Bentsson G, et al: Natural history of patients with untreated liver metastases from colorectal cancer. *Am J Surg* 1981; 141:586–589.

11. Gastrointestinal Tumor Study Group: Adjuvant therapy of colon cancer—results of a prospectively randomized trial. *N Engl J Med* 1984; 310:737–743.

12. Gastrointestinal Tumor Study Group: Prolongation of the disease-free interval in surgically treated rectal carcinoma. *N Engl J Med* 1985; 312:1465–1472.

13. Willet CG, et al: Failure patterns following curative resection of colonic carcinoma. *Ann Surg* 1984; 200:685–692.

14. Welch JP, et al: Detection and treatment of recurrent cancer of the colon and rectum. *Am J Surg* 1978; 135:505–511.

15. Pestana C, et al: The natural history of carcinoma of the colon and rectum. *Am J Surg* 1964; 108:826–829.

16. Moertel CG, et al: Alimentary tract cancer: Large bowel, in Holland J, et al (eds): *Cancer Medicine*. Philadelphia, Lea & Febiger, 1982, pp 1830–1859.

17. Lefor AT, et al: Intra-abdominal extrahepatic disease in patients with colorectal hepatic metastases. *Dis Colon Rectum* 1988; 31:100–103.

18. Kemeny M, et al: Preoperative staging with computerized axial tomography and biochemical laboratory tests in patients with hepatic metastases. *Ann Surg* 1986; 203:169–172.

19. Parker CP, et al: Cost effectiveness of liver scanning in the detection of hepatic metastasis in newly diagnosed colorectal carcinoma. *Prog Clin Biol Res* 1986; 216:191–197.

20. Colizza S, et al: Combined ultrasounds and CEA in preoperative assessment of hepatic metastases from gastrointestinal malignancies. *J Surg Oncol* 1985; 28:161–164.

21. Tartter PI, et al: Screening for liver metastases from colorectal cancer with carcinoembryonic antigen and alkaline phosphatase. *Ann Surg* 1981; 193:357–360.

22. August DA, et al: Lymphatic dissemination of hepatic metastases: Implications for the follow-up and treatment of patients with colorectal cancer. *Cancer* 1985; 55:1490–1494.

23. Steele G, et al: New surgical treatment for recurrent colorectal cancer. *Cancer* 1990; 65:723–730.

24. Minton JP, et al: Results of surgical excision of one to 13 hepatic metastases in 98 consecutive patients. *Arch Surg* 1989; 124:46–48.

25. August DA, et al: Hepatic resection of colorectal metastases: Influence of clinical factors and adjuvant intraperitoneal 5-fluorouracil via Tenckhoff catheter on survival. *Ann Surg* 1985; 201:210–218.

26. Lee YM: Metastatic cancer of the liver: Diagnosis with radiological and laboratory tests, in Gitnick G (ed): *Current Hepatology,* vol 8. St Louis, Mosby-Year Book, 1988, pp 303–326.

27. Mittal R, et al: Accuracy of computerized tomography in determining hepatic tumor size in patients receiving liver transplantation or resection. *J Clin Oncol* 1984; 2:637–642.

28. Steele G, et al: A prospective evaluation of hepatic resection for colorectal carcinoma metastases to the liver: Gastrointestinal Tumor Study Group Protocol 6584. *J Clin Oncol* 1991; 9:1105–1112.

29. Reinig JW, et al: Liver metastasis detection: Comparative sensitivities of MR imaging and CT scanning. *Radiology* 1987; 162:43–47.

30. Sitzmann JV, et al: Preoperative assessment of malignant hepatic tumors. *Am J Surg* 1990; 159:137–143.

31. Hughes KS, et al: Resection of the liver for metastatic solid tumors, in Rosenberg SA (ed): *Surgical Treatment of Metastatic Cancer.* Philadelphia, Lippincott, 1988, pp 125–164.

32. Gunven P, et al: Preoperative imaging of liver metastases. *Ann Surg* 1985; 202:573–579.

33. Fortner JG, et al: Multivariate analysis of a personal series of 247 consecutive patients with liver metastases from colorectal cancer. *Ann Surg* 1984; 199:306–316.

34. Hughes KS, et al: Extrahepatic tumor deposits mis-diagnosed as intrahepatic metastases. *Arch Surg* 1988; 123:1013–1015.

35. Rajpal S, et al: Extensive resections of isolated metastasis from carcinoma of the colon and rectum. *Surg Gynecol Obstet* 1982; 155:813–816.

36. Thompson HH, et al: Major hepatic resection: A 25-year experience. *Ann Surg* 1983; 197:375–388.

37. Iwatsuki S, et al: Experience with 150 liver resections. *Ann Surg* 1983; 197:247–253.

38. Tomas-dela Vega JE, et al: A ten year experience with hepatic resection. *Surg Gynecol Obstet* 1984; 159:223–228.

39. Kortz WJ, et al: Hepatic resection for metastatic cancer. *Ann Surg* 1984; 199:182–186.

40. Cady B, et al: Major hepatic resection for metachronous metastases from colon cancer. *Ann Surg* 1985; 201:204–209.

41. Gennari L, et al: Surgical treatment of hepatic metastases from colorectal cancer. *Ann Surg* 1986; 203:49–54.

42. Butler J, et al: Hepatic resection for metastases of the colon and rectum. *Surg Gynecol Obstet* 1986; 162:109–113.

43. Nordlinger B, et al: Hepatic resection for colorectal liver metastases: Influence on survival of preoperative factors and surgery for recurrences in 80 patients. *Ann Surg* 1987; 205:256–263.

44. Bozzetti F, et al: Pattern of failure following resection of colorectal cancer liver metastases: Rationale for a multimodal approach. *Ann Surg* 1987; 205:264–270.

45. Patt YZ, et al: Adjuvant perioperative hepatic arterial mitomycin C and floxuridine combined with surgical resection of metastatic colorectal cancer in the liver. *Cancer* 1987; 59:867–873.

46. Iwatsuki S, et al: Personal experience with 411 hepatic resections. *Ann Surg* 1988; 208:421–434.

47. Holm A, et al: Hepatic resection of metastasis from colorectal carcinoma: Morbidity, mortality, and pattern of recurrence. *Ann Surg* 1989; 209:428–434.

48. Savage AP, et al: Elective and emergency hepatic resection: Determinants of operative mortality and morbidity. *Ann Surg* 1991; 214:689–695.

49. Younes RN, et al: The influence of intraoperative hypotension and perioperative blood transfusion

on disease-free survival in patients with complete resection of colorectal liver metastases. *Ann Surg* 1991; 214:107–113.

49a. Niederhuber JE, et al: Surgical considerations in the management of hepatic neoplasia. *Semin Oncol* 1983; 10:135–147.

50. Fortner J, et al: Hepatic resection in the elderly. *Ann Surg* 1990; 211:141–145.

51. Hodgson WJB, et al: Hepatic resection for primary and metastatic tumors using the ultrasonic surgical dissector. *Am J Surg* 1992; 163:246–250.

52. Terblanche J, et al: Simplified hepatic resection with the use of prolonged vascular inflow occlusion. *Arch Surg* 1991; 126:298–301.

53. Wilson SM, et al: Surgical treatment of hepatic metastases from colorectal cancers. *Arch Surg* 1976; 111:330–334.

54. Attiyeh FF, et al: Hepatic resection for metastases from colorectal cancer. *Dis Colon Rectum* 1978; 21:160–162.

55. Foster JH: Survival after liver resection for secondary tumors. *Am J Surg* 1978; 135:389–394.

56. Registry of Hepatic Metastases: Resection of the liver for colorectal carcinoma metastases: A multi-institutional study of indications for resection. *Surgery* 1988; 103:278–288.

57. Wagner JS, et al: The natural history of hepatic metastases from colorectal cancer. *Ann Surg* 1984; 199:502–507.

58. Adson MA: The resection of hepatic metastases: Another view. *Arch Surg* 1989; 124:1023–1024.

59. Cobourn CS, et al: Examination of patient selection and outcome for hepatic resection for metastatic disease. *Surg Gynecol Obstet* 1987; 165:239–246.

60. Stehlin JS, et al: Treatment of cancer of the liver; twenty years experience with infusion and resection in 414 patients. *Ann Surg* 1988; 208:23–25.

61. Adson MA, et al: Resection of hepatic metastases from colorectal cancer. *Arch Surg* 1984; 119:647–651.

62. Stephenson KR, et al: Perioperative blood transfusions are associated with decreased time to recurrence and decreased survival after resection of colorectal liver metastases. *Ann Surg* 1988; 208:679–687.

63. Blumberg N, et al: Further evidence supporting a cause and effect relationship between blood transfusion and earlier cancer recurrence. *Ann Surg* 1988; 207:410–415.

64. Fernandez LA, et al: Immunologic changes after blood transfusion in patients undergoing vascular surgery. *Am J Surg* 1992; 163:263–269.

65. Steele G, et al: Resection of hepatic metastases from colorectal cancer: Biologic perspectives. *Ann Surg* 1989; 210:127–138.

CHAPTER 8

Complications of Portal Hypertension

Harold O. Conn, M.D.

Professor Emeritus, Yale University School of Medicine, New Haven, Connecticut; Department of Veteran's Affairs Medical Center, West Haven, Connecticut

All that glisters is not gold

The Merchant of Venice
William Shakespeare

We are in a logarithmic growth phase of publications that deal with portal hypertension and its complications. Indeed, there were so many articles about hemorrhage from esophagogastric varices, the most newsworthy complication, published in major, peer-reviewed medical journals that it is not possible to include all of them without simply listing the references. Therefore, we have cited and discussed only a small fraction of these articles—approximately 10%. Those selected included all that were intrinsically important and those that helped to define a new trend such as the sudden emergence of the transjugular intrahepatic portal-systemic stent-shunt (TIPS). In fact, I have emphasized TIPS as the *topic of the year* by discussing it first.

HEMORRHAGE FROM ESOPHAGOGASTRIC VARICES

Transjugular Intrahepatic Portal-Systemic Stent-Shunts

The big news in the management of portal hypertension this year is the emergence of TIPS. After a quarter of a century in the wings,[1-4] TIPS suddenly took over the spotlight at center stage as a clinical procedure.

TIPS are man-made, artificial fistulas between intrahepatic branches of the portal and the hepatic veins. They remain patent because of the introduction of an expandable stainless steel mesh stent between the vessels. The Palmaz stent[4] (Johnson & Johnson International Systems, Warren, NJ) and the Wallstent (Schneider, Minneapolis) are the two stents that are most widely used at present.

During 1992, a number of important articles about the early clinical results have been published,[5-8] but most of the literature consists of abstracts, many of which are cited in a review article published in January 1993.[9]

A TIPS functions as a side-to-side portacaval anastomosis (PCA) with similar indications, contraindications, effects, and complications as a surgical PCA.

Indications

TIPS reduces portal pressure and consequently is used in the *prevention of variceal hemorrhage* in patients with portal hypertension.[5, 8-13] They may be used to prevent recurrent hemorrhages after the bleeding from varices has been controlled, to control hemorrhage in patients who are actively bleeding,[5, 14] and even to prevent the initial hemorrhage from varices, although this last indication has not yet been reported.

One fascinating subgroup of such indications is the use of TIPS in patients who bleed while awaiting liver transplantation and who need temporary portal decompression until an appropriate liver can be found and implanted.[11, 15] Of course, TIPS is a much less invasive procedure than surgical PCA, which cannot be tolerated by many such critically ill patients. Furthermore, intrahepatic shunts do not increase the difficulty of transplantation surgery since the stent is completely removed when the recipient's liver is excised. Technical problems with the portal vein can usually be overcome by providing for the transplant surgeons a more generous segment of portal vein during its harvesting from the donor. The presence of surgical PCA, however, may complicate liver transplantation.[16-18]

Undoubtedly, prophylactic TIPS will be studied to determine whether this relatively benign procedure will be as effective as surgical PCA and safer.[19] Certainly, it must be compared with endoscopic sclerotherapy[20] and pharmacologic therapy such as propranolol[21] and/or nitrates.[22]

The second most important indication of TIPS is *ascites*.[6, 23-26] It has been used in intractable ascites in cirrhotic patients[23-25] and in at least one patient with the Budd-Chiari syndrome.[26] Because the insertion of TIPS is associated with improvement in renal function[23, 24] and because side-to-side PCA can reverse the hepato-renal syndrome (HRS),[27] a trial of TIPS in HRS is clearly an investigation that should be performed in the near future.

Contraindications

Contraindications to the performance of TIPS are anatomic abnormalities of the caval, hepatic, or portal venous systems or thromboses of any of these vessels. Severe coagulopathy, particularly disseminated intravascular coagulopathy (DIC), is a relative contraindication. Polycystic disease of the liver is a contraindication for fear of causing extra hepatic bleeding, i.e. hematuria.

Clinical Results

The procedure can be accomplished in well over 90% of patients[9, 14] with an acceptably low "operative" mortality. It appears to reduce the risks of recurrent hemorrhage from varices, and like PCA, it seems able to stop active variceal hemorrhage immediately.[14] It reduces portal venous pressure by about half, a mean reduction of approximately 10 mm Hg,[9,14] and it decreases the size of esophageal varices.

Ascites disappears or is ameliorated by TIPS,[7, 23–25] but its long-term effects have not been established. It is not possible to determine its effect on mortality until randomized clinical trials have been followed for a long period.

Complications

Portal-systemic encephalopathy (PSE) is the most common complication, and it has been reported in about 20% of patients.[9, 28–31] In general, the encephalopathy is mild and relatively responsive to therapy. Objective studies of the frequency and severity of PSE in comparison to cirrhosis *au natural* or to those with portal-systemic shunts have not yet been carried out. The relative infrequency and mildness of post-TIPS PSE probably reflects the small size of the shunts.[32, 33]

Stenosis

Stenosis and occlusion are common complications of TIPS and occur in 10% to 15% and 5% to 10%, respectively.[9] The stenosis is usually the consequence of intimal hypertrophy,[34] which appears to be an exaggeration of the normal endothelialization of steel stents that quickly converts them to true, blood-carrying, endothelium-lined blood vessels. The endothelialization process is usually complete within a month after implantation. This pseudointimal hyperplasia probably occurs more commonly than has been seen to present and may well be a function of the duration the stent remains in situ.

Intravascular hemolysis has been described in one dramatic case[35] in which the hemolysis appeared to represent traumatic, "Waring blender–like" hemolysis associated with trauma to erythrocytes by the exposed, nonendothelialized steel wires of the stent. Unpublished observations suggest that such hemolytic syndromes will probably be seen with increasing frequency.

Miscellaneous complications of stent implantation include rupture of the hepatic capsule with intra-abdominal hemorrhage,[13, 14] puncture of the gallbladder,[14] sepsis,[6, 14, 36] portal vein thrombosis,[36] "wandering stents,"[6] and pulmonary emboli. Others will be reported in time.

TIPS is an exciting new therapy that, it is hoped, will significantly change our approach to a variety of the complications of portal hypertension. Until the overall risks of implantation, late complications, and benefits are studied in randomized, controlled trials (RCTs), however, it will not be possible to state with assurance what the ultimate place of TIPS will be.

A complete review of TIPS through 1992 had been published by the author of this chapter.[9]

HEMORRHAGE FROM ESOPHAGEAL VARICES

Primary Prophylaxis

Prevention of the initial hemorrhage, which has a very high mortality rate, is the most rational approach to improving survival in cirrhotic patients with varices (Table 1). The most impressive of the investigations of primary prophylaxis, in which β-adrenergic blockade (BAB) was studied, has been discussed in detail previously.[37, 38]

Pagliaro et al. have recently reported a meta-analysis of the nonsurgical prevention of hemorrhage from esophageal varices (HEV).[39] This article, which summarizes the results of seven published RCTs that include 902 patients, concluded that BAB significantly decreases the risks of HEV in patients with large varices and corrected portal venous pressure levels ($>$12 mm Hg). Survival, however, was not significantly improved. A second meta-analysis based on the *individual* data from four of these seven RCTs showed similar results.[40] It can be inferred from these studies that the risks of HEV in cirrhotic patients with medium-sized or large varices by semiquantitative endoscopic grading, the red color endoscopic signs, and/or elevated portal venous pressure are significantly reduced by prophylactic propranolol therapy.

Similar meta-analyses of prophylactic *endoscopic sclerotherapy* (EST) of 15 published articles that included 1,498 patients demonstrated quite different results[39, 41] (Fig 1). These investigations, which reached conflicting conclusions, were very heterogeneous in a variety of ways: first, the high frequency of serious side effects of EST; second, the variations in technique (intravariceal vs. paravariceal, dosage, frequency of therapy, etc.); and third, the variable quality of the RCTs analyzed. Indeed, the early studies such as those of Paquet[42] and Witzel et al.,[43] which showed EST to be extremely beneficial in preventing bleeding and reducing mor-

TABLE 1.

Hemorrhage From Esophageal Varices

Primary prophylaxis
    Pharmacologic
        β-Adrenergic blockade
        Nitrates
    Endoscopic sclerotherapy
    Portal decompression
    Portal devascularization
Secondary prophylaxis
    Pharmacologic
        β-Adrenergic blockade
        Nitrates
        Somatostatin
        Octreotide
    Endoscopic therapy
        Sclerotherapy
        Variceal banding (ligation)
    Portal decompression
    Portal devascularization
Emergency
    Pharmacologic
    Endoscopic
    Portal decompression

tality rates, received relatively low quality scores.[39] As the design and execution of these investigations improved, however, the apparent efficacy of EST declined. This phenomenon may be considered a corollary of the aphorism that early therapeutic results are usually better than those observed by later investigators. It is interesting that the quality scores of the EST studies that were performed in the early 1980s were significantly lower than the scores of the RCTs of BAB, which were performed more recently[39] (Fig 2).

Prophylactic portal decompression operations have been shown in an earlier meta-analysis[44] to abolish bleeding from varices almost completely, but not to improve survival significantly. Indeed, prophylactic PCA *diminished* survival.[44, 45] No new RCT of primary prophylactic portal-systemic shunts has been reported in the past few years.

Prophylactic *portal nondecompressive devascularization* procedures have been shown to be beneficial in reducing HEV and mortality rates, but confirmation is needed.[46, 47]

Secondary Prophylaxis

Treatment with BAB has been shown to reduce significantly the incidence of HEV, but not of death.[21, 44] No new RCTs of BAB or beneficial reports of other therapeutic agents have been reported since.

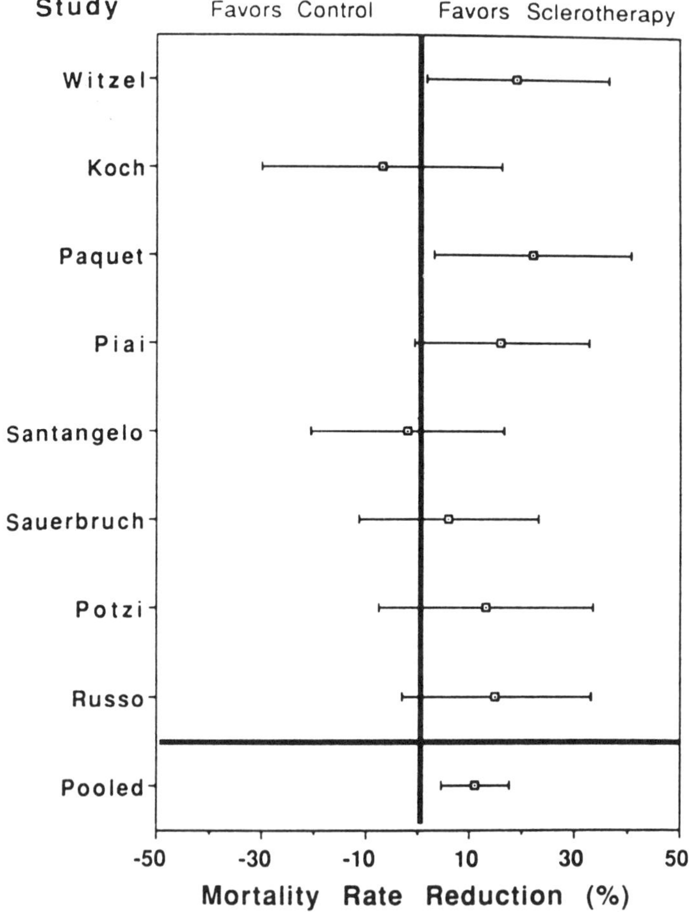

FIG 1.

Meta-analysis of mortality rate from randomized controlled trials of primary prophylaxis using endoscopic sclerotherapy. The 13-month mortality rate reduction is the mortality rate in the prophylactic sclerotherapy group minus the mortality rate in the control group. For each individual study *squares* represent the absolute mortality rate difference, and *error bars* represent 95% confidence intervals. (From Van Ruiswyk J, Byrd JC: *Gastroenterology* 1992; 102:587–597. Used by permission.)

Endoscopic Sclerotherapy

Previous analysis of secondary prophylactic (therapeutic) EST suggest that EST appeared to reduce the risks of recurrent HEV but did not improve survival.[44]

Endoscopic sclerotherapy was reviewed in 1,000 consecutive patients treated between 1982 and 1990 by Hashizume et al.[48] Variceal bleeding was controlled in 98% of the 215 actively bleeding patients. Varices were eradicated in 78% of the patients with the intensive, large-volume obliterative-type EST employed by this group.[49, 50] The 5-year cumulative rate of bleeding in those patients whose varices

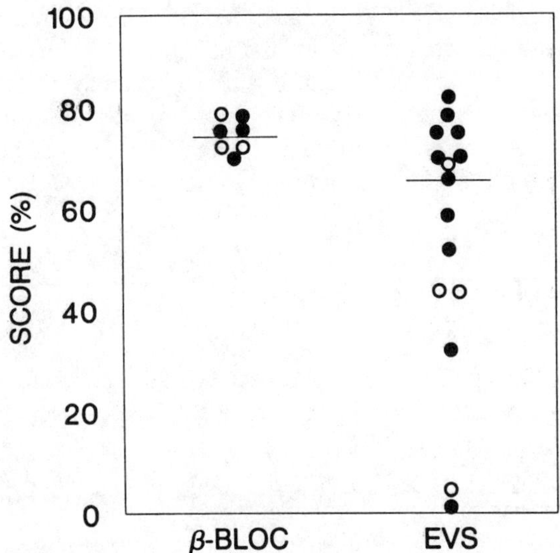

FIG 2.
Quality score of randomized clinical trials (RCTs) of the prevention of variceal hemorrhage. *Open circles* indicate RCTs in which a statistically significant favorable treatment effect was found. *Horizontal bars* represent median quality scores. β-BLOC = β-blockers; EVS = endoscopic variceal sclerotherapy. (From Pagliaro L, D'Amico G, Sorensen TIA: *Ann Intern Med* 1992; 117:59–70. Used by permission.)

had been eradicated was only 5%. Clearly, this intensive form of EST, which causes necrosis of the submucosal tissue and leaves behind dense submucosal scar, is effective. The data are complicated, however, since patients with active variceal bleeding, patients whose variceal hemorrhage had been controlled, and patients who had never bled from varices were included. Furthermore, more than 30% of the patients had hepatocellular carcinoma. Applicability to American patients is problematic since Japanese patients are more compliant and Japanese endoscopists appear to be more aggressive and more compulsive about EST.

One form of surgical therapy that has only rarely been used in the West is the *nondecompressive devascularization* procedure of Sugiura and Futagawa[51] that is commonly used in Japan. A modification of this procedure that excludes splenectomy, vagotomy, and pyloroplasty[52] was compared with EST in 100 patients 5 days after the index bleeding episode had been controlled.[53] In this RCT directed by the late David Triger, the two groups were similar in demographic and clinical features, i.e., predominantly middle-aged men with mild, alcoholic cirrhosis (Child's [Pugh] class A and B). There was a fascinating, hitherto unused exclusion criterion, i.e., patients who were hepatitis B surface antigen (HBsAg)-positive were excluded to prevent hepatitis B virus (HBV) exposure of the operating team for whom HBV vaccination was not available. Ninety-two patients were analyzed. Rebleeding occurred more frequently in the EST group (one half vs. one third in the surgical group) and required significantly more blood transfusions. Mortality was higher in the surgically treated patients, largely as a consequence of the operative mortality, but cumulative survival curves were similar thereafter. Costs were about four times greater for the surgical patients than for the EST-treated group ($P < .0001$). No cases of HBV hepatitis were mentioned. It is possible that the differences in results between EST and devascularization were in part a consequence of the modifications in the original devascularization operation since the latter procedure included splenectomy, which itself is a portal-decompressive procedure in patients with cirrhosis.

Emergency Pharmacologic Therapy

Pharmacologic therapy for bleeding varices started with posterior pituitary extract and advanced to vasopressin and then to triglycylvasopressin, glypressin, pharmacologic combinations of complementary drugs such as vasopressin plus nitroglycerin, somatostatin, and finally, octreotide, a synthetic analogue of somatostatin with advantageous properties. Although these various vasoconstrictive agents were effective to varying degrees in suppressing active bleeding, none was shown to improve survival. Indeed, it would be surprising if any such agent used in the active bleeding phase of variceal bleeding would be able to improve survival in patients in whom definitive therapy to prevent recurrences of bleeding had not yet been undertaken. Nothing published in 1992 has changed the status quo.

Emergency Endoscopic Therapy

Endoscopic Sclerotherapy

Endoscopic sclerotherapy is widely recognized as effective therapy for actively bleeding varices since it stops active bleeding in well over 90% of patients,[44, 48] although its use is associated with frequent severe complications.

Endoscopic Ligation

The introduction of endoscopic ligation of varices (ELV) occurred in 1986.[54] By 1990 a comparison of ELV and EST showed that the former was at least equal to EST in efficacy and survival.[55] In 1992 an RCT comparing the two endoscopic techniques was reported and suggested that ELV was superior.[56] In this study of 129 patients, 27 of whom were actively bleeding, it was found that ELV resulted in better control of active bleeding than did EST (86% vs. 77%; $P > .05$), fewer recurrences of bleeding varices (36% vs. 48%; $P > .05$), a lower complication rate (2% vs. 22%; $P < .001$), and a lower mortality rate (28% vs. 45%; $P < .05$) (Fig 3). The lower complication and mortality rates suggest that this new technique is superior to sclerotherapy. Can other endoscopists do as well with the elastic banding technique as the originators? This multicenter trial suggests that they can.

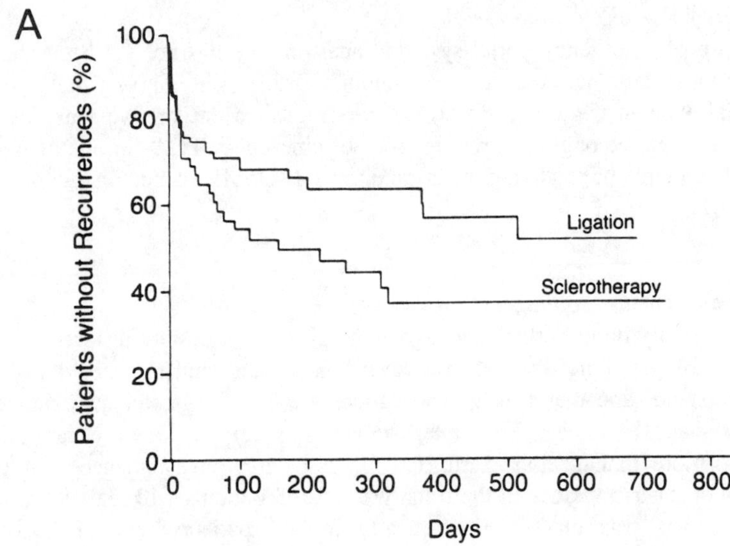

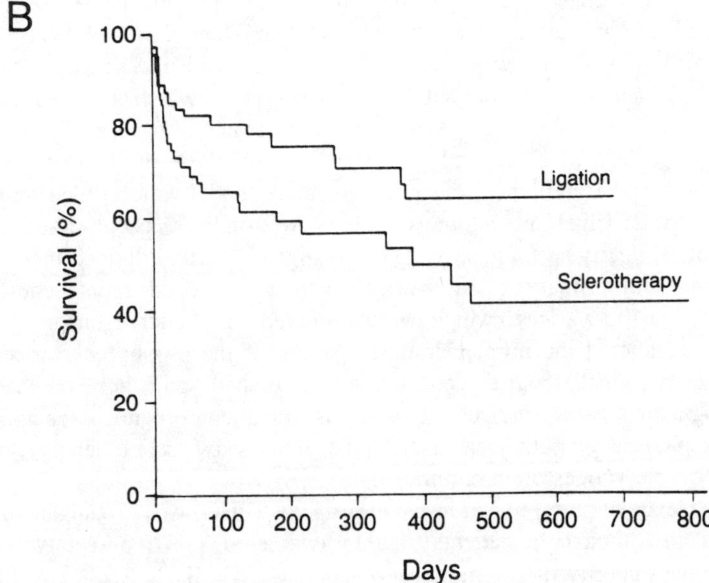

FIG 3.
A, absence of recurrent bleeding after initial treatment of variceal bleeding by endoscopic sclerotherapy or endoscopic ligation in patients with cirrhosis. The difference between groups was not statistically significant ($P = .072$). **B,** survival in patients with cirrhosis and bleeding esophageal varices treated with endoscopic sclerotherapy or endoscopic ligation. The survival rate in patients treated with endoscopic ligation was significantly higher ($P = .041$) than that in patients treated with endoscopic sclerotherapy. (From Stiegmann G, Goff JS, Sun JH: *Am J Surg* 1990; 159:21–26. Used by permission.)

Emergency Portal Decompression

The use of emergency portal-systemic anastomoses has not yet been shown to be superior to emergency EST,[57, 58] although Orloff et al. suggest that it may be beneficial even in Child's C cirrhosis.[59] As indicated earlier, we must await the results of objective ongoing investigations of emergency PCA, in one of which at least 100 patients have already been randomized (Orloff M, personal communication).

Gastric and Gastroesophageal Varices

It is generally thought that esophageal and gastric varices are different anatomic variations of the same disorder. However, physicians tend to fear what they do not understand, and therefore gastric varices are held in greater awe and respect than esophageal varices. The latter somehow seem to be more familiar and therefore more manageable. Sarin and his associates have enhanced our understanding of gastric varices in their analysis of 568 patients with gastric varices.[60] The diagnosis was made endoscopically in 301 patients with cirrhosis, 115 patients with noncirrhotic portal hypertension, 117 patients with extrahepatic portal vein obstruction, and 35 patients with hepatic vein obstruction. Of the 568, 363 had bled from varices and 175 had not bled. They classified gastric varices anatomically (Fig 4) as *gastroesophageal varices* or (isolated) *gastric varices*. Gastroesophageal varices were subdivided into type 1, which involved the lesser curvature, and type 2, which extended to the greater curvature. Type 2 had a greater propensity to bleed and to do so severely. Gastric varices were also divided into type 1 and type 2. Type 1, which are fundal varices, bled frequently, whereas type 2, which are ectopic varices, were usually seen only after EST and did not bleed nearly so frequently. The investigators further divided their patients into those with primary gastric varices, which developed spontaneously, and secondary gastric varices, which were observed only after esophageal sclerotherapy had altered the normal drainage pattern of the esophageal varices. This classification, which requires confirmation, may shed some light on the pathophysiology of gastric varices as well as on their prognosis and therapy. Gastroesophageal varices can usually be treated by sclerotherapy, whereas isolated gastric varices often require surgery.

The presence of portal hypertensive gastropathy (PHG) was investigated by Vigneri et al. in 136 cirrhotic patients[61] and by Iwao et al. in 47 consecutive cirrhotic patients, the majority of whom had posthepatitic cirrhosis.[62] About two thirds of both groups had gastropathy, in about half of whom it was mild and in half severe. The presence of PHG was independent of age, sex, etiology, severity of the cirrhosis, or the grade of esophageal varices. The hepatic vein pressure gradient (HVPG) was significantly greater in patients with severe PHG than in those with mild PHG or in those without PHG. Clearance of indocyanine green was decreased in patients with PHG. These studies suggest that as the severity of the cirrhosis increases, the presence and severity of PHG increases as well.

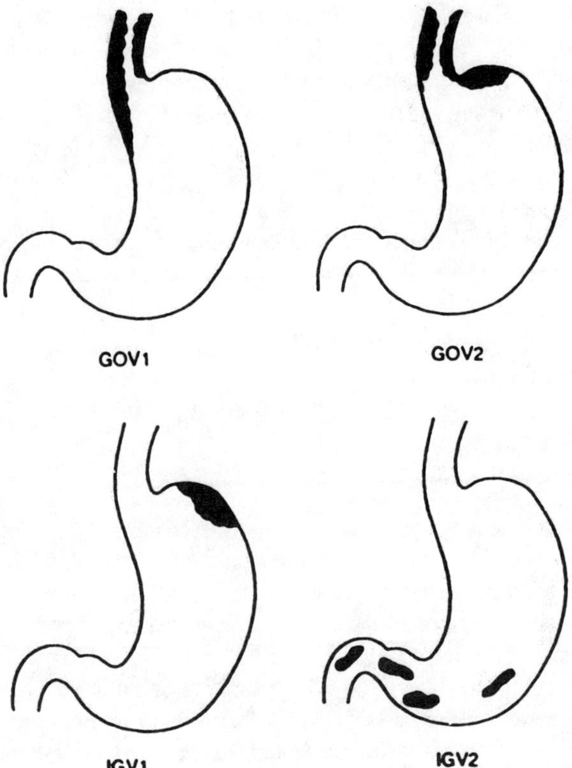

FIG 4.
Diagrams of the distribution of gastric varices. GOV_1 (gastroesophageal varices type 1) are continuous with esophageal varices and extend 2 to 5 cm below the gastroesophageal junction along the lesser curve of the stomach. GOV_2 (gastroesophageal varices type 2) are continuous with esophageal varices that extend into the fundus of the stomach. IGV_1 (isolated gastric varices type 1) are restricted to the fundus of the stomach. IGV_2 (isolated gastric varices type 2) may be seen anywhere in the stomach including the body, antrum, or varices. (From Sarin SK, Lahoti D, Saxena SP: *Hepatology* 1992; 16:1343–1349. Used by permission.)

Pharmacologic Therapy for Esophagogastric Varices in the Future

Pharmacologic treatment of portal hypertension over the past 40 years has progressed from one vasoconstrictor to another: first posterior pituitary extract, then vasopressin, then somatostatin, followed by its synthetic analogue octreotide and, later, BAB. Nitroglycerin, a vasodilator, was first introduced to antagonize some of the undesirable vasoconstrictive effects of vasopressin.[63] Since then other combinations of vasoconstrictors and vasodilators, such as vasopressin plus ketanserin, have been introduced and show similar or perhaps superior effects.[64] New vasodilators such as *molsidomine* have been used alone in patients with portal hypertension and show portal pressure–reducing effects.[65] This agent, which is free of the tolerance that develops with other organic nitrates, may be a treatment of the future since only small decrements in portal venous pressure may be sufficient to prevent hemorrhage from varices. *Nipradilol* is another exciting new drug. It is a potent antihypertensive, antianginal, noncardioselective β-adrenergic blocker that does not reduce cardiac output in cirrhotic patients.[66] Its isopropyl-amino-propranolol side chain and nitroester group provide competing vasoconstrictive and vasodilatory effects that simulate the combination of vasopressin and nitroglycerin. Soon we will be reading about RCTs with some of these agents alone and in combination.

ASCITES

Pathophysiology

Ascites is the most common and probably the most complex of the adverse consequences of portal hypertension. Its appearance is often an unwelcome harbinger of other complications to come—hemorrhage from varices, spontaneous bacterial peritonitis (SBP), and HRS. The last major advance in our understanding of ascites was the recognition by multiple investigators at multiple places around the globe that peripheral arterial vasodilation is the primary abnormality in the formation of ascites.[67] Dudley has written a thoughtful review that cites virtually all the articles worth citing that had been published through 1990.[68]

Mysteries persist, however. Ascitic cirrhotic patients have been reported to have circulating levels of atrial natriuretic peptide (ANP) that were increased,[69] normal,[70] and decreased.[71]

Sometimes ANP seems to exhibit paradoxical plasma concentrations. As has been recently shown again by Angeli et al., ANP concentrations in plasma are higher in cirrhotic patients than in control subjects (71 ± 47 vs. 42 ± 16 pg/mL; $P < .025$).[72] Levels of ANP were higher in patients who subsequently exhibited spontaneous diuresis than in those who required diuretic therapy (213 ± 194 vs. 72 ± 41 pg/mL; $P < .025$). In addition, ANP concentrations were higher in those who responded to spironolactone therapy (500 mg daily) than in those who were more resistant to diuretic therapy and required furosemide as well as spironolactone (76 ± 49 vs. 51 ± 19 pg/mL; $P < .05$). Keep in mind that the ANP and renal function measurements in these studies were made before diuretic therapy and are therefore not the effects of diuretic therapy. The investigators interpret these data to mean that patients who diurese spontaneously exhibit "filled" or "overfilled" plasma volumes but that those who tend to be less responsive, i.e., more resistant to diuretic therapy, become progressively more "underfilled" as an antinatriuretic state progressively develops, as reflected by increasing ANP levels.

I personally view the response to spironolactone alone as the result of optimal, logical therapy directed primarily against the elevated aldosterone levels and activity. Indeed, spironolactone not only inhibits sodium reabsorption by the renal tubules but also inhibits aldosterone synthesis in the zona glomerulosa of the adrenal gland.[73] I think of the use of furosemide as less logical, more hostile therapy since such diuretic agents may be considered to be tubular toxins. Admittedly, they are mild toxins, but they are toxins, nevertheless.

Atrial natriuretic peptide appears to compensate for vasoconstrictive, sodium-retaining factors such as the renin-angiotensin-aldosterone and the sympathetic nervous systems. However, when ANP is most needed in advanced ascites, cirrhotic patients appear to become resistant to it. Morali et al. suggested that this phenomenon is a consequence of the fact that sodium reabsorption occurs proximal to the site at which ANP acts.[74] They confirmed this hypothesis by showing that the administration of mannitol causes more distal delivery of sodium to the inner medullary collecting tubules and greater natriuresis. These observations indicate that the intracellular signaling mechanisms remain intact and suggest new therapeutic approaches. Not all patients respond in this way, however; it appears that those who have the most severe cirrhosis do not, and, therefore, have the worst prognosis.

Some of the variability in ANP concentrations may reflect variations in the diurnal pattern of ANP levels in plasma. Panos and his associates disclosed a pronounced diurnal pattern in cirrhotic subjects.[75] Urinary sodium excretion in normal subjects is highest between 4:00 P.M. and midnight, while they are mobile, and lowest between midnight and 8:00 A.M., when they are recumbent. Plasma ANP levels parallel sodium excretion from 4:00 P.M. until 8:00 A.M. and peak between midnight and 8:00 A.M., but not during the early part of the day (8:00 A.M. to 4:00 P.M.) (Fig 5). Plasma renin activity (PRA) and plasma aldosterone concentrations, which were always much higher in cirrhotic patients than in control subjects, tended to peak between noon and 8:00 P.M.. In control subjects ANP, PRA, and plasma aldosterone all remain relatively constant except for peaks in aldosterone at noon and at 4:00 A.M. These observations suggest that ANP contributes to the nocturnal diuresis of cirrhosis, perhaps a consequence of reduced PRA and plasma aldosterone during recumbency.

Mineralocorticoid escape is the phenomenon of becoming unresponsive to the sodium-retaining effects of mineralocorticoids such as α_2-fluorohydrocortisone despite continued administration of the steroid.[76] It is common in patients with compensated cirrhosis. This unresponsiveness appears to be related to inadequate expansion of effective plasma volume, which is in turn a consequence of the accumulation of ascites that tends to occur in patients with severe, peripheral, arteriolar vasodilation. Thus, failure to escape occurs almost exclusively in compensated cirrhotic patients who are not at risk for the development of ascites. What came first, the chicken or the egg?

Salis-Herrazo et al. have shown that the metabolic clearance of arginine vasopressin is decreased in cirrhosis and, furthermore, that this abnormal metabolism appears to be a consequence of diminished hepatic function.[77] These investigations do not themselves solve any major ascitic problems, but they do contribute to our

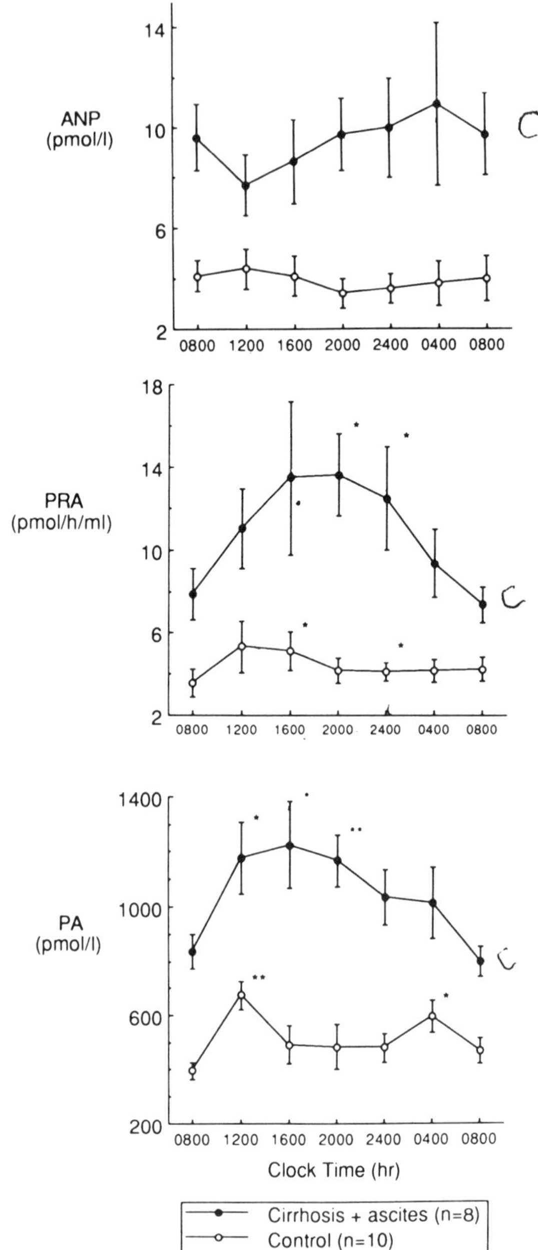

FIG 5.

Circadian rhythm in ten control and eight cirrhotic patients with ascites. ANP = atrial na-triuretic peptide; PRA = plasma renin activity; PA = plasma aldosterone. (From Panos MZ, Anderson JV, Payne N: *Hepatology* 1992; 16:42–48. Used by permission.)

overall understanding and ultimately will eventually contribute to the solution of such refractory syndromes.

It has recently been reported that concentrations of *interleukin-6* (IL-6) are increased in ascitic patients with cirrhosis (1,700 ± 2,100 pg/mL) and with malignant ascites (4,000 ± 1,500 pg/mL).[78] Interleukin-1 was not found. The ascitic fluid concentration was approximately 100 times greater than in serum in cirrhosis and almost 600-fold greater in malignant ascites. The authors concluded that the IL-6 was produced in the peritoneal cavity. The explanation for the increased synthesis is not known. None of the patients studied had bacterial infection. Endotoxins are a possible cause. It was suggested that the presence of IL-6 in ascitic fluid could explain the fever that often occurs with ascites reinfusions and after opening peritoneovenous shunts. Unfortunately, the investigators did not indicate whether the malignant ascitic fluid was due to intrahepatic or to intraperitoneal metastases (or whether there was a difference in IL-6 levels between these two types of "malignant" ascitic fluid). Conceivably, the concentration of IL-6 might parallel that of albumin, as do complement levels. (I would predict so.)

The introduction of cardiologists and cardiac hemodynamics into the assessment of patients with cirrhosis is long overdue. Friedman and Fernando in a small, simple study of 20 cirrhotic patients demonstrated that cirrhotic patients had higher heart rates, left ventricular end-diastolic volume, left ventricular ejection fractions, and cardiac outputs and lower mean arterial pressures than normal subjects.[79] These hemodynamic abnormalities correlated well with the estimated volume of ascites. They concluded that the presence of ascites is not simply the accumulation of lymph fluid in the peritoneal cavity but represents intense vasodilation with a hyperdynamic circulation. That is what hepatologists have been saying for years.

Diagnosis

The diagnosis of ascites can be considered on many levels.[80] *Is ascites present or not?* In the distant past this question was answered by physical examination. More recently it has been made by ultrasonography. When all else fails, it is settled by trial by needle. When ascitic fluid appears in the syringe, the answer is clear. When it is not, we may still be uncertain.

Is Neoplastic Ascites Caused by Chronic, Intrinsic Liver Disease or by Neoplasm?

Runyon and Mauer and their coworkers have shown that the *serum ascites-albumin gradient (SAAG)* is the simplest and most precise way of separating a transudate from an exudate.[81-83] By calculating the SAAG from paired specimens of serum and ascitic fluid in more than 900 patients Runyon et al. were able to differentiate patients with portal hypertension from those without. Using a cutoff gradient of 11 g/L (1.1 g/dL), they could make this differentiation in 97% of their patients (Table 2). The SAAG is closely correlated with portal venous pressure.[81] They argue persuasively that the albumin concentration of ascitic fluid is no longer tenable as a functional concept and that SAAG gradients greater than 10 g/L indicate that these patients will respond to diuretic therapy. However, patients with an ascitic fluid albumin concentration less than 10 g/L are extremely susceptible to SBP.[84]

It has long been difficult to understand why some patients with neoplastic ascites respond to diuretic therapy and some do not. A recent investigation by Pockros et al. applied the SAAG to malignant ascites and makes this differentiation relatively simple.[85] They classified their patients as having chylous malignant ascites (CMA), peritoneal carcinomatosis (PC), or massive hepatic metastases (MHM). They found that patients with MHM had SAAG values greater than 11 g/L and are in a high renin-aldosterone state that is responsive to conventional diuretic therapy (spironolactone alone or with furosemide). All patients were treated with the lowest dosage of diuretic drugs that caused a weight loss of at least 0.5 kg/day. The patients with MHM exhibited weight loss twice as large and a mean daily decrease in ascitic fluid volume five times as great as those in the other two categories. These studies were interpreted to mean that obstructed outflow of lymphatic vessels by tumor is responsible for the accumulation of ascitic fluid in patients with CMA and PC.[86] Ascitic fluid in cirrhosis, however, forms largely as a consequence of increased renin-aldosterone secretion.[87]

On the basis of these observations Pockros et al. constructed an algorithm for the rational treatment of neoplastic ascites. If the ascitic fluid cytologic examination for malignant cells is positive, the SAAG is less than 11 g/L, and the ascitic fluid appears chylous, diuretic therapy will not be effective and may induce renal dysfunction or orthostatic hypotension. If the cytologic examination is negative, the SAAG is greater than 11 g/L, and the ascitic fluid is not chylous, diuretic therapy is indicated.

Lee et al. demonstrated that a SAAG of 15 g/L differentiated malignant ascitic fluid from that of chronic liver disease.[88] They did not differentiate between intrahepatic and peritoneal metastases, however.

TABLE 2.
Serum Ascites-Albumin Gradient in Different Types of Ascites*

Disorder	No. Patients	SAAG > 11 g/L
Cirrhotic ascites	202	84%–97%
Cardiac ascites	28	80%–100%
Intrahepatic metastases	20	100%
Peritoneal metastases	54	0%–7%

*Adapted from Runyon BA, Montano AA, Akrivialis FA, et al: *Ann Intern Med* 1992; 117:215–220.

Treatment

For many years before effective diuretic drugs became available, the periodic performance of *large paracenteses* was the standard means of treating cirrhotic patients with severe ascites. This therapy was not without hazard, however, although careful follow-up of patients in large "paracentesis clinics" was neither performed nor described. As reported in recent studies, hypotension, azotemia, hepatic encephalopathy (HE), and hyponatremia almost certainly must have been common consequences.[89, 90] Such abnormalities are not always seen[91] but probably occur only when the ascites is completely mobilized[92] or when the patients have no edema fluid to replenish the constricting plasma volume. At present, plasma volume has been maintained by the intravenous infusion of albumin, dextran or polygeline (hemocel) (6 g/L of ascites removed).[93, 94] In two studies Terg et al. and Fassio et al. recently compared dextran 70 with albumin following paracenteses of 11 to 13 L.[96, 97] They found dextran 70 to be clinically efficacious and cost-effective. Albumin costs 25 times as much as dextran 70 ($365 vs. $15). However, more patients showed an increase in PRA with dextran 70 than with albumin, thus suggesting that dextran does not maintain plasma volumes as well as albumin.

The half-life of these *synthetic plasma expanders* ranges from 6 to 28 hours. Presumably the substance lasts long enough to compensate for the transient hemodynamic changes induced by large taps. Indeed, they may be avoided by the infusion of isotonic saline.[98] The use of dextran 40, which is composed of smaller molecules that have a shorter half-life, however, is associated with frequent hyponatremia and renal impairment.[99] These observations suggest that "small" dextran has too short a half-life to protect plasma volume after large paracenteses.

Although large paracenteses appear to be safe and are almost always uncomplicated,[100] severe intraperitoneal bleeding may occasionally occur[101] (Fig 6). Although large umbilical collateral vessels can be detected by ultrasonography and computed tomography,[101, 102] it would not be cost-effective to perform such examinations in all patients scheduled to have paracentesis. On the other hand, such examinations are indicated if large hypogastric or umbilical abdominal collaterals are visible or if arterial bruits or venous hums are audible. Certainly, if one plans to insert a large peritoneal dialysis catheter[103] or if liver biopsy is also planned, it is the better part of valor to take a quick ultrasonic listen to the abdominal wall.

The treatment of ascites is well reviewed in a recent article by Arroyo et al.[92]

There is little new information about HRS since it was suggested in the last volume of *Current Hepatology* that octopressin might cause peripheral arterial vasoconstriction and renal arterial dilatation,[104] a theoretically ideal therapy for HRS.

The findings of Moore et al. of plasma levels of *endothelins* almost 10 times normal in HRS may provide some insight into the renal arterial vasoconstriction.[105] Endothalins are 21–amino acid peptides that are cleaved to form "big" endothelin and, later, to form smaller, active endothelin peptides. Endothelin, which is formed in the vascular endothelium, is a renoselective vasoconstrictor substance. Endothe-

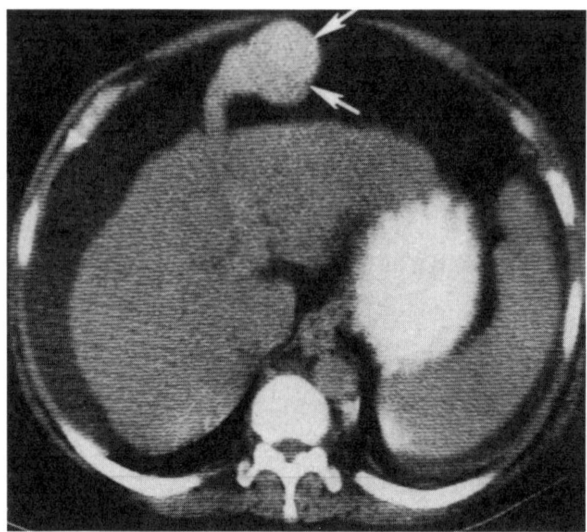

FIG 6.
Axial computed tomography reveals ascites and splenomegaly with an enhanced venous varix *(arrows)* fed by the left portal vein. (From Qureshi WA, Harshfield D, Shah H: *Am J Gastroenterol* 1992; 87:1209–1211. Used by permission.)

lin 1 levels are not elevated in cirrhotic patients with normal renal function, in patients with acute or chronic renal failure, or in patients with hepatic disease and renal impairment other than HRS. Since calcium antagonists inhibit the vasoconstrictive effects of endothelin, new therapy may already be available for the latest putative cause of HRS.[106] Another hormone has been heard from, and it should be looked at.

We should not lose sight of the fact that liver transplantation is the final court of appeal for the treatment of HRS. Indeed, Starzl et al. established this important point over 20 years ago,[107] and it is periodically brought back to mind.[108]

SPONTANEOUS BACTERIAL PERITONITIS

Clinical Picture

It is remarkable how rapidly SBP has become an integral part of medical life. Thirty years ago it was an unknown entity.[109] In fact, it was first named SBP in 1971.[110] At present it appears that this syndrome develops in at least 20% of cirrhotic patients.

Its clinical picture is still being defined. In a recent communication SBP was reported as having occurred in a young, *noncirrhotic* woman who had previously been completely well.[112] Such cases are very rare. Although this report may be such a case, as an aficionado of this disease, I believe not. First, there was apparently no preexisting ascites, a prerequisite that I believe is an obligate sine qua non of the syndrome. Second, the organisms cultured from the ascitic fluid and blood were *Bacteroides,* which are rarely recovered from patients with classic SBP. Indeed, anaerobic bacteria are rarely responsible in *spontaneous* peritonitis, although they are characteristic of *secondary* SBP. Third, the patient had had cryosurgery for cervical dysplasia 3 weeks before the infection. I suspect that the infection was introduced into the uterine cervix at the time of surgery, silently passed through the lumen of the uterus, climbed up a fallopian duct, and gently dropped into the peritoneal cavity where it caused a *purulent* peritonitis. Pus is also very rare in SBP. Most cases of secondary SBP are the result of perforation of an intra-abdominal viscus,[113] but oviduct trekkers leave no clues. Actually, this case may represent a variant of the Fitz-Hugh–Curtis syndrome.[114]

Another report described a woman who had had non-A, non B (NANB) hepatitis but not cirrhosis and in whom SBP developed 60 hours after laparotomy and appendectomy for lower abdominal pain.[115] This case, too, is almost certainly secondary bacterial peritonitis. By definition, iatrogenic invasion of the peritoneal cavity that antedates the appearance of the typical symptoms, signs, and laboratory abnormalities excludes the diagnosis of *spontaneous* bacterial peritonitis. The syndrome is broadening nicely on its own without bringing in false positive cases.

Spontaneous bacterial peritonitis in noncirrhotic, ascitic patients with acute viral hepatitis is reported in a remarkable article by Chu et al. from Taiwan.[116] Of 82 consecutive admissions for acute viral hepatitis to their hospital during a 1-year period, 26 had SBP (32%). None had a history or findings indicative of underlying chronic liver disease. The ascites usually developed 1 to 2 months after the onset of illness. The great majority (85%) were HBsAg positive and IgM anti-HBC negative, which is characteristic of acute viral hepatitis in Taiwan, and were considered to be HBV carriers with acute hepatitis. The paracenteses were performed when the ascites became clinically evident. The organisms cultured were largely aerobic, gram-negative bacteria, typical of those seen in SBP in cirrhosis. These were sick patients! They were deeply jaundiced, had mean alanine aminotransferase (ALT) levels of over 600 IU/L, mean albumin concentrations of 2.1 g/dL, and prothrombin times greater than 5 seconds prolonged. Almost 90% had ascitic fluid protein levels of less than 1.0 g/dL. Actually, these same characteristics were seen in the 56 patients whose ascitic fluid cultures were negative. Bacteremia was common (60%), as was renal failure (60%) and gastrointestinal bleeding (40%), and almost three fourths of the patients died. Cirrhosis was apparently not found at autopsy; no postmortem hepatic histopathology was presented, however.

Although SBP in acute viral hepatitis has been reported before,[117, 118] this is a unique series. Obviously, patients with mild, acute hepatitis are not routinely admitted to this hospital, but even so, this terrible prognosis is striking. It would be of interest to know how many cases of less severe hepatitis had occurred in the same area during the same period. Why were the albumin levels in both serum and ascitic fluid so low? The authors comment that opsonic activity of the ascitic fluid was extremely low, but they present no data. Since the ascites did not develop until the patients had been ill for a month or longer, it is reminiscent of the syndrome of late-onset, (subacute) fulminant hepatic failure (FHF).[119] Is this a regional syndrome seen in Taiwanese carriers of HBV, is it a random cluster of cases, or does it represent an epidemic of an especially fulminant hepatitis virus. I suspect that it is the former, but further studies are needed to provide some answers.

Spontaneous bacterial peritonitis continues to attract attention around the world as indicated by reports of series of patients from various countries—Chile,[120] Germany,[121] India,[122] and Spain.[123] Clinically, the disease is similar or identical to American SBP in these different series. The disorder is frequently silent and is highly lethal. In at least 20% of ascitic cirrhotic patients in these different series SBP appears to develop. I believe that if these patients were followed for any period of time, the cumulative incidence would be much higher—perhaps 40%.

Pathogenesis

The hypothesis proposed for the pathogenesis of SBP in 1971 presupposed four components.[110] First, ascites, the sine qua non of the syndrome, often develops in cirrhotic patients. Second, portal-systemic collateral vessels that act like holes in the hepatic reticuloendothelial filter that normally clears bacteria from the bloodstream usually develop in cirrhotic patients with portal hypertension. Third, the ascitic fluid is a hospitable medium for bacteria in which they can flourish and cause bacterial peritonitis. Fourth, extrinsic factors such as bacterial infections, gastrointestinal bleeding, diagnostic or therapeutic procedures (for example, endoscopic or dental examinations), or diarrhea give rise to bacteremias that are prolonged by the presence of the portal-systemic collaterals.

This pathogenesis suggests that SBP is a serendipitous disease. Serendipity is often defined as "chance and the prepared mind." I believe that SBP represents a chance bacteremia and an abnormal ("prepared") peritoneal cavity. A recent paper illustrates this phenomenon in reporting the development of SBP shortly after colonoscopy.[124]

An abnormality that renders the ascitic fluid especially susceptible to bacterial infection is associated with a decreased concentration of albumin.[125] Decreased albumin levels appear to parallel decreased complement levels and thereby diminished opsonic activity in the ascitic fluid.[126]

This hypothesis, which appears to be withstanding the test of time, was assessed in an interesting prospective clinical trial by Llach and his colleagues at the University of Barcelona.[127] They performed long-term follow-up (mean of 22 months) on 127 consecutive cirrhotic patients with ascites who had been admitted to the clinical research unit and who had not previously had SBP. They analyzed 34 variables that they considered to be potential predictors of SBP (Table 3). Using uni-

TABLE 3.

Variables Analyzed as Possible Predictors of the
Development of the First Episode of Spontaneous
Bacterial Peritonitis*

Age
Sex
Cause of cirrhosis
Previous history of ascites
Previous history of hepatic encephalopathy
Previous history of gastrointestinal hemorrhage
Time since the first episode of ascites
Physical examination
  Hepatic stigmata
  Hepatomegaly
  Splenomegaly
  Nutritional status (good, regular, or poor)
Standard liver and kidney function tests
  Serum bilirubin
  Serum albumin
  Prothrombin activity
  Serum AST†
  Serum ALT†
  Serum alkaline phosphatase
  Serum γ-glutamyltranspeptidase
  Serum cholesterol
  Serum γ-globulin
  Platelet count
  WBC count
  Blood urea nitrogen
  Serum creatinine
  Serum sodium
  Urinary sodium excretion
  Glomerular filtration rate
Other
  Child-Pugh classification (A, B, and C)
  Total protein concentration in ascitic fluid
  Esophageal varices (presence or absence; small
    or large)
  Arterial pressure
  Portal pressure (hepatic venous pressure
    gradient)
  Treatment of ascites (diuretics, paracentesis, or
    LeVeen shunt)

*From Llach J, Rimola A, Navasa M: *Hepatology* 1992;
16:724–727. Used by permission.
†AST = aspartate aminotransferase; ALT = alanine
aminotransferase.

variate and multivariate regression analysis, they found that only a low concentration of protein in the ascitic fluid correlated independently with the development of SBP ($P < .002$). They noted that SBP developed during the first year of follow-up in 11% of the patients followed and in 15% during the first 3 years. These percentages are lower that the 20% reported in recent series.[120–123, 127] The patients studied had only mild or moderately advanced cirrhosis (Child-Pugh classes A and B) at the time the follow-up period started, and some of them had received oral, nonabsorbable antibiotics in an attempt to prevent SBP after gastrointestinal hemorrhage. (Therapy that may affect the prevalence of a disease represents a flaw in the design of an investigation undertaken to study the natural history of that disease.) Furthermore, those patients who had previously had SBP, a group that is destined to have many recurrences of SBP (>70%),[128] had been excluded from the study of Llach and associates. Finally, these investigators noted that SBP developed in 25% of the patients with ascitic fluid protein concentrations less than 1.0 g/dL as compared with 4% of those with ascitic fluid protein levels over 1.0 g/dL ($P < .005$) (Fig 7).

The efficacy of oral antibiotics in the prevention of SBP has been established in several categories of cirrhotic patients who are at high risk of the development of SBP.[128–132] The use of oral antibiotics directed at aerobic gram-negative bacteria has been termed *selective bacterial decontamination*. Rimola[129] and Soriano and associates[130] demonstrated in RCTs that the frequency of SBP and other gram-negative, aerobic, bacterial infections in cirrhotic patients after gastrointestinal bleeding was reduced by the prophylactic administration of norfloxacin. In the most

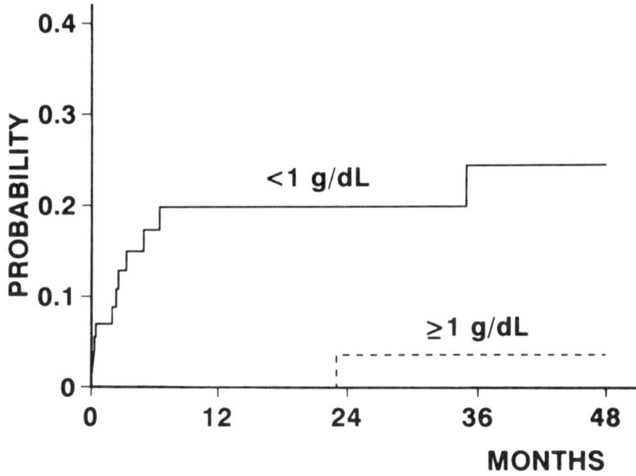

FIG 7.

Probability of the initial episode of spontaneous bacterial peritonitis developing in cirrhotic patients with ascites divided into two groups according to the concentration of protein in ascitic fluid: <1 g/dL and >1 g/dL. (From Llach J, Rimola A, Navasa M: *Hepatology* 1992; 16:724–727. Used by permission.)

recent of these investigations, norfloxacin (400 mg given twice daily), starting immediately after emergency endoscopy, was compared in 60 patients and in 59 control patients who received placebo. In addition to SBP, the frequency of bacteremia and urinary tract infections was reduced (Table 4). Although mortality was lower in the treated patients, this difference was not significant statistically. The frequency of gram-positive coccal infections was not significantly reduced by antibiotic therapy in any of these investigations.

In an earlier investigation Soriano et al. showed that norfloxacin reduced the rate of SBP in cirrhotic patients whose ascitic fluid protein concentrations were less than 1.5 g/dL from 23% in the placebo group to 0% in the antibiotic-treated group.[130] Other infections were reduced from 20% to 3% ($P < .05$). The mortality rate was decreased by prophylactic antibiotic therapy, but not significantly.

Selective intestinal decontamination (SID) has also been shown to be effective in treating leukopenic patients with leukemia.[133] If SID can prevent infection in cirrhotic patients who are unusually susceptible to SBP, why not in acute liver failure in which bacterial infections are very common?[134, 135] Salmeron and his associates, who include the authors of many of the other articles on bacterial peritonitis that originated in Barcelona, studied the effect of neomycin (1 g), colistin (1×10^6 units), and nystatin (1.5×10^6 units) every 6 hours, which were used in 15 patients, or norfloxacin (400 mg every 12 hours) and nystatin (1×10^6 units every 6 hours), which was used in 19 patients.[136] These 34 patients were admitted after 1985. The control group of 57 patients had been admitted between 1972 and 1985.

TABLE 4.

Bacterial Infections Diagnosed in Patients Treated With Norfloxacin (Group 1) or Placebo (Group 2)*

	Group 1 ($n = 60$)		Group 2 ($n = 59$)		
	No. of Infections	No. of Patients	No. of Infections	No. of Patients	P†
Infections	6	6	26	22‡	<.001
Bacteremia or SBP/CNNA§	2	2	10	10	<.05
Bacteremia	0	0	6	6	<.05
SBP/CNNA	2	2	4	4	NS
Urinary	0	0	11	11	<.001
Respiratory	4¶	4	4	4	NS
Perianal abscess	0	0	1	1	NS
Possible infections	6	6	6	6	NS

*From Soriano G, Guarner C, Tomas A: *Gastroenterology* 1992; 103:1267–1271. Used by permission.
†With respect to the number of patients.
‡Two infections developed in four patients each.
§SBP = spontaneous bacterial peritonitis; CNNA = culture-negative neutrocytic ascites.
¶One case of pyopneumothorax.

The selection of therapy was determined temporally by the year of admission. How the antibiotic combination was selected is not mentioned. Presumably, it was not determined randomly. Infections occurred in 58% of the control patients (group 1) and in 35% of the treated patients (group 2) ($P < .05$) (Table 5). Urinary tract infections, bacteremia, pneumonia, and bacterial peritonitis developed in fewer treated patients, but these differences were not statistically significant. Fewer treated patients died. Because these patients were not randomized, however, we must await confirmatory experiments before we can consider this study to be valid and this therapy to be established.

Miscellaneous Aspects

Culture-positive SBP was compared with culture-negative SBP (neutrocytic ascites) in 64 patients.[137] The two groups were similar on admission in demographic and clinical features, although there was a higher percentage of blood culture–positive patients in the culture-positive group (70% vs. 10%). Mortality rates and SBP recurrence rates were similar in the two groups. Previous comparisons of culture-positive SBP and culture-negative neutrophilic ascites suggested that the prognosis tended to be worse in the former group.[138, 139] Because of the clinical and prognostic similarity, Terg et al. considered the two syndromes to be variants of the SBP syndrome.[137]

A reproducible rodent model of SBP has been created.[140] Carbon tetrachloride was used to induce cirrhosis. Ascites developed in 93% of the cirrhotic animals,

TABLE 5.

Bacterial Infections Recorded in Patients Who Did (Group 1) and Did Not Receive (Group 2) Oral Poorly Absorbable Antibiotics*

	Group 1 ($n = 34$)	Group 2 ($n = 57$)
Patients with infection	12 (35%)	33 (58%) $P < .05$
Patients with		
Urinary tract infection	5 (15%)	18 (32%)
Bacteremia	5 (15%)†	14 (25%)‡
Pneumonia	3 (9%)	9 (16%)
Peritonitis§	3 (9%)	0
Soft tissue infection	1 (3%)	0

*From Salmeron JM, Tito L, Rimola A: *J Hepatol* 1992; 14:280–285. Used by permission.
†Bacteremia was secondary to urinary tract infection, pneumonia, and soft tissue infection in one case each and primary in the remaining two cases.
‡Bacteremia was secondary to urinary tract infection in five cases and to pneumonia in one case and primary in the remaining eight cases.
§Percentage related to the number of patients with ascites (22 in group 1 and 29 in group 2).

and SBP developed in more than 50% of these ascitic rats. This model should be very helpful in resolving some of the many mysteries of SBP.

HEPATIC ENCEPHALOPATHY

Pathogenesis

The pathogenesis of HE remains like Russia after World War II, a riddle wrapped in a mystery inside an enigma.[141] In the center of the HE enigma is ammonia.

Hepatic encephalopathy is in part, at least, *ammonia intoxication,* and therefore the role of hepatic glutamine metabolism is critical in the pathogenesis of this protean syndrome. The work of Häussinger has emphasized the importance of glutamine synthetase, which is found in about 7% of the hepatocytes segregated in the innermost certrilobular rings of cells.[142-144] Indeed, this localization of functional activity in a specific anatomic area is the basis of the perihepatic venous ammonia scavenger cell hypothesis (Fig 8). These cells, which are virtually devoid of urea cycle enzymes, are capable of taking up α-ketoglutarate, glutamate, and aspartate and converting them to glutamate, glutamine, and asparagine, respectively. Glutaminase, on the other hand, is a mitochondrial enzyme found in most hepatocytes throughout the acinus, but primarily in the periportal areas. This low-affinity, high-capacity enzyme system controls carbamoyl-phosphate synthesis and urea cycle flux. These cells, which have great gluconeogenic and ureagenic potential, take up alanine, glutamine, and proline and form glycogen. This reciprocal anatomic-functional configuration provides an extremely efficient ammonia-utilizing system. However, hepatotoxic substances that specifically induce pericentral necrosis and eradicate the ammonia "scavenger" function can cause hyperammonemia even though urea synthetic function persists unimpaired.[144]

The ammoniacal hypothesis of HE is supported by elevated arterial ammonia levels, increased cerebral extraction of ammonia, the development of abnormal astrocytes known as Alzheimer type II cells, and the reversal of these metabolic and histopathologic abnormalities by ammonia-reducing therapy.[145] Localization of glutamine synthetase in the astrocytes of the brain appears to account for the localization of these histologic abnormalities of the astrocytes.

Lockwood et al. have shown that ammonia intoxication is associated with an increased cerebral metabolic rate for ammonia and an increased permeability–surface area product that favors the passage of ammonia into the brain.[146] In a later study they showed that there was decreased cerebral blood flow and a decreased metabolic rate in the cortex, but not in the cerebellum, thalamus, and caudate lobes.[147] These observations emphasize the need for antiammonia-oriented therapy in HE.

The importance of *portal-systemic shunting* in the pathogenesis of HE is shown

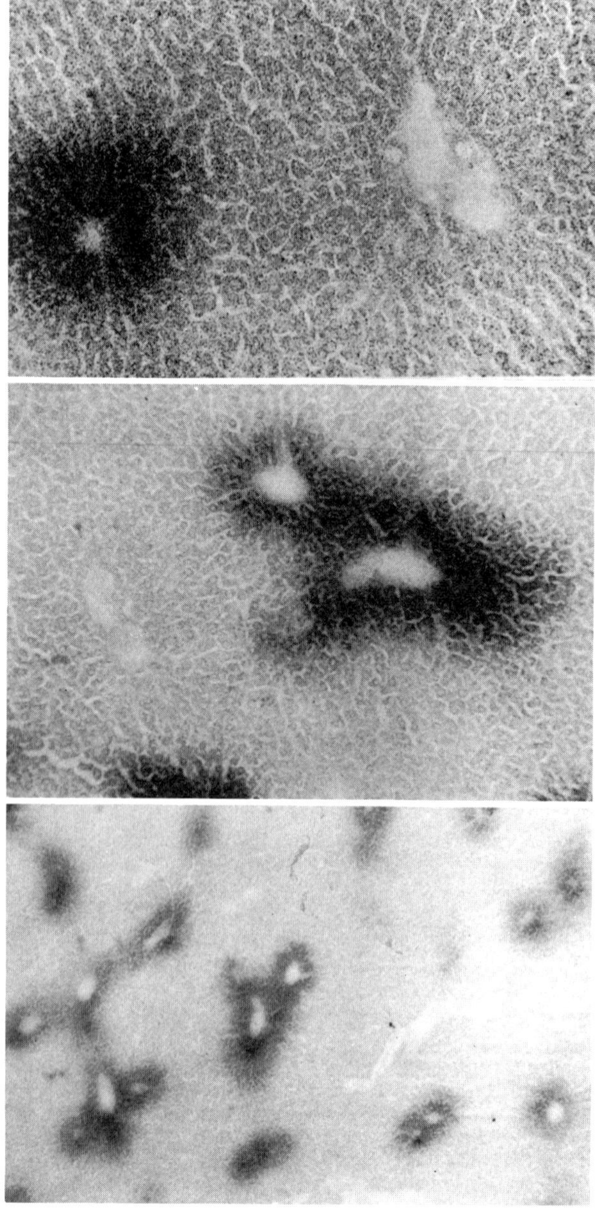

FIG 8.

Histoautoradiograms of rat livers after a bolus injection of [^{3}H]glutamate. Livers were perfused in either the retrograde (from the hepatic to the portal vein) *(top, center)* or antegrade direction (from the portal to the hepatic vein) *(bottom)* in a medium containing unlabeled glutamate. (From Stoll B, McNeilly S, Buscher HP, et al: *Hepatology* 1991; 13:247–253. Used by permission.)

by the report of Haskal et al.[148] They noted that 10 of 93 patients (11%) who had had TIPS implanted following variceal bleeding required a second, parallel stent to reduce persistent portal hypertension (8 patients) or because of shunt malfunction (2 patients). All the stents implanted were Wallstents, and 80% of them had been dilated to 10-mm diameter and the remainder to only 8 mm. The mean prestent portal venous pressure gradient was 16.5 mm Hg. The mean poststent pressure gradient in the 83 patients after a single stent was 10.2 mm Hg, whereas it was 19.1 mm Hg in the 10 patients who required second stents. After placement of the second stents, which were all distended to 8-mm diameter, the mean pressure gradient was 12.5 mm Hg. Chronic recurrent HE developed in 2 of these 10 patients for the first time after implantation of the second stent. Except for transient episodes of HE during active bleeding or other such acute, comagenic events, HE developed in none of the patients with single stents. The addition of an 8-mm stent to an existing 10-mm stent increases the volume of shunted blood by 40% according to Poiseuille's equation, assuming that all other things are equal. Thus the delivery of increased amounts of portal blood containing large amounts of ammonia and/or other potentially comagenic substances is the critical factor in the pathogenesis of HE.

A recently described rat model for hyperammonemia promises a way of performing simple, inexpensive studies in an animal that reacts biochemically much like humans.[149]

One interesting report analyzed the *branched-chain amino acid (BCAA)*/aromatic amino acid (AAA) *(BCAA/AAA) molar ratios* in patients with cirrhosis of varying degrees of severity[150] and confirmed that the ratio falls as the cirrhosis progresses (Table 6). Unfortunately, the authors did not assess the degree of portal-systemic shunting, which also inversely parallels the BCAA/AAA ratio.[151]

In Volume 13 of *Current Hepatology* I discussed in detail the study of Marchesini et al.,[152] which showed that BCAA-supplemented diets were superior to diets with an equinitrogenous amount of casein in chronic HE. In a retrospective follow-up Bianchi et al. reported that *prolactin levels* were not altered in those patients who

TABLE 6.

Association of the Branched-Chain Amino Acid/Aromatic Amino Acid Ratio With the Severity of Cirrhosis*

Cirrhosis	Mean BCAA/AAA Ratio
No cirrhosis	3.9
Stable cirrhosis	2.9
Unstable cirrhosis	1.7
Cirrhosis with hepatic encephalopathy	0.8

*Adapted from Campollo O, Sprengers D, McIntyre N: *Rev Invest Clin* 1992; 44:513–518.

received BCAAs and showed clinical benefit.[153] Prolactin has been implicated in the pathogenesis of HE.[154]

In the patients who received casein, plasma prolactin levels increased by 50% during the 3 months of therapy. Similarly, estradiol levels did not change in the BCAA-treated group but increased in the casein-treated patients. Estradiol has not been considered an encephalopathogenic substance. Since the benefits of BCAA therapy were attributed to improved nutrition, as suggested by higher serum albumin and transferrin levels, one can conclude, but without great confidence, that prolactin did not play a role in these patients' HE. Conceivably but unlikely, the BCAA treatment prevented a gradual rise in prolactin levels, which induced relative worsening in the casein-treated patients in whom prolactin levels rose and HE persisted. Probably these phenomena are coincidental and unrelated.

Zinc deficiency as a cause of HE comes as something of a surprise.[155, 156] Although it has been known for many years that serum zinc levels are often abnormally low in patients with cirrhosis and alcoholism, these relationships in HE have been recognized relatively recently. It is now known that zinc concentrations are reduced in leukocytes and liver tissue. Other evidence of zinc deficiency occurring in cirrhotic patients is hypogeusia, i.e., loss of smell and therefore of taste. In addition, visual acuity is diminished and vitamin A levels are decreased, as is retinol-binding pigment. Albumin binding of zinc is also decreased in cirrhosis. The low zinc levels reflect increased urinary loss and decreased intestinal absorption.[157] Zinc deficiency is most marked in those patients with advanced cirrhosis, usually alcoholic, that is characterized by both hepatic dysfunction and portal-systemic shunting.[157]

What is the function of zinc in the body? Zinc is a component of many enzymes, among which is ornithine transcarbamoylase (OTC), which is a key enzyme of urea synthesis. It is not surprising, therefore, that decreased serum zinc levels develop in patients receiving zinc-deficient diets. It is surprising, however, that these patients exhibit increased blood ammonia levels. Indeed, induced zinc deficiency causes increased ammonia levels in normal subjects.[157] These, too, are reversible phenomena. Zinc therapy has been proved to be therapeutically effective in zinc deficiency with encephalopathy.[158]

Zinc deficiency has been implicated in the pathogenesis of HE on circumstantial grounds. Grungreiff and coworkers studied 148 cirrhotic and 20 control subjects.[156] Abnormally low zinc concentrations were observed in all patients with decompensated cirrhosis. Furthermore, they found a close inverse correlation between serum zinc and plasma ammonia concentrations (Fig 9), whereas there was no relationship between zinc levels and albumin or individual amino acid levels. Zinc levels were lowest and ammonia concentrations highest in cirrhotic patients with HE, intermediate in cirrhotic patients without HE, and highest and lowest, respectively, in normal subjects. In these investigations serum albumin and BCAA levels were reduced, whereas AAA concentrations were elevated. Scholmerich and his associates suggested that zinc deficiency is associated with portal-systemic shunting.[157]

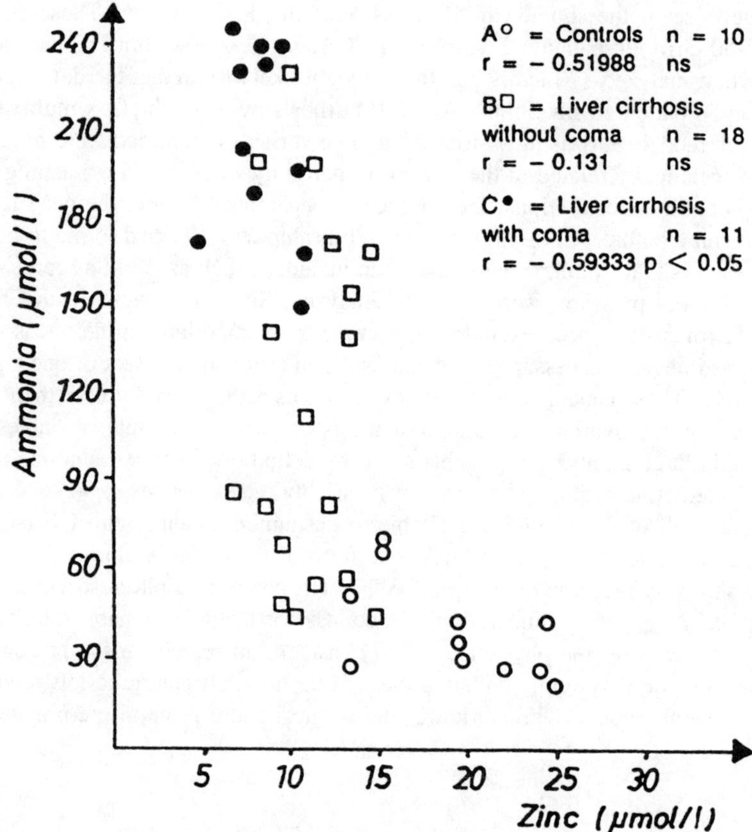

FIG 9.

Relationship of plasma ammonia and serum zinc concentrations in cirrhotic patients and normal control subjects (Spearman's rank correlation test). (From Grungreiff K, Franke D, Lebner B: *Gastroenterology* 1991; 29:101–106. Used by permission.)

The fact that glutamic dehydrogenase and carbamoylphosphate synthetase (CPA) are zinciferous enzymes suggests that zinc deficiency may exert its effects via impaired ammonia fixation and excretion. The report of Riggio et al. indicates that in rats with experimental cirrhosis and reduced zinc and increased ammonia levels, dietary zinc supplementation restores zinc and ammonia levels to normal and causes an increase in hepatic OTC activity.[159]

Prognosis

When I read the title of the article by Planas et al.,[160] "Prognostic factors of hepatic encephalopathy after portacaval anastomosis: A multivariate analysis in 50 patients," I thought I could predict most of the factors that the article would identify: age, size of the shunt, Child's class, etc. But I was wrong! These authors studied 50 cirrhotic patients 2 years after PCA, in 43% of whom HE had developed. They analyzed 37 factors that they thought likely to predict the development of HE in 50 patients with Child's A and B cirrhosis by using the Cox multivariate regression model. Surprisingly, four of the five variables identified were mundane and not specifically related to the liver or to portal hypertension, i.e., hemoglobin and γ-globulin concentrations, the absence of hepatomegaly, and the need for diuretic therapy before PCA. Only the serum bilirubin level seemed to me to be relevant. Factors that I think should have been included, such as Child's score, shunt size, and portal pressure, were not even analyzed. Since all patients with Child's class C cirrhosis had been excluded, the single most important variable was missing. Sometimes it is necessary to evaluate such an article by the seat of one's pants and to say, "These conclusions are irrelevant or misleading," and ignore them. Besides, every multivariate regression analysis in which multiple variables are screened in large numbers of patients must, by definition, identify some factors as having "predictive" value. They are not invariably of real value.

Although all of the therapies available to unshunted patients with HE (see below) are available to those with PCA, one form of treatment is unique to patients with shunts—*obliteration of the shunt*. When HE persists despite restriction of dietary protein and the administration of lactulose (or lactitol), nonabsorbed antibiotic agents, or both, the physician should consider and search for the presence of spontaneous portal-systemic collateral vessels such as left gastric-to-left renal venous collateral vessels. Obliteration of the surgical shunt promptly terminates the HE.[161]

Diagnosis

The Number Connection Test[162] is a widely used psychometric test in the grading of HE and in the detection of *subclinical hepatic encephalopathy* (SHE).[163] It is, however, only a rough index of the presence or severity of disordered intellectual capability. It is affected by a number of variables, among which are age and education. Zeneroli and her associates have recently reported on a large sample of 210 normal subjects from 15 to 89 years of age who had spent from 8 to 16 years in school.[164] They established that the NCT time increased with increasing age and decreased with years of education (Fig 10). They attempted to calculate correction factors and found that such factors might require arbitrary reduction to 18% of the measured time, a factor greater than fivefold. Obviously, correction factors must be established, but it is important that such factors be based on large numbers of patients so that age, education, and other factors that could affect such tests, including ethnic and national origin and native intelligence, would be taken into account.

Attempts to diagnose SHE by electroneurologic methods continue.[165] It is well

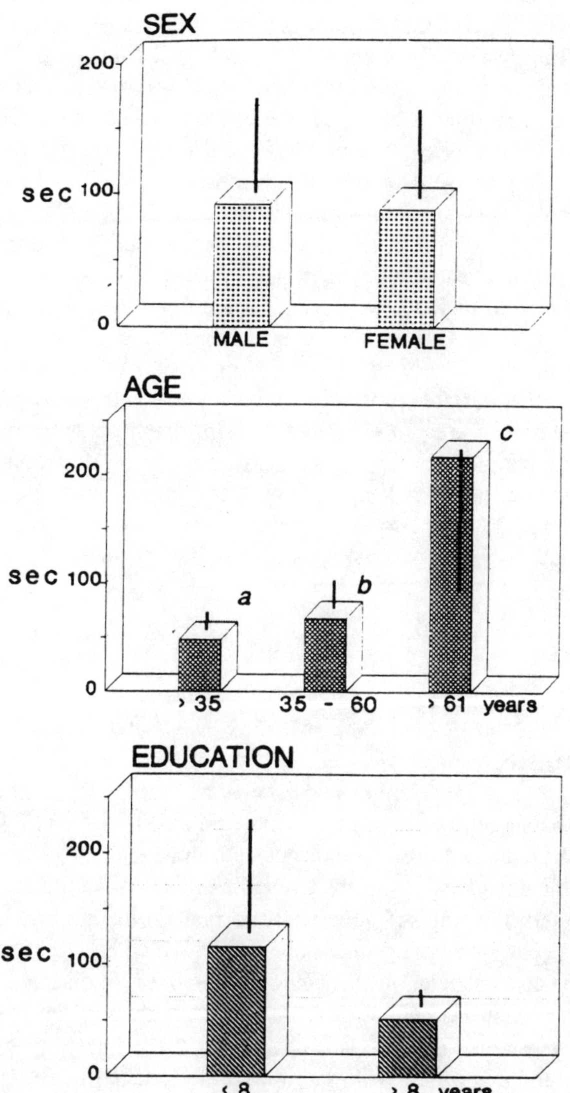

FIG 10.

Correlation of mean Number Connection Test times with sex, age, and education. Scores are means ± SD of the Number Connection Test (part A) in healthy subjects ($n = 210$) in relation to sex, age and education. *t*-Test: sex, not significant; age, *a* vs. *b* and *b* vs. *c*, $P < .001$; education, $P < .001$. (From Zeneroli ML, Cioni G, Ventura P: *J Hepatol* 1992; 15:263–264. Used by permission.)

established that semiquantitative electroencephalographic (EEG) analysis correlates closely with the degree of HE.[166] Various types of evoked potentials have been studied, but only the two that require patient participation, *pattern reversal* and *auditory p 300* event-related potentials,[167] can be used to assess SHE. These two electrophysiologic methods in turn correlated with spectral analysis of EEG,[166, 167] thus giving them a reason for credence. Pattern reversal detected SHE in only 10% of patients with clinically established SHE, and p 300 potentials did so in 18%. This percentage of positive detection is far too low to be of clinical value and can, therefore, only be used in establishing frames of reference. The "gold standard" for making the diagnosis of SHE is the use of psychomotor tests—the NCT[162] and a variety of other established methods.[163] Since the NCT can at present be considered only "gold plated," we must, if we are honest with ourselves, consider such correlations to be sand castles to be taken with a grain of sand. First, we must improve the NCT, perhaps by finding appropriate correction factors for age, education, and other variables and/or by devising new and better tests. Second, we may then, after having created reliable criteria of diagnosis, ideally by using fast, simple, inexpensive methodologies, reassess a variety of electrophysiologic tests. Furthermore, we must always keep in mind that correlation coefficients are among the least powerful statistical tools available. In a sense we must avoid building new sand castles on the unstable foundations of earlier ones.

Treatment

Nonabsorbed Disaccharides

For almost 15 years *lactulose* has been considered to be the treatment of choice, with nonabsorbable antibiotics such as neomycin a distant second.[168, 169] *Lactitol,* which is identical to lactulose in concept and almost identical in its pharmacology[170] and clinical response,[171] is not available in the United States. Consequently, I will use the term "lactulose" generically to include lactitol and even *lactose* in lactase-deficient patients.[172] *Crystalline lactulose,* which is better tolerated than lactulose syrup, is also included in this acidogenous group of disaccharides.[173] These carbohydrates, which are neither degraded nor absorbed in the upper bowel, are metabolized by bacteria in the lower bowel and cause intestinal luminal acidosis by trapping ammonia, which with the aid of acid-induced intestinal propulsion is excreted as feces.

The mechanisms by which lactulose performs its wonders remain a mystery. It is well established that lactulose, which cannot be cleaved into its component monosaccharides in the small bowel, is metabolized in the large bowel where it is converted to short-chain fatty acids (SCFAs), carbon dioxide, and hydrogen, thus acidifying the lower intestinal lumen. The laws of physics require the passage of gaseous ammonia across semipermeable membranes from the alkaline to the acid compartment. Thus, the transport of ammonia from the blood into the lumen of the bowel reduces the concentration of ammonia in the blood. This transfer of ammonia is therapeutically beneficial in HE since the uptake of ammonia by the brain is proportional to the arterial ammonia concentration.[174] Early in the short history of lactulose it had been assumed that the ammonia was trapped in the luminal contents and excreted as a consequence of acid-stimulated peristalsis. Paradoxically, however, the concentration of ammonia in stool water was found to be very low.[175] Apparently other mechanisms are involved. One such mechanism is the incorporation of intestinal ammonia into bacterial protein, which is then excreted as a component of feces.[176] Thus the wisdom of the body allows lactulose to induce the excretion of nitrogen, the substrate from which ammonia is formed, rather than excretion of ammonia, the comagenic substance itself. Such biochemical algebra provides insight into how the body solves its metabolic problems, but it does not indicate why it does so in such a way.

Lactulose works in other mysterious ways as well. During lactulose administration ammonia production, urea synthesis, and the urea pool are all decreased.[176] As Mortenson has shown in his latest report, orally administered lactulose is degraded to the shortest SCFA, acetate, which is nontoxic, rather than to three-, four-, and five-carbon acids, i.e., butyric, valeric, and isovaleric acids,[177] which are progressively more comagenic the longer the carbon chain of these SCFAs. Furthermore, lactulose affects the degradation of proteins, amino acids, and other carbohydrates similarly by favoring their metabolism to nontoxic acetate rather than to the longer BCAAs.[178]

In another study of SCFAs, Peters and his associates in New Zealand compared portal and peripheral venous concentrations after the injection of lactulose (10 g) into the cecum during cholecystectomy.[179] The metabolism of lactulose occurred very rapidly, SCFA levels peaking within 15 to 45 minutes (Table 7). Mean portal plasma levels of acetate, propionate, and butyrate doubled within 30 to 45 minutes of the instillation of lactulose. In the peripheral blood, acetate levels increased from 75 to 130 μmol/L within 45 minutes. Propionate levels, which were very low (<4 μmol/L), did not change. Butyrate was not detectable in the plasma of peripheral blood.

These data indicate that SCFAs in the portal venous blood are derived from in-

TABLE 7.

Short-Chain Fatty Acid Concentrations in Portal and Peripheral Venous Plasma Before and After Intracecal Lactulose (10 g)*

	Portal Vein Levels		Peripheral Vein Levels	
	Basal	Peak	Basal	Peak
Acetate	128 ± 71†	241±142	75±17	130±74
Propionate	34 ± 23	39± 18	4± 1	4± 2
Butyrate	18 ± 18	27± 18	Not detectable	Not detectable

*Adapted from Peters SG, Pomare EW, Fisher CA: *Gut* 1992; 33:1249–1252.
†Values are micromoles per liter.

gested carbohydrates and are promptly metabolized in the liver. In the peripheral blood, however, acetate, which is endogenous in origin, remains relatively constant and is only transiently affected by the ingestion of nonabsorbed carbohydrates.

Even though lactitol is not available everywhere, it seems to have been studied everywhere, usually in comparison with lactulose. A meta-analysis of such studies that included patients with acute, chronic, and subclinical HE reported that the two disaccharides were therapeutically equal.[180] The abstract of this study ended in an unintentionally very funny line, "However, flatulence was significantly more frequent with lactulose, and therefore, lactitol should be used in preference. . ." Can a little flatus be that bad?

Incidentally, it has been reported that both lactulose and lactitol induce mild to moderate steatorrhea in cirrhotic patients[181] and that this previously unnoted adverse effect should be considered in patients who require long-term therapy.

Nonabsorbed Antibiotics

A long-awaited RCT in which a nonabsorbable antibiotic agent was compared with a placebo in the treatment of HE has been published.[182] Unfortunately, there is not much to cheer about. Treatment failure and death occurred as frequently in the *neomycin*-treated (6 g/day) as in the placebo group—approximately 20% in each group. Responses to therapy occurred about 25% faster in the treatment group (a mean of 39 vs. 49 hours), but this difference is neither statistically nor clinically significant. Personally, I am so convinced of the efficacy of antibiotic therapy in HE that I harbor doubts about the conclusions of this investigation, even though it was performed by Dr. Edna Strauss, who is a competent investigator and a good friend. I suspect a type II error.

My only alternative is to discard many clinical observations that I made during almost 40 years of clinical investigation and practice. It is especially difficult for me to accept that neomycin has no beneficial effect in HE because it means that logically I must also accept that the benefits of lactulose, lactitol, and lactose (in lactase-deficient patients) in HE, which have been found in RCTs to be approximately as effective as neomycin in my own studies and in others, do not exist. Since I have devoted my professional life to the RCT, I cannot disavow this cornerstone of clinical science. Therefore, I credit the naysayers with one point. I assume that other RCTs will contradict (or explain) the results of Strauss et al. and that after a sufficient number of RCTs have been reported, meta-analysis will indicate that both antibiotic treatment, and disaccharide therapy are effective therapies for HE. It is pertinent that I confess that very recently I heard another friend, H. Michel of Marseilles, who is also a respected clinical hepatologist, state without out data or discussion that he believes that neither neomycin nor lactulose is effective in the treatment of HE. I hate to be forced to choose between my beliefs and my friends.

Other recent studies of nonabsorbed antibiotics in the treatment of HE have recently been reported by Festi et al.[183] They point out that *rifaximin*, a nonabsorbed, nonaminoglyosidic, topical antibiotic agent,[184] has potent antimicrobial activity in vivo and in vitro against gram-negative and gram-positive bacteria. This agent appears to be as efficacious as neomycin[185, 186] and paromomycin.[187] Most important, rifaximin appears to be essentially free of the renal side effects that occur with neomycin and another aminoglycoside, metronidazole, which is also effective in HE. Metronidazole is limited in its antibiotic spectrum to obligative anaerobic bacteria and has little effect on aerobic bacteria, which are responsible for most bacterial infections in cirrhotic patients and for much of the ammonia generated in the intestinal tract.

Other Therapeutic Agents

Alternative therapeutic agents are now competing with lactulose for a piece of the action. Several clinical trials have been reported in which *sodium benzoate* (or *sodium phenylacetate*) has been shown to be effective in chronic HE.[188–190] Unfortunately, the first of these has no control group,[188] and the second has been reported so far only in abstract form.[189] The third, however, is an RCT performed in 74 consecutive patients with acute HE in which lactulose syrup, given orally or by gastric tube three times daily, was compared with an oral sodium benzoate solution.[190] The lactulose was given in a dosage (67 mL or 50 g/day) that induced two or three semiformed stools per day, whereas the benzoate was given in a dosage of 5 g as an aqueous solution twice per day. The majority of the patients had cirrhosis, primarily posthepatic; a few had had portal-systemic anastomoses for idiopathic portal hypertension. The two groups were similar in demographic characteristics, in clinical and laboratory features, and in Child's classification. (About half of both groups were class B and one third was class C.) The duration and severity of HE were similar. The mean PSE index was 0.65. Dietary protein was restricted to 20 g/day, and antibiotic agents were administered to treat infections as indicated.

Both therapies were quite effective. The mean PSE index fell from 0.68 to 0.19 in the lactulose group and 0.61 to 0.20 in the benzoate-treated patients. Both drugs were about equally efficacious, and equivalent numbers of patients died in both groups (about 20%). Side effects occurred with about equal frequency in the two groups, but with lactulose diarrhea and flatulance were reported, whereas benzoate caused nausea, vomiting, and/or epigastric distress. Benzoate costs about one thirtieth as much as lactulose. Evoked potentials were not helpful, and psychometric tests were too sensitive for use in acute HE.

The study was designed to be performed in a double-blinded manner, but the physical characteristics and the side effects of the therapeutic solutions are so different that only single-blinded trials are possible, and even that cannot be taken for granted. Indeed, comparisons of lactulose, a syrup, with tablets or powdered preparations are possible but require double- or even triple-drug therapy.[191] Clearly, however, sodium benzoate and lactulose appear to be equally efficacious.

L-*Ornithine-*L-*Aspartate*

L-Ornithine is the key amino acid in urea synthesis, which is carried out largely in the periportal hepatocytes.[142, 144] Ornithine activates ornithine carbamoyltransferase and CPS[192] and also serves as the primary substrate for urea synthesis.

L-Aspartate is the key amino acid in glutamine synthesis, which is carried out largely in centrilobular hepatocytes[193] (see Fig 8). Aspartate, α-ketoglutarate, and other citric decarboxylates (malate, oxalacetate, benzoate) are taken up almost exclusively by the small number of hepatocytes in the two most central rings of hepatocytes.[144, 193] They are not taken up by the periportal liver cells.[144] In pathologic states such as acute and chronic liver injury, aspartate and other dicarboxylates stimulate increased glutamine synthesis by these perivenous scavenger cells.[194, 195]

Deficiencies in dicarboxylates and ornithine have been implicated in the pathogenesis of HE.[196] Replacement of these substances has been used therapeutically.[197, 198]

Recently, RCTs have been reported in which L-ornithine-L-aspartate (OA) has been used in a variety of hyperammonemic states.[199–203] These investigations have been published in the German literature and are not well known elsewhere. They have been summarized by Kircheis et al.[204]

Henglein-Ottermann reported on hyperammonemia induced by the intravenous infusions of NH_4Cl in ten normal and ten cirrhotic patients.[199] As expected, blood ammonia levels were higher in the cirrhotic patients than in the noncirrhotic patients and were prevented or reduced by the addition of OA to the NH_4Cl infusions.

Leweling et al. in a double-blind RCT showed that the level of hyperammonemia induced in ten cirrhotic patients by the ingestion of an oral protein solution could be diminished by intravenous infusions of OA.[200] The increment in blood ammonia concentration was reduced by infusions of 5 and 20 g of OA and completely abolished by infusions of 40 g of OA. The BCAA/AAA ratio, which was reduced by placebo infusions after protein ingestion, was increased by OA infusions. These phenomena suggest an anabolic effect of OA. Unfortunately, the grades of HE were not reported in this study.

In a double-blind, multicenter trial, Nilius et al. studied 114 cirrhotic patients with HE and hyperammonemia.[201] Improvement in mental state occurred more frequently and to a greater degree after the intravenous infusion of 20 g of OA daily for 7 days than after placebo infusions ($P < .001$). Mean NCT times were faster after OA ($P < .001$). Both fasting and postprandial ammonia levels were lower after OA than after placebo ($P < .01$ and $P < .05$, respectively). Plasma urea levels tended to increase after OA administration. Nausea and vomiting required discontinuation of OA therapy in about 5% of patients.

Stauch and Rosch in another double-blind, multicenter, placebo-controlled RCT investigated the effects of oral OA in 63 cirrhotic patients with HE and hyperammonemia.[202] Half received placebo and half received 18 g of OA per day for 2 weeks. Although mental state improved in the OA-treated group, the differences were not statistically significant. The NCT time was significantly shortened by OA ($P < .01$), and both fasting and postprandial, venous, plasma ammonia levels decreased ($P < .01$ and $P < .05$, respectively).

L-Ornithine-L-aspartate (27 g/day) was compared with lactulose (50 mL three times per day) by Liehr et al. in 42 cirrhotic patients with HE and hyperammonemia.[203] Hepatic encephalopathy, NCT times, and venous ammonia levels improved in the majority of patients with both treatments. Treatment with OA appeared to be slightly but insignificantly more effective than lactulose and to be better tolerated by the patients. Lactulose induced diarrhea in 45%, whereas OA caused dyspepsia in only 5%. Unfortunately, this article exists only in abstract form, and detailed analysis is not yet possible.

L-Ornithine-L-aspartate appears to be a promising addition to the antiammonia armamentarium. It will require rigorous comparison with lactulose, lactitol, benzoate, etc. Conceivably, combinations of these agents may be more effective than any of them individually.

Grisolia's group has reported that in rats diets that are completely free of protein paradoxically cause an increase in blood ammonia levels.[205, 206] This phenomenon is associated with decreased activity of CPS and one of its activators, acetylglutamate, and consequently, a decrease in urea synthesis. Restoration of normal protein intake reverses these phenomena. Reasoning that if a decrease in acetylglutamate enhances blood ammonia concentrations, the stimulation of CPS activity might decrease blood ammonia levels. Because acetylglutamate is rapidly degraded by a decylase in the cytosol, it cannot be used, but *carbamoylglutamate,* which is not so degraded and which stimulates CPS activity, has been used instead. Grau et al. gave carbamoylglutamate (1 mmol/L) in the drinking water to rats fed standard or protein-free diets.[207] Furthermore, this agent, which is nontoxic and well tolerated,[208] can reduce these adverse effects of a protein-free diet in experimental animals by stimulating urea synthesis. Since CPS activity has been reported to be reduced in cirrhotic patients,[209, 210] it seems reasonable to stimulate it by the administration of carbamoylglutamate. Perhaps in a year or two I will be writing about the therapeutic success (or lack thereof) of carbamoylglutamate in HE.

Investigators at various institutions in the United States and Japan have collaborated to publish an article describing successful *liver transplantation* to correct genetic *deficiencies* of *urea cycle enzymes.*[211] One patient, a 14-day-old boy with carbamoylphosphate synthetase-1 (CPS-1) deficiency, and a young man with argininosuccinic acid deficiency were reported. The latter is the first case of a patient with this enzyme deficiency to receive a transplant. They report that 5 patients with OTC deficiency have already successfully received transplants, as has one other with CPS-1 deficiency. Thus, three of the enzyme deficiencies of the urea cycle have been corrected. The other two, which are much more rare, will almost certainly be corrected by liver transplantation as soon as they are detected near a liver transplant center. These diverse syndromes, all of which show HE as their major manifestation and all of which are ultimately lethal, can now be considered correctable lesions.

Acute Liver Failure

Fulminant hepatic failure is often complicated by increased intracranial pressure (ICP), which is responsible for death in a high percentage of such patients.[212] Liver transplantation has improved survival rates in patients with FHF from 25% to 60% or 70%.[213] Now that such effective treatment is available, it is essential to monitor the ICP so that patients awaiting liver transplantation can be treated promptly when intracranial hypertension develops. Unfortunately, increased ICP is the only way of identifying patients who required computed or ultrasonic tomography to detect cerebral edema.[214] To assess the efficacy of ICP monitoring and the treatment of intracranial hypertension in FHF Lidofsky et al. at the University of California, San Francisco, studied 23 patients.[213] In 10 of them (43%) ICP greater than 25 mm Hg developed, and were treated with mannitol, barbiturates, or both. In 4 of the 10 a sustained reduction in ICP was accomplished, and 3 of the 4 survived. The 6 in whom the elevated ICP was refractory to treatment all died of brain stem herniation. Furthermore, ICP often increases during transplant surgery in such patients, and ICP monitoring makes detection of the ICP and treatment much more efficient. On the other hand, ICP monitoring is not completely benign. Intracranial hemorrhage developed in 5 of these patients, and in 2 of them it contributed to their deaths. Prospective controlled trials are obviously needed.

Why is it that the ICP increases so dramatically in FHF and is not part of the clinical picture of chronic HE despite the hyperammonemia and increased brain levels of glutamine? Does it occur at all in the chronic disorder? Yes, it does! Crippin et al. have recently reported intracranial hypertension and HE in two cirrhotic patients with chronic liver disease.[215] In these patients the ICP was measured with an epidural ICP monitor and was found to be 42 and 24 mm Hg, respectively. In chronic HE hyperammonemia and one of its consequences, the intracerebral accumulation of glutamine,[216, 217] may cause an increase in ICP. Glutamine is an osmolyte, i.e., a highly oncotic substance that draws water into the tissues. Indeed, if the accumulation of glutamine in the brain of experimental animals can be prevented, the cerebral edema that accompanies FHF may be abolished.[217, 218]

Sussman and his coworkers have reported their results with an experimental, extracorporeal liver assist device (ELAD) that may help tide patients over acute episodes of FHF.[218] Such "artificial livers" may provide time for patients to regenerate their liver and, it is hoped, to obviate the need for liver transplantation entirely. The ELAD is a cartridge (Fig 11) that consists of semipermeable, hollow-fiber capillaries that permit the passage of plasma and its component substances to the outside of the capillaries where hepatocytes grow in tissue culture. Such "simple" devices that permit cultured hepatocytes to act as accessary livers may eventually prove to be of real clinical value.

Why does symptomatic cerebral hypertension develop in a few patients with chronic HE and not in the great majority? One of the patients of Crippin et al.[215]

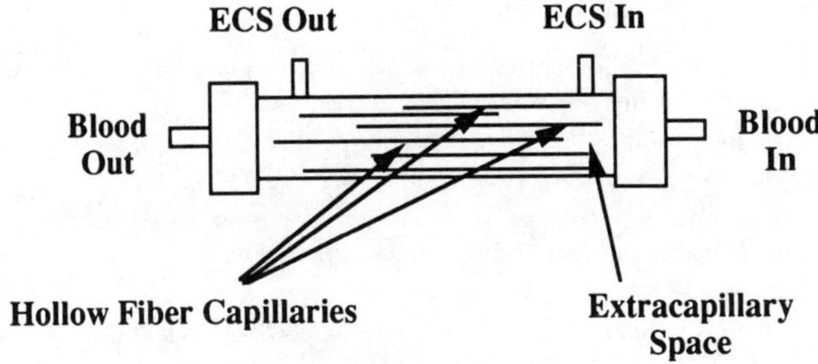

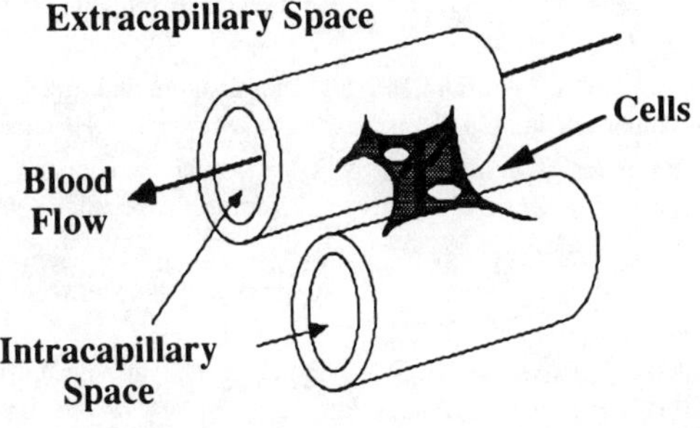

FIG 11.
Diagram of a hollow-fiber, extracorporeal cartridge device used in the treatment of experimental fulminant hepatic failure. Cells are cultured on the extracapillary side *(ECS)* of the semipermeable fibers while blood or medium flows through the lumen. The devices used in these studies contain 10,000 individual fibers and provide a growth surface of approximately $2\ m^2$. The nominal molecular weight cutoff is 70,000, and each device supports the growth of an estimated 200 g of C3A cells. (From Sussman NL, Chong MG, Koussayer T: *Hepatology* 1992; 16:60–65. Used by permission.)

had PBC, and the other had alcoholic cirrhosis. Neither displayed extremely abnormal liver function, except that the arterial ammonia concentration in both was enormously elevated (about 16 times the upper limit of normal). Both exhibited seizure activity. It may mean that glutamine synthesis is linearly proportional to the degree of hyperammonemia. Perhaps it has to do with the rate at which severe hyperammonemia develops. In FHF many other hepatic functions are impaired, and blood ammonia levels are not so greatly increased. Indeed, in FHF the increase in ICP appears to be a function of increased permeability of the blood-brain barrier. In Reye's syndrome in which cerebral hypertension and its complications are common, both increased permeability of the blood-brain barrier and enormous elevations of blood ammonia concentration coexist.

I predict that increased ICP will now be shown to be a common finding in chronic HE. As is true of so many other dramatic syndromes like SBP, primary sclerosing cholangitis, Reye's syndrome, and acquired immunodeficiency syndrome (AIDS), once these disorders have been recognized, they become ubiquitous.

REFERENCES

1. Rosch J, Hanafee WN, Snow H: Transjugular portal venography and radiological portosystemic shunt: An experimental study. *Radiology* 1969; 92:1112–1114.

2. Gutierrez OH, Burgener FA: Production of nonsurgical portosystemic venous shunts in dogs by transjugular approach. *Radiology* 1969; 130:507–509.

3. Colapinto RF, Stronell RD, Gildiner M, et al: Formation of an intrahepatic portosystemic shunt using balloon dilatation catheter. Preliminary clinical experience. *AJR Am J Roentgenol* 1983; 140:709–714.

4. Palmaz J, Sibbitt RR, Reuter SR, et al: Expandable intrahepatic portocaval shunt stents: Early experience in the dog. *AJR Am J Roentgenol* 1985; 145:821–825.

5. LaBerge JM, Ring EJ, Lake JR: Transjugular intrahepatic portosystemic shunts (TIPS): Preliminary results in 25 patients. *J Vasc Surg* 1992; 16:258–267.

6. Zemel G, Katzen BT, Becker GJ, et al: Percutaneous transjugular portosystemic shunt. *JAMA* 1991; 266:390–393.

7. Sanyal AJ, Freedman AF, Purdum PP: Use of transjugular intrahepatic porto-caval stent shunt (TIPSS) for treatment of intractable ascites: A case report. *Am J Gastroenterol*, in press.

8. Bilodeau M, Bioux L, Willems B, et al: Transjugular intrahepatic portacaval stent shunt as a rescue treatment for life-threatening variceal bleeding in a cirrhotic patient with severe liver failure. *Am J Gastroenterol* 1992; 87:369–371.

9. Conn HO: Transjugular intrahepatic portal-systemic shunts: The state of the art. *Hepatology* 1993; 17:148–158.

10. Rossle M, Noldge G, Pararnau JM: Transjugular intrahepatic portosystemic stent-shunt (TIPSS): Experience with an improved technique (abstract). *Hepatology* 1991; 14:96.

11. Garcia-Villarreal L, Zozaya JM, Quiroza J, et al: TIPS for portal hypertension and liver cirrhosis (abstract). *J Hepatol* 1992; 16(suppl):91.

12. Sanyal AJ, Freedman AM, Luketic VA: Transjugular intrahepatic porto-systemic shunt (TIPS) and pathophysiology of portal hypertension (PH): Endoscopic, radiologic and biochemical correlations. *Am J Gastroenterol* 1992; 87:1305.

13. Fenyves K, Willems B, Lafortune M, et al: Hemodynamic effects of transjugular intrahepatic porto-systemic stent shunt (TIPSS) in cirrhotic patients (abstract). *J Hepatol* 1992; 16(suppl):36.

14. LaBerge JM, Ring EJ, Gordon RL, et al: Creation of transjugular intrahepatic portosystemic shunts (TIPS) with the Wallstent endoprosthesis: Results in 100 patients. *Radiology,* 1993; 187:413–420.

15. Ring EJ, Lake JR, Roberts JP: Using transjugular intrahepatic portosystemic shunts to control variceal bleeding before liver transplantation. *Ann Intern Med* 1992; 116:304–309.

16. Brems JJ, Hiatt JR, Klein AS: Effect of a prior portasystemic shunt on subsequent liver transplantation. *Ann Surg* 1989; 209:51–56.

17. Mazzaferro V, Todo S, Tsakis AG: Liver transplantation in patients with previous portasystemic shunt. *Am J Surg* 1990; 160:111–116.

18. Langnas AN, Marujo WC, Stratta RJ: Influence of a prior porta-systemic shunt on outcome after liver transplantation. *Am J Gastroenterol* 1992; 87:714–718.

19. Conn HO, Lindenmuth WW, May CJ: Prophylactic portacaval anastomosis. A tale of two studies. *Medicine (Baltimore)* 1972; 51:27–40.

20. The Veterans Affairs Cooperative Variceal Sclerotherapy Group: Prophylactic sclerotherapy for esophageal varices in men with alcoholic liver disease: A randomized, single-blind, multicenter clinical trial. *N Engl J Med* 1991; 324:1779–1784.

21. Conn HO, Grace ND, Bosch J: Propranolol in the prevention of the first hemorrhage from esophageal varices: A multicenter, randomized clinical trial. *Hepatology* 1991; 13:902–912.

22. Ikegami M, Toyonaga A, Tanikawa K: Reduction of portal pressure by chronic administration of isosorbide dinitrate in patients with cirrhosis: Effects on systemic and splanchnic hemodynamics and liver function. *Am J Gastroenterol* 1992; 87:1160–1164.

23. Sanyal AJ, Freedman AM, Shiffman ML: Transjugular intrahepatic porto-systemic shunt for ascites: A preliminary report. *Am J Gastroenterol* 1992, in press.

24. Ochs A, Sellinger M, Haag K: Transjugular intrahepatic portosystemic stent-shunt (TIPS) for the treatment of refractory ascites and hepatorenal syndrome: Results of a pilot study (abstract). *Gastroenterology* 1992; 102:862.

25. Garcia-Villarreal L, Zozaya JM, Quiroga J, et al: Transjugular intrahepatic portosystemic shunt (TIPS) for intractable ascites (IA)—Preliminary results (abstract). *J Hepatol* 1992; 16(suppl):36.

26. Rossle M, Noeldge G, Ochs A: Feasibility of transjugular intrahepatic portosystemic stent shunt (TIPS) in the treatment of fulminant Budd-Chiari syndrome (BCS) (abstract). *Gastroenterology* 1992; 102:875.

27. Pladson TR, Parrish RM: Hepatorenal syndrome: Recovery after peritoneovenous shunt. *Arch Intern Med* 1977; 137:1248–1249.

28. Sellinger M, Haag K, Ochs A, et al: Factors influencing the incidence of hepatic encephalopathy in patients with transjugular intrahepatic portosystemic stent-shunt (TIPS) (abstract). *Hepatology* 1992; 16:122.

29. Somberg KA, Riegler JL, Doherty M, et al: Hepatic encephalopathy following transjugular intrahepatic portosystemic shunts (TIPS): Incidence and risk factors (abstract). *Hepatology* 1992; 16:122.

30. Sanyal AJ, Freedman AM, Shiffman ML: Portosystemic encephalopathy (PSE) following transjugular intrahepatic portosystemic shunt (TIPS): A controlled study (abstract). *Hepatology* 1992; 16(suppl):86.

31. Sellinger M, Ochs A, Haag K: Incidence of hepatic encephalopathy and follow-up of liver function in patients with transjugular intrahepatic portosystemic stent-shunt (TIPS) (abstract). *Gastroenterology* 1992; 102:883.

32. Rypins EB, Sarfeh IJ: Small-diameter portacaval H-graft for variceal hemorrhage. *Surg Clin North Am* 1990; 70:395–404.

33. Johansen K: Partial portal decompression for variceal hemorrhage. *Am J Surg* 1989; 157:479–482.

34. LaBerge JM, Ferrell LB, Ring EJ: Histopathologic study of transjugular intrahepatic portosystemic shunts. *J Vasc Intervent Radiol* 1991; 2:549–556.

35. Sanyal AJ: Hemolysis after TIPS (letter). *Ann Intern Med* 1992; 117:443.

36. Klastenburg DM, Munoz SJ: Complications of transjugular intrahepatic portal systemic shunting (TIPS) (abstract). *Am J Gastroenterol* 1992; 87:1300.

37. Conn HO, Grace ND, Bosch J: Propranolol in the prevention of the first hemorrhage from esophageal varices: A multicenter, randomized clinical trial. *Hepatology* 1991; 13:902–912.

38. Groszmann RJ, Bosch J, Grace ND: Hemodynamic events in a prospective randomized trial of propranolol vs placebo in the prevention of the first variceal hemorrhage. *Gastroenterology* 1990; 99:1401–1407.

39. Pagliaro L, D'Amico G, Sorensen TIA: Prevention of first bleeding in cirrhosis. A meta-analysis of randomized trials of nonsurgical treatment. *Ann Intern Med* 1992; 117:59–70.

40. Poynard T, Cales P, Pasta L: Beta-adrenergic–antagonists in the prevention of first gastrointestinal bleeding in patients with cirrhosis and oesophageal varices. An analysis of data and prognostic factors in 589 patients from four randomized clinical trials. *N Engl J Med* 1991; 324:1532–1538.

41. Van Ruiswyk J, Byrd JC: Efficacy of prophylactic sclerotherapy for prevention of a first variceal hemorrhage. *Gastroenterology* 1992; 102:587–597.

42. Paquet HJ: Prophylactic endoscopic sclerosing treatment of the esophageal wall in varices: A prospective controlled randomized trial. *Endoscopy* 1982; 14:4–5.

43. Witzel L, Wolbergs E, Merki H: Prophylactic endoscopic sclerotherapy of oesophageal varices: A prospective controlled trial. *Lancet* 1985; 1:773–775.

44. Pagliaro L, Burroughs AK, Sorensen TI: Therapeutic controversies and randomized controlled trials (RCTs): Prevention of bleeding and rebleeding in cirrhosis. *Gastroenterol Int* 1989; 1:71–84.

45. Conn HO, Lindenmuth WW, May CJ, et al: Prophylactic portacaval anastomosis. A tale of two studies. *Medicine (Baltimore)* 1972; 51:27–40.

46. Inokuchi K, Cooperative Study Group of Portal Hypertension of Japan: Improved survival following prophylactic portal nondecompression surgery for esophageal varices. *Hepatology* 1990; 12:1–6.

47. Conn HO: Why is prophylactic portal nondecompressive surgery effective in preventing hemorrhage from esophageal varices? *Hepatology* 1990; 12:166–169.

48. Hashizume M, Kitano S, Koyanagi N: Endoscopic injection sclerotherapy for 1000 patients with esophageal varices: A nine-year prospective study. *Hepatology* 1992; 15:69–75.

49. Kitano S, Koyanagi N, Iso N: Prevention of recurrence of esophageal varices after endoscopic injection sclerotherapy with ethanolamine oleate. *Hepatology* 1987; 7:810–815.

50. Higashi H, Kitano S, Hashizume M: A prospective randomized trial of schedules for sclerosing esophageal varices: 1- versus 2-week intervals. *Hepatogastroenterology* 1989; 36:337–340.

51. Sugiura M, Futagawa S: Results of six hundred and thirty six esophageal transections with paraesophagogastric devascularization in the treatment of esophageal varices. *J Vasc Surg* 1984; 1:254–260.

52. Spence RA, Johnston GW: Results in 100 consecutive patients with stapled esophageal transection for varices. *Surg Gynecol Obstet* 1985; 160:323–329.

53. Triger DR, Johnson AG, Brazier JE: A prospective trial of endoscopic sclerotherapy v oesophageal transection and gastric devascularisation in the long term management of bleeding oesophageal varices. *Gut* 1992; 33:1553–1558.

54. Stiegmann G, Cambre T, Sun JH: A new endoscopic elastic band ligating device. *Gastrointest Endosc* 1986; 32:230–233.

55. Stiegmann G, Goff JS, Sun JH: Endoscopic ligation of esophageal varices. *Am J Surg* 1990; 159:21–26.

56. Stiegmann G, Goff JS, Michaletz-Onody PA: Endoscopic sclerotherapy as compared with endoscopic ligation for bleeding esophageal varices. *N Engl J Med* 1992; 326:1527–1532.

57. Rikkers IF, Burnett DA, Volentine GD: Shunt surgery versus endoscopic sclerotherapy for long-term treatment of variceal bleeding: Early results of a randomized trial. *Ann Surg* 1987; 206:261–271.

58. Spina GP, Santambrogio R, Opocher E: Distal splenorenal shunt versus endoscopic sclerotherapy in the prevention of variceal rebleeding: First stage of a randomized, controlled trial. *Ann Surg* 1990; 211:178–186.

59. Orloff MJ, Orloff MS, Rambotti M, et al: Is portal-systemic shunt worthwhile in Child's class C cirrhosis? *Ann Surg* 1992; 216:256–268.

60. Sarin SK, Lahoti D, Saxena SP: Prevalence, classification and natural history of gastric varices: A long-term follow-up study in 568 portal hypertension patients. *Hepatology* 1992; 16:1343–1349.

61. Vigneri S, Termini R, Piraino A: The stomach in liver cirrhosis. Endoscopic, morphological, and clinical correlations. *Gastroenterology* 1991; 101:472–478.

62. Iwao T, Toyonaga A, Sumino M: Portal hypertensive gastropathy in patients with cirrhosis. *Gastroenterology* 1992; 102:2060–2065.

63. Groszmann RJ, Kravetz D, Bosch J: Nitroglycerin improves the hemodynamic response to vasopressin in portal hypertension. *Hepatology* 1982; 2:757–762.

64. Lee F-Y, Tsai Y-T, Lin H-C: Hemodynamic effects of a combination of vasopressin and ketanserin in patients with hepatitis B-related cirrhosis. *J Hepatol* 1992; 15:54–58.

65. Ruiz del Arbol L, Garcia-Pagan JC, Feu F: Effects of molsidomine, a long acting venous dilator, on portal hypertension. A hemodynamic study in patients with cirrhosis. *J Hepatol* 1991; 13:179–186.

66. Aramaki T, Sekiyama T, Katsuta Y: Long-term haemodynamic effects of a 4-week regimen of nipradilol, a new beta-blocker with nitrovasodilating properties, in patients with portal hypertension due to cirrhosis. A comparative study with propranolol. *J Hepatol* 1992; 15:48–53.

67. Schrier RW, Arroyo V, Bernardi M: Peripheral arterial vasodilation hypothesis: A proposal for the initiation of renal sodium and water retention in cirrhosis. *Hepatology* 1988; 8:1151–1157.

68. Dudley FJ: Pathophysiology of ascites formation. *Gastroenterol Clin North Am* 1992; 21:215–232.

69. Warner LC, Campbell PJ, Morali GA: The response of atrial natriuretic factor and sodium excretion to dietary sodium challenges in patients with chronic liver disease. *Hepatology* 1990; 12:460–466.

70. Gerbes A, Wernze H, Arendt RM: Atrial natriuretic factor and renin-aldosterone in volume regulation of patients with cirrhosis. *Hepatology* 1989; 9:417–422.

71. Bankovsky HL, Hartle DK, Mellen BG: Plasma concentrations of immunoreactive atrial natriuretic peptide in hospitalized cirrhotic and non-cirrhotic patients: Evidence for a role of deficient atrial natriuretic peptide in pathogenesis of cirrhotic ascites. *Am J Gastroenterol* 1988; 83:531–535.

72. Angeli P, Caregaro L, Menon F: Variability of atrial natriuretic peptide plasma levels in ascitic cirrhotics: Pathophysiological and clinical implications. *Hepatology* 1992; 16:1389–1394.

73. Conn JW, Hinerman DL: Spironolactone-induced inhibition of aldosterone biosynthesis in primary aldosteronism. Morphological and functional studies. *Metabolism* 1977; 26:1293–1307.

74. Morali GA, Tobe SW, Skorecki KL, et al: Refractory ascites: Modulation of atrial natriuretic factor unresponsiveness by mannitol. *Hepatology* 1992; 16:42–48.

75. Panos MZ, Anderson JV, Payne N: Plasma atrial natriuretic peptide and renin-aldosterone in patients with cirrhosis and ascites: Basal levels, changes during daily activity and nocturnal diuresis. *Hepatology* 1992; 16:82–88.

76. La Villa G, Salmeron JM, Arroyo V: Mineralocorticoid escape in patients with compensated cirrhosis and portal hypertension. *Gastroenterology* 1992; 102:2114–2119.

77. Solis-Herruzo JA, Gonzalez-Gamarra A, Castellano G, et al: Metabolic clearance rate of arginine vasopressin in patients with cirrhosis. *Hepatology* 1992; 16:974–979.

78. Andus T, Gross V, Holstege A: Evidence for the production of high amounts of interleukin-6 in the peritoneal cavity of patients with ascites. *J Hepatol* 1992; 15:378–381.

79. Friedman HS, Fernando H: Ascites as a marker for the hyperdynamic heart of Laënnec's cirrhosis. *Alcoholism* 1992; 16:968–970.

80. Conn HO: The diagnosis and examination of ascitic fluid, in Beker S (ed): *Hepatic Diseases*. New York, ARUSS, 1983, pp 529–565.

81. Runyon BA, Montano AA, Akriviadis EA, et al: The serum-ascites albumin gradient is superior to the exudate-transudate concept in the differential diagnosis of ascites. *Ann Intern Med* 1992; 117:215–220.

82. Mauer K, Manzione NC: Usefulness of the serum-ascites albumin concentration gradient in separating transudative from exudative ascites: Another look. *Dig Dis Sci* 1988; 33:1208–1212.

83. Hoefs JC: Serum protein concentration and portal pressure determine the ascitic fluid protein concentration in patients with chronic liver disease. *J Lab Clin Med* 1983; 102:260–273.

84. Runyon BA: Low-protein-concentration ascitic fluid is predisposed to spontaneous bacterial peritonitis. *Gastroenterology* 1986; 91:1343–1346.

85. Pockros PJ, Esrason KT, Nguyen C, et al: Mobilization of malignant ascites with diuretics is dependent on ascitic fluid characteristics. *Gastroenterology* 1992; 103:1302–1306.

86. Feldman GB: Lymphatic obstruction in carcinomatous ascites. *Cancer Res* 1975; 35:325–332.

87. Chonko AM, Bay BH, Stein JH, et al: The role of renin and aldosterone in the salt retention of edema. *Am J Med* 1977; 63:881–885.

88. Lee C-M, Changchien C-S, Shyu W-C, et al: Serum-ascites albumin concentration gradient and ascites fibronectin in the diagnosis of malignant ascites, *Cancer* 1992; 70:2057–2060.

89. Simon DM, McCain JR, Bonkovsky HL: Effects of therapeutic paracentesis on systemic and hepatic hemodynamics and on the renal and hormonal function. *Hepatology* 1987; 7:423–429.

90. Panos MZ, Moore K, Vlavianos P: Single, total paracentesis for tense ascites: sequential hemodynamic changes and right atrial size. *Hepatology* 1990; 11:662–667.

91. Gentile S, Angelico M, Bologna E: Clinical, biochemical, and hormonal changes after a single large-volume paracentesis in cirrhosis with ascites. *Am J Gastroenterol* 1989; 84:279.

92. Arroyo V, Gines P, Planas R: Treatment of ascites in cirrhosis. *Gastroenterol Clin North Am* 1992; 21:237–256.

93. Gines P, Tito LL, Arroyo V: Randomized comparative study of therapeutic paracentesis with and without intravenous albumin in cirrhosis. *Gastroenterology* 1988; 94:1493–1505.

94. Planas R, Gines P, Arroyo V: Dextran-70 versus albumin as plasma expanders in cirrhotic patients with tense ascites treated with total paracentesis: Results of a randomized study. *Gastroenterology* 1990; 99:1736–1741.

95. Salerno F, Badalamenti S, Lorenza E: Randomized comparative study of hemaccel vs albumin infusion after total paracentesis in cirrhotic patients with refractory ascites. *Hepatology* 1991; 13:707–713.

96. Terg R, Romero G, Berreta J: Dextran administration avoids hemodynamic changes following paracentesis in cirrhotic patients. A safe and inexpensive option. *Dig Dis Sci* 1991, in press.

97. Fassio E, Terg R, Landeira G: Paracentesis with dextran 70 vs. paracentesis with albumin in cirrhosis with tense ascites. Results of a randomized study. *J Hepatol* 1992; 14:310–316.

98. Cabrera J, Inglada L, Quintero E: Large-volume paracentesis and intravenous saline: effects on the renin-angiotensin system. *Hepatology* 1991; 14:1025–1028.

99. Salerno F: Large-volume paracentesis and volume re-expansion: Can synthetic plasma expanders safely replace albumin? *J Hepatol* 1992; 14:143–145.

100. Runyon BA: Paracentesis of ascitic fluid: A safe procedure. *Arch Intern Med* 1986; 146:2259–2261.

101. Qureshi WA, Harshfield D, Shah H: An unusual complication of paracentesis. *Am J Gastroenterol* 1992; 87:1209–1211.

102. Ditchfield MR, Gibson RN, Donlan JD, et al: Duplex Doppler ultrasound signs of portal hypertension: Relative diagnostic value of examination of paraumbilical vein, portal vein and spleen. *Australas Radiol* 1992; 36:102–105.

103. Wilcox CM, Woods BL, Mixon HT: Prospective evaluation of a peritoneal dialysis catheter system for large volume paracentesis. *Am J Gastroenterol* 1992; 87:1443–1446.

104. Lenz K, Hortnagl H, Druml W: Beneficial effect of 8-ornithine vasopressin on renal dysfunction in decompensated cirrhosis. *Gut* 1989; 30:90–96.

105. Moore K, Wendon J, Frazer M: Plasma endothelin immunoreactivity in liver disease and the hepatorenal syndrome. *N Engl J Med* 1992; 327:1774–1778.

106. Loutzenhiser R, Epstein M, Hayashi K, et al: Direct visualization of the effects of endothelin on the renal microvasculature. *Am J Physiol* 1990; 258:61–68.

107. Iwatsuki S, Corman J, Popovtzer M, et al: Recovery from hepatorenal syndrome after successful orthotopic liver transplantation. *Surgical Forum* 1973; 24:348–350.

108. Detroz G, Honore P, Monami B: Combined treatment of liver failure and hepatorenal syndrome with orthotopic liver transplantation. *Acta Gastroenterol Belg* 1992; 55:350–357.

109. Conn HO: Spontaneous peritonitis and bacteremia in cirrhotic patients caused by enteric bacteria. *Ann Intern Med* 1964; 60:568–580.

110. Conn HO, Fessel JM: Spontaneous bacterial peritonitis in cirrhosis. Variations on a theme. *Medicine (Baltimore)* 1971; 50:161–197.

111. Garcia-Tsao G: Spontaneous bacterial peritonitis. *Gastroenterol Clin North Am* 1992; 21:257–275.

112. Alpern HD, Zulick LC, Reese RE: Spontaneous bacterial peritonitis (letter). *J Clin Gastroenterol* 1992; 15:89–90.

113. Runyon B, Hoefs J: Ascitic fluid analysis in the differentiation of spontaneous bacterial peritonitis from gastrointestinal tract perforation into ascitic fluid. *Hepatology* 1984; 4:447–450.

114. Francis TI, Osoba AO: Gonococcal hepatitis (Fitz-Hugh–Curtis syndrome) in a male patient. *Br J Vener Dis* 1972; 48:187–188.

115. Brase R, Kuckelt W, Manhold C, et al: Spontaneous bacterial peritonitis without ascites. *Anasth Intensivether Notfallmed* 1992; 27:325–327.

116. Chu C-M, Chiu K-W, Liaw Y-F: The prevalence and prognostic significance of spontaneous bacterial peritonitis in severe acute hepatitis with ascites. *Hepatology* 1992; 15:799–803.

117. Valla D, Flejou JF, Lebrec D, et al: Portal hypertension and ascites in acute hepatitis: Clinical, hemodynamic and histological correlations. *Hepatology* 1989; 10:482–487.

118. Thomas FB, Fromkes JJ: Spontaneous bacterial peritonitis associated with acute viral hepatitis. *J Clin Gastroenterol* 1982; 4:259–262.

119. Gimson AE, O'Grady J, Ede RJ: Late onset hepatic failure: Clinical serological and histological features. *Hepatology* 1986; 6:288–294.

120. Chesta J, Brahm J, Poniachik J: Spontaneous bacterial peritonitis: A frequent and recurrent complication in cirrhotic patients with ascites. *Rev Med Chile* 1991; 119:273–278.

121. Press AG, Meyer zum Buschenfelde KH, Ramadori G: Spontaneous bacterial peritonitis. *Z Gastroenterol* 1992; 30:543–552.

122. Amarapurkar DN, Viswanathan N, Parikh SS: Prevalence of spontaneous bacterial peritonitis. *J Assoc Physicians India* 1992; 40:236–238.

123. Gomez-Jimenez J, Ribera E, Martinez-Vasquez JM: Bacterial peritonitis in cirrhosis. Prospective study of 80 episodes. *Med Clin* 1992; 99:493–497.

124. Thornton JR, Losowsky MS: Septicaemia after colonoscopy in patients with cirrhosis. *Gut* 1991; 32:450–451.

125. Runyon BA: Low-protein-concentration ascitic fluid is predisposed to spontaneous bacterial peritonitis. *Gastroenterology* 1986; 91:1343–1346.

126. Runyon BA: Patients with deficient ascitic fluid opsonic activity are predisposed to spontaneous bacterial peritonitis. *Hepatology* 1988; 8:632–635.

127. Llach J, Rimola A, Navasa M: Incidence and predictive factors of first episode of spontaneous bacterial peritonitis in cirrhosis with ascites: Relevance of ascitic fluid protein concentration. *Hepatology* 1992; 16:724–727.

128. Rimola A: Infections in liver disease, in McIntyre N, Benhamou J-P, Bircher J (eds): *Oxford Textbook of Clinical Hepatology*. Oxford, Oxford Medical Press, 1991, pp 1272–1284.

129. Tito LL, Rimola A, Gines P: Recurrence of spontaneous bacterial peritonitis in cirrhosis: Frequency and predictive factors. *Hepatology* 1988; 8:27–31.

130. Soriano G, Guarner C, Tomas A: Norfloxacin prevents bacterial infection in cirrhotics with gastrointestinal hemorrhage. *Gastroenterology* 1992; 103:1267–1272.

131. Gines P, Rimola A, Planas R: Norfloxacin prevents spontaneous bacterial peritonitis recurrence in cirrhosis: Results of a double-blind, placebo-controlled trial. *Hepatology* 1990; 12:716–724.

132. Soriano G, Guarner C, Teixido M: Selective intestinal decontamination prevents spontaneous bacterial peritonitis. *Gastroenterology* 1991; 100:477–481.

133. Karp JE, Merz WG, Hendricksen C: Oral norfloxacin for prevention of gram-negative bacterial infections in patients with acute leukemia and granulocytopenia. A randomized, double-blind, placebo-controlled trial. *Ann Intern Med* 1987; 106:1–7.

134. Wyke RJ, Canalese JC, Gimson AES: Bacteraemia in patients with fulminant hepatic failure. *Liver* 1982; 2:45–52.

135. Rolando N, Harvey F, Brahm J: Prospective study of bacterial infection in acute liver failure: An analysis of fifty patients. *Hepatology* 1990; 11:49–53.

136. Salmeron JM, Tito L, Rimola A: Selective intestinal decontamination in the prevention of bacterial infection in patients with acute liver failure. *J Hepatol* 1992; 14:280–285.

137. Terg R, Levi D, Lobez P: Analysis of clinical course and prognosis of culture-positive spontaneous bacterial peritonitis and neutrocytic ascites. Evidence of the same disease. *Dig Dis Sci* 1992; 37:1499–1504.

138. Runyon BA, Hoefs JC: Culture-negative neutrocytic ascites: A variant of spontaneous bacterial peritonitis. *Hepatology* 1984; 4:1209–1211.

139. Pelletier G, Salmon D, Ink O: Culture-negative neutrocytic ascites: A less severe variant of spontaneous bacterial peritonitis. *J Hepatol* 1990; 10:327–331.

140. Runyon BA, Sugano S, Kanel G, et al: A rodent model of cirrhosis, ascites, and bacterial peritonitis. *Gastroenterology* 1991; 100:489–493.

141. Churchill WLS, Radiotalk, October 1939: *Into Battle,* 1941, p 131.

142. Haussinger D: Liver glutamine metabolism. *JPEN J Parenter Enteral Nutr* 1990; 14(suppl 4):56–62.

143. Haussinger D: Hepatocyte heterogeneity in glutamine and ammonia metabolism and the role of an intercellular glutamine cycle during ureagenesis in perfused rat liver. *Eur J Biochem* 1983; 133:269–274.

144. Stoll B, McNeilly S, Buscher HP, et al: Functional hepatocyte heterogeneity in glutamate, aspartate and α-ketoglutarate uptake: A histoautoradiographical study. *Hepatology* 1991; 13:247–253.

145. Butterworth RF: Pathogenesis and treatment of portal-systemic encephalopathy: An update. *Dig Dis Sci* 1992; 37:321–327.

146. Lockwood AH, Yap EWH, Wong W-H: Cerebral ammonia metabolism in patients with severe liver disease and minimal hepatic encephalopathy. *J Cereb Blood Flow Metab* 1991; 11:337–341.

147. Lockwood AH, Yap EWH, Rhoades BA, et al: Altered cerebral blood flow and glucose metabolism in patients with liver disease and minimal encephalopathy. *J Cereb Blood Flow Metab* 1991; 11:331–336.

148. Haskal ZJ, Ring EJ, LaBerge JM: Role of parallel transjugular intrahepatic portosystemic shunts in patients with persistent portal hypertension. *Radiology* 1992; 185:813–817.

149. Azorin I, Minana M-D, Felipo V: A simple animal model of hyperammonemia. *Hepatology* 1989; 10:311–314.

150. Campollo O, Sprengers D, McIntyre N: The BCAA/AAA ratio of plasma amino acids in three different groups of cirrhotics. *Rev Invest Clin* 1992; 44:513–518.

151. Eriksson LS, Conn HO: Branched chain amino acids in the management of hepatic encephalopathy: An analysis of variants. *Hepatology* 1989; 10:228–246.

152. Marchesini G, Dioguardi FS, Bianchi GP: Long-term oral branched-chain amino acid treatment

in chronic hepatic encephalopathy. A randomized double-blind casein-controlled trial. *J Hepatol* 1990; 11:1–10.

153. Bianchi GP, Marchesini G, Zoli M: Oral BCAA supplementation in cirrhosis with chronic encephalopathy: Effects on prolactin and estradiol levels. *Hepatogastroenterology* 1992; 39:443–446.

154. McClain CJ, Krombout JP, Elson MK: Hyperprolactinemia in portal systemic encephalopathy. *Dig Dis Sci* 1976; 26:353–357.

155. Van Rijt CCD, Schalm SW: Zina deficiency and hepatic encephalopathy, in Conn HO, Bircher J (eds): *Hepatic Encephalopathy: Syndromes and Therapies*. East Lansing, Mich, Medi-Ed Press, 1994, pp 365–372.

156. Grungreiff K, Franke D, Lobner B: Zinc deficiency—a factor in the pathogenesis of hepatic encephalopathy? *Z Gastroenterol* 1991; 29:101–106.

157. Scholmerich J, Becher MS, Kottgen E: The influence of porto-systemic shunting on zinc and vitamin A deficiency in liver cirrhosis. *Hepatogastroenterology* 1983; 30:143–147.

158. Reding P, Duchateau J, Bataille C: Oral zinc supplementation improves hepatic encephalopathy. *Lancet* 1984; 2:493–494.

159. Riggio O, Merli M, Capocaccia L: Zinc supplementation reduces blood ammonia and increases liver ornithine transcarbamylase activity in experimental cirrhosis. *Hepatology* 1992; 16:785–789.

160. Planas R, Gomes-Vieira MC, Cabre E, et al: Prognostic factors of hepatic encephalopathy after portacaval anastomosis: A multivariate analysis in 50 patients. *Am J Gastroenterol* 1992; 87:1792–1796.

161. Ito T, Ikeda N, Watanabe A: Obliteration of portal systemic shunts as therapy for hepatic encephalopathy in patients with non-cirrhotic portal hypertension. *Gastroenterol Jpn* 1992; 27:759–764.

162. Conn HO: The trailmaking and balloon connection tests in assessing mental state in portalsystemic encephalopathy. *Am J Dig Dis* 1977; 22:541–550.

163. Conn HO. Subclinical hepatic encephalopathy, in Conn HO, Bircher J (eds): *Hepatic Encephalopathy: Syndromes and Therapies*. East Lansing, Mich, Medi-Ed Press, 1994, p 27–42.

164. Zeneroli ML, Cioni G, Ventura P: The number connection test: Corrections for age and education (letter). *J Hepatol* 1992; 15:263–264.

165. Van der Rijt CCD, Schalm SW: Quantitative EEG analysis and evoked potentials to measure (latent) hepatic encephalopathy. *J Hepatol* 1992; 14:141–142.

166. Van der Rijt CCD, Schalm SW, DeGroot GH: Objective measurement of hepatic encephalopathy by means of automated EEG analysis. *Electroencephalogr Clin Neurophysiol* 1984; 57:423–426.

167. Weissenborn K, Scholz M, Hinrichs H: Neurophysiological assessment of early hepatic encephalopathy. *Electroencephalogr Clin Neurophysiol* 1990; 75:289–295.

168. Conn HO, Lieberthal MM: *The Hepatic Coma Syndromes and Lactulose*. Baltimore, Williams & Wilkins, 1979.

169. Conn HO, Bircher J: *Hepatic Encephalopathy: Syndromes and Therapies*. East Lansing, Mich, Medi-Ed Press, 1994.

170. Van Velthuijsen JA: Lactitol: Chemical and biological properties, in Conn HO, Bircher J (eds): *Hepatic Encephalopathy: Syndromes and Therapies*. East Lansing, Mich, Medi-Ed Press, 1994, pp 219–242.

171. Morgan MY: Lactitol for the treatment of hepatic encephalopathy, in Conn HO, Bircher J (eds): *Hepatic Encephalopathy: Syndromes and Therapies*. East Lansing, Mich, Medi-Ed Press, 1994, pp 243–264.

172. Uribe M: Management of PSE with lactose in patients with lactase deficiency, in Conn HO, Bircher J (eds): *Hepatic Encephalopathy: Syndromes and Therapies*. East Lansing, Mich, Medi-Ed Press, 1994, pp 311–330.

173. Vendemiale G, Palasciano G, Cirelli G: Crystalline lactulose in the therapy of hepatic cirrhosis. *Arzneimittelforschung* 1992; 42:969–972.

174. Lockwood AH, McDonald JM, Reiman RE: The dynamics of ammonia metabolism in man. Effects of liver disease and hyperammonemia. *J Clin Invest* 1979; 63:449–460.

175. Agostini L, Down PF, Murison J: Faecal ammonia and pH during lactulose administration in man: Comparison with other cathartics. *Gut* 1972; 13:859–866.

176. Vince A, Killingley M, Wrong OM: Effect of lactulose on ammonia production in a fecal incubation system. *Gastroenterology* 1978; 74:544–549.

177. Mortensen PB: The effect of oral-administered lactulose on colonic nitrogen metabolism and excretion. *Hepatology* 1992; 16:1350–1356.

178. Mortensen PB, Holtug K, Bonnen H: The degradation of amino acids, proteins and blood to short-chain fatty acids is prevented by lactulose. *Gastroenterology* 1990; 98:353–360.

179. Peters SG, Pomare EW, Fisher CA: Portal and peripheral blood short chain fatty acid concentrations after caecal lactulose instillation at surgery. *Gut* 1992; 33:1249–1252.

180. Blanc P, Daures JP, Rouillon JM, et al: Lactitol of lactulose in the treatment of chronic hepatic encephalopathy: Results of a meta-analysis. *Hepatology* 1992; 15:222–228.

181. Merli M, Caschera M, Piat C: The effect of lactulose and lactitol administration on fecal fat excretion in patients with liver cirrhosis. *J Clin Gastroenterol* 1992; 15:125–127.

182. Strauss E, Tramote R, Silva EP: Double-blind randomized clinical trial comparing neomycin and placebo in the treatment of exogenous hepatic encephalopathy. *Hepatogastroenterology* 1992; 39:542–545.

183. Festi D, Mazzella G, Parini P: Treatment of hepatic encephalopathy with non-absorbable antibiotics. *Ital J Gastroenterol* 1992; 24(suppl 2):14–16.

184. Cellai L, Cerrini S, Brufani M: Structure-activity relationship in a new rifamycin: L 105. A potential topical intestinal antibiotic (abstract). *Chemioterapia* 1982; 1(Suppl 4):217.

185. DiPiazza S, Filippazzo MG, Valenza LM: Rifaximin versus neomycin in the treatment of porto-systemic encephalopathy. *Ital J Gastroenterol* 1991; 23:403–407.

186. Pedretti G, Calzetti C, Missale G: Rifaximin versus neomycin on hyperammoniemia in chronic portal systemic encephalopathy of cirrhotics. A double blind, randomized trial. *Ital J Gastroenterol* 1991; 23:175–178.

187. Parini P, Cipolla A, Ronchi M: Effect of rifaximin and paromomycin in the treatment of portal-systemic encephalopathy. *Curr Ther Res* 1992; 51:1–6.

188. Mendenhall CL, Rooster S, Marshall L: A new therapy for portal systemic encephalopathy. *Am J Gastroenterol* 1986; 81:540–543.

189. Uribe M, Marin E, Cervera E: Sodium benzoate versus disaccharides: A controlled multicenter clinical trial (abstract). Presented at the Bien Sci Mtg International Association for Study of the Liver. Gold Coast, Australia, Sept 1990.

190. Sushma S, Dasarathy S, Tandon RK: Sodium benzoate in the treatment of acute hepatic encephalopathy: A double-blind randomized trial. *Hepatology* 1992; 16:138–144.

191. Conn HO, Leevy CM, Vlacevic ZR: A comparison of lactulose and neomycin in the treatment of portal-systemic encephalopathy: A double blind controlled trial. *Gastroenterology* 1977; 72:573–583.

192. Banko G, Zollner H: Does ornithine stimulate carbamoylphosphate synthetase? *Int J Biochem* 1985; 17:503–507.

193. Stoll B, Haussinger D: Functional hepatocyte heterogeneity: Vascular oxoglutarate is almost exclusively taken up by perivenous glutamine-synthetase–containing hepatocytes. *Eur J Biochem* 1989; 181:709–716.

194. Haussinger D, Gerok W: Hepatocyte heterogeneity in ammonia metabolism: Impairment of glu-

tamine synthetase in CCl_4-induced liver cell necrosis with no effect on urea synthesis. *Chem Biol Interact* 1984; 48:191–194.

195. Kaiser S, Gerok W, Haussinger D: Ammonia and glutamine metabolism in human liver slices: New aspects of the pathogenesis of hyperammonemia in chronic liver disease. *Eur J Clin Invest* 1988; 18:535–542.

196. Batshaw ML, Walser M, Brusilow SW: Plasma α-ketoglutarate in urea cycle enzymopathies and its role as a harbinger of hyperammonemic coma. *Pediatr Res* 1980; 14:1316–1319.

197. Zieve L, Lyftogt C, Raphael D: Ammonia toxicity: Comparative protective effect of various arginine and ornithine derivatives, aspartate, benzoate, and carbamyl glutamate. *Metab Brain Dis* 1986; 1:25–35.

198. Batshaw ML, Thomas GH, Brusilow SW: New approaches to the diagnosis and treatment of inborn errors of urea synthesis. *Pediatrics* 1981; 68:290–297.

199. Henglein-Ottermann D: Der einflus von Ornithin-Aspartat auf die experimentell erzeugte Hyperammoniamie. Klinisch experimentelle Studie. *Ther Gegenw* 1976; 115:1504–1518.

200. Leweling H, Kortsik C, Gladisch R: Effects of ornithine aspartate on plasma ammonia and plasma amino acids in patients with liver cirrhosis. A double-blind, randomized study using a four-fold cross-over design, in Bengtsson F, et al (eds): *Progress in Hepatic Encephalopathy and Metabolic Nitrogen Exchange*. Boca Raton, Fla, CRC Press, 1991 pp 377–389.

201. Nilius R, Kircheis G: Plazebokontrollierte Doppelblindstudie zur therapeutischen Wirksamkeit von L-Ornithin-L-Aspartat-Infusionskonzentrat bei Patienten mit Leberzirrhose und hepatischer Enzephalopathie, in Kuntz E (ed): *Die Hepatische Enzephalopathie. Aspekte der Diagnose und Behandlung* Jena, Germany, Univ-Verlag 1992, pp 99–117.

202. Stauch S, Rosch W: Ornithin-Aspartat in der Therapie der hepatischen Enzephalopathie. Eine plazebokontrollierte Doppelblindstudie, in Kuntz E (ed): *Die Hepatische Enzephalopathie. Aspekte der Diagnose und Behandlung*. Jena, Germany, Univ-Verlag 1992, pp 89–98.

203. Liehr H, Huth M, Kircheis G, et al: A comparison of L-ornithine-L-aspartate and lactulose in the management of chronic liver disease and hepatic encephalopathy (HE) (abstract). *J Gastroenterol Hepatol* 1992; 7(Suppl 1):106.

204. Kircheis G: L-Ornithine-L-aspartate, in Conn HO, Bircher J (eds): *Hepatic Encephalopathy: Syndromes and Therapies*. East Lansing, Mich, Medi-Ed Press, 1994, pp 373–383.

205. Felipo V, Minana MD, Grisolia S: Paradoxical protection of both protein-free and high protein diets against acute ammonium intoxication. *Biochem Biophys Res Commun* 1988; 156:506–510.

206. Felipo V, Minana MD, Grisolia S: Control of urea synthesis and ammonia utilization in protein deprivation and refeeding. *Arch Biochem Biophys* 1991; 285:351–356.

207. Grau E, Felipo V, Minana M-D: Treatment of hyperammonemia with carbamylglutamate in rats. *Hepatology* 1991; 15:446–448.

208. Brown R, Manning R, Delp M: Treatment of hepatocerebral intoxication. *Lancet* 1958; 1:591–592.

209. Ugarte G, Pino ME, Valenzuela J: Urea cycle enzymatic abnormalities in patients in endogenous hepatic coma. *Gastroenterology* 1963; 45:182–188.

210. Khatra BS, Smith RB III, Millikan WJ: Activities of Krebs-Henseleit enzymes in normal and cirrhotic human liver. *J Lab Clin Med* 1974; 84:708–715.

211. Todo S, Starzl TE, Tzakin A: Orthotopic liver transplantation for urea cycle enzyme deficiency. *Hepatology* 1992; 15:419–422.

212. Ede RJ, Williams R: Hepatic encephalopathy and cerebral edema. *Semin Liver Dis* 1986; 6:107–118.

213. Lidofsky SD, Bass NM, Prager MC: Intracranial pressure monitoring and liver transplantation for fulminant hepatic failure. *Hepatology* 1992; 16:1–7.

214. Munoz SJ, Robinson M, Northrup B: Elevated intracranial pressure and computed tomography of the brain in fulminant hepatocellular failure. *Hepatology* 1991; 13:209–212.

215. Crippin JS, Gross JB Jr, Lindor KD: Increased intracranial pressure and hepatic encephalopathy in chronic liver disease. *Am J Gastroenterol* 1992; 87:879–882.

216. Kreis R, Ross BD, Farrow NA: Metabolic disorders of the brain in chronic hepatic encephalopathy detected with H-1 MR spectroscopy. *Radiology* 1992; 182:19–27.

217. Takahashi H, Koehler RC, Brusilow SL: Inhibition of brain glutamine accumulation prevents cerebral edema in hyperammonemic rats. *Am J Physiol* 1991; 261:825–829.

218. Sussman NL, Chong MG, Koussayer T: Reversal of fulminant hepatic failure using an extracorporeal liver assist device. *Hepatology* 1992; 16:60–65.

CHAPTER 9

Bile Acid Abnormalities in Biliary Tract Diseases

Gerald Salen, M.D.

Professor of Medicine, University of Medicine and Dentistry of New Jersey-New Jersey Medical School, Newark, New Jersey; Gastrointestinal Research Laboratory, Veterans Administration Medical Center, East Orange, New Jersey

Ashok K. Batta, Ph.D.

Associate Professor of Medicine, University of Medicine and Dentistry of New Jersey-New Jersey Medical School, Newark, New Jersey

G. Stephen Tint, Ph.D.

Professor of Medicine, University of Medicine and Dentistry of New Jersey-New Jersey Medical School, Newark, New Jersey; Gastrointestinal Research Laboratory, Veterans Administration Medical Center, East Orange, New Jersey

Recently, increased attention has focused on the role of bile acids as either cause or treatment of a number of important gastrointestinal or hepatic diseases. This article reviews the most important advances.

PRIMARY BILIARY CIRRHOSIS

Introduction

Primary biliary cirrhosis (PBC), most often diagnosed in middle-aged women, is a progressive, often fatal cholestatic liver disease characterized by destruction of interlobular bile ducts with resultant cirrhosis and eventual liver failure. The disease may take several years to diagnose, and the initial symptoms are usually pruritus followed by xanthelasmas and mild hepatomegaly in many cases. Serum alkaline phosphatase and γ-glutamyltranspeptidase levels are markedly increased, and as the disease progresses, the serum transaminases are also increased. Pruritus may sometimes recede, but antimitochondrial antibodies are now demonstrated in almost all cases. Histologically, PBC is classified into four stages: stage I is characterized by marked infiltration of periportal tracts and proliferation of bile ducts. In stage II, the inflammatory infiltrations extend to the liver parenchyma, and in stage III, the proliferation of bile ducts is reduced. In stage IV, liver cirrhosis occurs, hepatic tissue is indurated by connective tissue, and the bile ducts are rarified.

The etiology of the disease is not known, but altered immune mechanisms are thought to lead to the initial bile duct damage[1] that results in impaired hepatic clearance of bile acids and their retention in the blood and liver.[2-5] The occurrence of concomitant immune diseases like keratoconjunctivitis sicca, arthropathies, thyroiditis, etc., also results from the expression of immunoreactions. Histologically there is augmentation of T_4 and T_8 lymphocytes. So far there has been no effective treatment for PBC, and drugs like azathioprine, corticosteroids, D-penicillamine, chlorambucil, phenobarbital, and rifampicin are of questionable benefit and limited by toxicity.[6-15] Improvement in liver biochemical tests but not in symptoms or histology has been demonstrated after colchicine and methotrexate therapy.[16-20] Hepatic transplantation has thus far been the only definitive treatment for PBC,[21-23] but the transplanted liver has also shown early damage.[24] With the advent of new drugs that may improve life expectancy, it has become important to predict survival in patients with PBC. It is imperative that all patients with PBC be treated as early as possible since the life expectancy of even asymptomatic patients may be shortened and it has been shown that there is a higher survival rate in symptomatic patients than in asymptomatic patients.[25] Increased bilirubin levels, which usually occur in the later stage of the disease, may be a useful criterion for selection of patients for liver transplantation[26] but not for survival in the initial stage of disease. A combination of laboratory, clinical, and histologic data can be helpful,[6, 26-28] but these require liver biopsy. The Mayo model, proposed recently and based on five clinical and laboratory variables to predict survival at any stage of PBC,[29] has now been shown to accurately predict survival of patients with PBC only when measured at a point more than 2 years before death and may not be reliable for patients with end-stage disease.[30] Thus this model may be useful early in the disease when therapies are considered, but not for timing of liver transplantation.

As a result of impaired bile formation and secretion, endogenous detergent bile acids such as chenodeoxycholic acid (CDCA) and cholic acid (Fig 1) accumulate in the hepatocyte and may dissolve hepatocyte membranes composed of phospholipid and cholesterol and lead to hepatocellular necrosis.[31-33] Ursodiol (3α,7β-dihydroxy-5β-cholan-24-oic acid, ursodeoxycholic acid), the 7β-hydroxy derivative of CDCA, is more hydrophilic and less detergent than CDCA and less toxic to cellular membranes. In vitro and in vivo studies have demonstrated cytoprotective benefit of ursodeoxycholic acid in blocking injury induced by cholic acid or CDCA.[27, 34, 35] The administration of ursodiol has recently been shown to improve liver function test results and symptoms in patients with early stages of PBC.[36-42] Also, adjuvant treatment with this bile acid for liver transplant patients seems to reduce the frequency of acute rejection episodes.[43]

Effect of Ursodiol in Primary Biliary Cirrhosis

Clinical Symptoms and Liver Function

The origin of pruritus, the major disabling symptom in PBC, is controversial. High concentrations of plasma bile acids are associated with pruritus,[44-46] although recently opiate agonists have been suggested to cause pruritus.[47, 48] Several drugs like cholestyramine, phenobarbital, rifampin, and androgens have been used for treatment of pruritus but with only partial success.[13, 49-53] Recently Borgeat et al. showed that subhypnotic doses of propofol are effective for short-term symptomatic relief of pruritus associated with liver disease, with minimal side effects.[54] Ursodiol has been shown to consistently reduce pruritus, and the effect is seen as early as after 1 month of therapy.[38] However, the effects of ursodiol acid treatment of patients with PBC on liver histology are not completely known. Although some studies have shown histologic stability or even reduced inflammation with ursodiol, others have suggested that there is no improvement in the histologic progression of the disease.[55-58] In a recent report, Perdigoto and Wiesner presented three patients with symptomatic, noncirrhotic PBC who after 1 to 2 years of ursodiol treatment showed histologic progression to cirrhosis despite improvement in liver function test results and pruritus.[59] However, missing from the report was measurement of serum and biliary bile acids to ascertain whether sufficient ursodiol fluxed through the liver.

It has been shown that as early as 4 weeks after initiation of ursodiol therapy, elevated serum alkaline phosphatase, aminotransferase, and γ-glutamyltranspeptidase levels are significantly lowered in patients with PBC and the changes are even more significant after prolonged treatment. In some patients, ursodiol also reduces elevated serum bilirubin levels, and serum IgM levels, which are often increased, decline significantly, thus suggesting improvement in immune reactions in PBC.[42] However, as mentioned above,[59] improvement in biochemical liver test

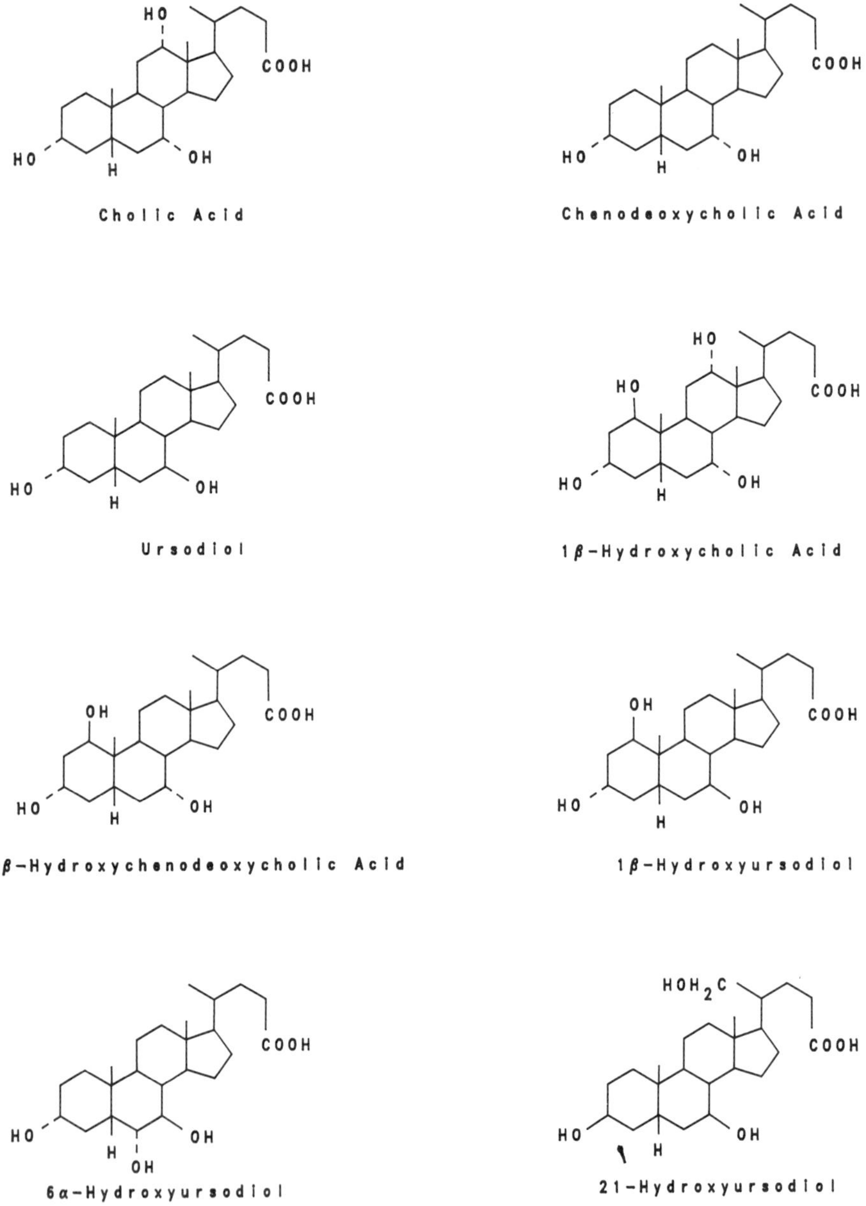

FIG 1.

Major bile acids in patients with primary biliary cirrhosis before and during treatment with ursodiol.

results may not necessarily be associated with halting histologic progression, and further long-term controlled ursodiol trials are needed to establish the effect of ursodiol on histologic improvement and prolonging survival in these patients.

Bile Acids

In PBC, cholic acid synthesis is decreased and biliary secretion of both primary bile acids, CDCA and cholic acid, is impaired. The accumulation of bile acids in hepatocytes and their overflow into the blood[60] lead to abnormally high serum bile acid concentrations and proportionately high urinary excretion. Biliary bile acid composition has been found to parallel that in the serum rather than the urine (Tables 1 to 3), and a number of unusual bile acids (Fig 1) are preferentially excreted in the urine.[38, 61] Apparently because of reduced bile acid synthesis in this disease, more taurine is available for conjugation and the glycine/taurine ratio of endogenous bile acids is significantly lower than in healthy controls (approximately 1.2 vs. 3 in healthy controls) (Table 4).[62, 63] After administration, ursodiol becomes a major biliary bile acid, and the proportion of cholic acid is reduced whereas that of CDCA is virtually unchanged (Table 3).[62] Biliary enrichment with ursodiol

TABLE 1.

Effect of Ursodiol Treatment on Serum Bile Acids in Patients With Primary Biliary Cirrhosis‡‡

	Bile Acids (μM)				
Treatment	Endogenous*	Hydroxylated†	Ursodiol	Others‡	Total
Patients					
Pretreatment§	46 ± 15	2.4 ± 0.4	1.4 ± 0.4	2.9 ± 0.2	53 ± 13
Placebo¶	53 ± 16	2.4 ± 0.5	1.7 ± 0.3	3.5 ± 0.2	61 ± 14
Ursodiol‖ (6 mo)	20 ± 4**	3.5 ± 0.6	20 ± 7**	5.4 ± 2.8	49 ± 9
Ursodiol‖ (12 mo)	23 ± 4**	3 ± 0.4	27 ± 8**	6 ± 2.7	59 ± 11
Ursodiol‖ (24 mo)	23 ± 4**	3.5 ± 0.4	31 ± 8**	3.2 ± 2.2	60 ± 10
Controls††					
Pretreatment	3.4 ± 0.5	—	0.2 ± 0.1	—	3.6 ± 0.6
Ursodiol (2 wk)	0.6 ± 0.3	0.2 ± 0.1	7.2 ± 0.8	0.3 ± 0.1	8.3 ± 0.6

*Chenodeoxycholic acid, cholic acid, deoxycholic acid, lithocholic acid.
†1β,3α,12α-Trihydroxy-5β-cholanoic acid; 1β,3α,7β-trihydroxy-5β-cholanoic acid; 1β,3α,7α,12α-tetrahydroxy-5β-cholanoic acid.
‡Iso-ursodeoxycholic acid, ursocholic acid, hyocholic acid, ω-muricholic acid.
§Fasting serum was obtained immediately pretreatment. Values reported are means ± SD.
¶Fasting serum was obtained every month from patients receiving placebo. Values reported are means ± SD (n = 11).
‖Fasting serum was obtained every month from patients receiving 900 mg/day of ursodiol. Values reported are means ± SD.
**P < .001.
††Fasting serum was obtained from four healthy subjects. Ursodiol (900 mg/day) was fed for 10 days and serum collected before and on the last day of bile acid feeding.
‡‡From Batta AK, et al: *Am J Gastroenterol* 1993; 88:691–700. Used by permission.

TABLE 2.

Effect of Ursodiol Treatment on Urinary Bile Acids in Patients with Primary Biliary Cirrhosis§§

Treatment	Bile Acids (μM/g Creatinine)				
	Endogenous*	Hydroxylated†	Ursodiol	Others‡	Total
Patients					
Pretreatment§	37 ± 17	14 ± 10	2.9 ± 0.5	7.8 ± 2.8	62 ± 22
Placebo¶	36 ± 15	12 ± 9	2.7 ± 0.6	8.1 ± 2.4	59 ± 19
Ursodiol‖ (6 mo)	24 ± 9**	14 ± 5	78 ± 20††	24 ± 8	140 ± 29††
Ursodiol‖ (12 mo)	25 ± 8**	15 ± 5	120 ± 34††	39 ± 13	199 ± 43††
Ursodiol‖ (24 mo)	19 ± 5**	12 ± 5	97 ± 24††	35 ± 9	163 ± 35††
Controls‡‡					
Pretreatment	1.7 ± 0.3	—	0.3 ± 0.1	0.5 ± 0.1	2.5 ± 0.4
Ursodiol (2 wk)	2.5 ± 0.5	2.1 ± 0.3	33 ± 7	11 ± 2	49 ± 7

*Chenodeoxycholic acid, cholic acid, deoxycholic acid, lithocholic acid.
†1β,3α,12α,Trihydroxy-5β-cholanoic acid; 1β,3α,7β-trihydroxy-5β-cholanoic acid; 1β,3α,7α,12α-tetrahydroxy-5β-
  cholanoic acid.
‡Iso-ursodeoxycholic acid, ursocholic acid, hyocholic acid, ω-muricholic acid.
§Early morning urine was obtained immediately pretreatment. Values reported are means ± SD.
¶Early morning urine was obtained every month from patients receiving placebo. Values reported are means ± SD (n
  = 11).
‖Early morning urine was obtained every month from patients receiving 900 mg/day of ursodiol. Values reported are
  means ± SD.
**P = NS.
††$P < .001$.
‡‡Early morning urine was obtained from four healthy subjects. Ursodiol (900 mg/day) was fed for 10 days and
  serum collected before and on the last day of bile acid feeding.
§§From Batta AK, et al: *Am J Gastroenterol* 1993; 88:691–700. Used by permission.

is less in patients with PBC than that obtained when similar doses are given to patients with gallstones and normal hepatic function.[64] This may reflect an inability of the abnormal liver to take up the fed bile acid efficiently in PBC since it has recently been shown that less than 5% of administered ursodiol is excreted in the urine.[40]

Significant amounts of unconjugated bile acids have been reported in the serum and bile of patients with PBC.[62, 65, 66] The proportion of unconjugated bile acids did not change after ursodiol treatment (Table 5). It is therefore suggested that hypercholeresis via a cholehepatic circulation mechanism[67] related to the biliary secretion of unconjugated bile acids does not play a role in the beneficial effects of ursodiol therapy.[66]

Bile Alcohols

The occurrence of large quantities of bile alcohols, the obligate intermediates in the biosynthesis of bile acids, reflects abnormal bile acid synthesis. Thus, because of defective oxidation of the cholesterol side chain in cerebrotendinous xanthomatosis, large quantities of C_{27} bile alcohols are found in the serum, urine, bile, and feces.[68] Several C_{26} and C_{27} bile alcohol glucuronides were reported in the urine

TABLE 3.

Effect of Ursodiol on Biliary Bile Acids in Primary Biliary Cirrhosis¶¶

	Patients			Controls§	
Bile Acid	Pre*	Placebo† (%)	Ursodiol‡	Pretreatment	Ursodiol
CDCA¶	33 ± 8‖	41 ± 2	29 ± 8	24 ± 5	18 ± 3
CA	62 ± 8	57 ± 2	33 ± 9**	49 ± 8	15 ± 2††
UDCA	0.3 ± 0.2	0.1 ± 0.1	31 ± 12‡‡	1 ± 1	55 ± 7‡‡
LCA	0.7 ± 0.3	0.5 ± 0.2	1 ± 1	1 ± 0.2	2 ± 0.4
DCA	3 ± 3	0.4 ± 0.2	5 ± 3	25 ± 6	9 ± 0.3
Others§§	1 ± 0.2	1 ± 0.4	1 ± 1	—	1 ± 0.2

*Values reported are means ± SD for the pretreatment bile samples ($n = 6$).

†Duodenal bile was obtained from patients receiving placebo. Two measurements were averaged to obtain means ± SD ($n = 3$).

‡Duodenal bile was obtained from patients receiving 900 mg/day of ursodiol. Two values were averaged to obtain means ± SD ($n = 3$).

§Bile was collected from four healthy subjects. Ursodiol (900 mg/day) was fed for 10 days and bile collected before and on the last day of bile acid feeding.

¶CDCA = chenodeoxycholic acid; CA = cholic acid; UDCA = ursodiol; LCA = lithocholic acid; DCA = deoxycholic acid.

‖The values represent total bile acids in the pretreatment, placebo, or ursodiol-treated bile samples.

**$P < .002$.

††$P < .001$.

‡‡$P < .0001$.

§§Iso-ursodiol; ursocholic acid; hyocholic acid; 1β,3α,12α-trihydroxy-5β-cholanoic acid; 1β,3α,7α,12α-tetrahydroxy-5β-cholanoic acid; 1β,3α,7β-trihydroxy-5β-cholanoic acid; ω-muricholic acid.

¶¶From Batta AK, et al: *Am J Gastroenterol* 1993; 88:691–700. Used by permission.

of patients with PBC,[69–72] and Huijghebaert et al. found consistently increased urinary excretion of 27-nor-5β-cholestane-3α,7α,12α,24,25-pentol in these patients.[69] We have also detected small amounts of C_{25} bile alcohols, 5β-homocholane-3α,7α,25-triol, and 5β-homocholane-3α,7α,12α,25-tetrol in the urine and bile of patients with PBC (Fig 2).[73] The biological significance of bile alcohols is not clear. Huijghebaert et al. found increased amounts of urinary bile alcohols in patients with cholestatic liver disease but not in patients with noncholestatic liver diseases like chronic active hepatitis.[69] They suggested that patients with cholestatic liver disease have decreased biliary secretion of bile alcohols that may result in their spillover into the urine. However, whether or not the presence of bile alcohols in PBC is of diagnostic value can only be demonstrated after screening a large number of patients with various degrees of the disease.

Mechanism of Action of Ursodiol

Increased amounts of cholic acid and CDCA in the liver tissue of patients with PBC may cause hepatocyte injury,[5] and the hydrophilic ursodiol may protect against cell injury caused by these detergent bile acids.[74] Beuers et al. studied the effect of ursodiol on the kinetics of deoxycholic acid and CDCA, the major hydrophobic bile acids, and found that the pools of these two bile acids did not decrease despite

TABLE 4.

Effect of Ursodiol on the Biliary Bile Acid Conjugation Pattern in Patients With Primary Biliary Cirrhosis* **

Treatment	GCA†	TCA	GCDCA	TCDCA	GUDCA	TUDCA	G:T‡ Endo
Patients							
Pretreatment	35 ± 3§	29 ± 3	20 ± 3	15 ± 2	—	—	1.2
Ursodiol (6 mo)	22 ± 3	9 ± 3	23 ± 5	12 ± 5	29 ± 11	4 ± 1	2.1
Control							
Pretreatment¶	33 ± 5	10 ± 3	18 ± 3	6 ± 2	3 ± 1	—	3.4
Ursodiol¶	13 ± 2	3 ± 1	15 ± 3	3 ± 1	50 ± 5	5 ± 1	4.7

*Ursodiol (900 mg/day) was fed and duodenal bile collected before and at the end of the trial.

†GCA = glycocholic acid; TCA = taurocholic acid; GCDCA = glycochenodeoxycholic acid; TCDCA = taurochenodeoxycholic acid; GUDCA = glycoursodiol; TUDCA = tauroursodiol.

‡Glycine:taurine ratio of the conjugated endogenous bile acids (conjugated chenodeoxycholic acid and conjugated cholic acid).

§Values are percentages of total bile acids.

¶Ursodiol (900 mg/day) was fed for 10 days to four healthy subjects and bile collected before and on the last day of bile acid feeding.

**From Batta AK, et al: *Am J Gastroenterol* 1993; 88:691–700 . Used by permission.

improvement in serum liver test results.[75] Thus they concluded that the beneficial effect of ursodiol is not caused by displacement of hydrophobic endogenous bile acids. However, since cholic acid is partially displaced by the more hydrophilic ursodiol, overall hydrophilicity of the bile does occur during ursodiol treatment, and since hydrophilic bile acids are relatively less toxic, this mechanism may still operate.[66]

Poda et al. suggested that ursodiol may act to increase the overall hydrophilicity of the bile acid pool in cholestatic liver disease.[76] The β-configuration of the hydroxyl group at C_7 is considered responsible for the hydrophilicity of ursodiol and its cytoprotective effect. β-Muricholic acid (3α,6β,7β-trihydroxy-5β-cholanoic acid), the 6β-hydroxy derivative of ursodiol, has a similar chemical structure and is more hydrophilic than ursodiol. Tauro-β-muricholate has recently been shown to preserve choleresis and prevent taurocholate-induced cholestasis in colchicine-treated rat liver[77] and prevents taurochenodeoxycholic acid–induced liver damage in the rat.[78] Ursocholic acid, the 7β-hydroxy epimer of cholic acid (Fig 1) and a highly hydrophilic bile acid, has been shown to possess litholytic properties.[79–81] We studied the effect of administering ursocholic acid, 900 mg/day, to two patients with PBC and an equal dose of tauroursocholate to another two patients with PBC for a period of 1 month.[82] Neither ursocholic acid nor tauroursocholate improved liver function test results in these patients, whereas a similar dose of ursodiol administered immediately afterward showed a reduction of 30% to 40% in the abnormal liver function values in all four patients. This may be due to efficient clearance of this bile acid by the kidney together with its bacterial 7β-dehydroxylation to deoxycholic acid formation.[83, 84] Formation of the hydrophobic deoxycholic acid may more than offset the hydrophilic effect of ursocholic acid.

TABLE 5.

Unconjugated Bile Acids as a Percentage of the Total Biliary Bile Acids in Patients With Primary Biliary Cirrhosis**

Patient	Treatment	Free Bile Acids as Percentage of Total Bile Acids*			
		CDCA	CA	DCA	UDCA
1	Pretreatment†	0.4‡	5.1	0.5	—
	Placebo§	1.8	2.4	1.8	—
2	Pretreatment	0.2	0.4	—	—
	Placebo	0.1	0.1	—	—
3	Pretreatment	7.4	9.5	0.4	—
	Placebo	4.1	13	0.3	—
4	Pretreatment	1.3	2.4	0.4	—
	UDCA¶	0.2	0.7	0.6	4.9
5	Pretreatment	0.1	1.2	—	—
	UDCA	0.3	0.4	0.1	0.5
6	Pretreatment	2.6	5.4	0.5	—
	UDCA	2.2	2.6	0.9	2.7
Control‖	Pretreatment	—	0.5	—	—
	UDCA	—	—	—	0.6

*CDCA = chenodeoxycholic acid; CA = cholic acid; UDCA = ursodiol; DCA = deoxycholic acid.
†Values reported are means ± SD for the pretreatment bile samples ($n = 6$).
‡Values represent percent of total bile acids in the pretreatment, placebo, or ursodiol-treated bile samples.
§Duodenal bile was obtained from patients receiving placebo. Two measurements were averaged to obtain means ± SD ($n = 3$).
¶Duodenal bile was obtained from patients receiving 900 mg/day of ursodiol. Two values were averaged to obtain means ± SD ($n = 3$).
‖Bile was collected from four healthy subjects. Ursodiol (900 mg/day) was fed for 10 days and bile collected before and on the last day of bile acid feeding.
**From Batta AK, et al: *Am J Gastroenterol* 1993; 88:691–700. Used by permission.

Recent studies suggest that ursodiol could have immunoregulating properties.[85-87] Thus ursodiol treatment decreases expression of HLA class I antigens on hepatocytes.[85] However, aberrant expression of HLA class II antigens on biliary tract cells is not observed, which suggests continued failure of immune regulation even after ursodiol treatment and calls for combination therapy with anti-inflammatory drugs.

FIG 2.
Novel bile alcohols in bile and urine of patients with primary biliary cirrhosis.

PRIMARY SCLEROSING CHOLANGITIS

Introduction

Primary sclerosing cholangitis (PSC) is another autoimmune hepatobiliary disease of unknown etiology that is characterized by obliterative, inflammatory fibrosis of the extrahepatic and intrahepatic bile ducts and results in their stricturing and eventual liver failure.[88, 89] The disease affects men slightly more than women. As many as 75% of patients have associated ulcerative colitis, and therefore immunologic mechanisms are implicated in PSC. An immune mechanism is also supported by the inhibition of leukocyte migration by biliary antigens and the presence of circulating immune complexes and their decreased clearance in these patients.[90–92] T lymphocytes have been shown to be involved in the destruction of bile ducts, further suggesting immunologically mediated damage.[93, 94] Like PBC, the disease is characterized by elevation of liver enzyme levels, e.g., alkaline phosphatase, γ-glutamyltranspeptidase, glutamic oxaloacetic transaminase (GOT), and glutamic pyruvic transaminase (GPT). However, unlike PBC, the antimitochondrial antibody test is negative in PSC. In addition to ulcerative colitis, patients with PSC are at increased risk of cholangiocarcinoma developing. Liver biopsy or cholangiography is the only sure way to diagnose the disease. Liver biopsy is recommended not only for diagnosis but also for staging of the disease; thus it helps in determining prognosis as well as the decision to proceed with liver transplantation.

Orthotopic liver transplantation is the definitive treatment for PSC,[95, 96] although complications can result, especially in patients with associated ulcerative colitis.[97] Other than ursodiol, of the various therapeutic drugs tried for the treatment of PSC, only low-dose methotrexate seems to show some promise.[98–104] Ursodiol improves liver biochemistry and pruritus in this disease, and several pilot studies of clinical trials of treating PSC with ursodiol have been initiated.[105–108]

Effect of Ursodiol

Clinical and Biochemical Symptoms

Symptoms of fatigue and pruritus are reduced with ursodiol.[108] In patients with associated ulcerative colitis, diarrhea is a common complaint.[75, 109] Serum alkaline phosphatase, amino transpeptidase, and aminotransferase levels are all dramatically lowered. Discontinuation of ursodiol is promptly associated with aggravation of the liver test results, which are again lowered after ursodiol is reinstituted.[108] As observed in PBC, ursodiol lowers bilirubin levels.[110] However, the drug seems to have no beneficial effect on histology or survival. The goal for ursodiol therapy seems to be to slow the rate of disease progression, lessen mortality risk, and improve the quality of life. Lebovics et al. showed resolution of extensive intrahepatic biliary and pancreatic duct strictures in a patient with PSC.[111] In a recent prospective, randomized, double-blind, placebo-controlled trial, Beuers et al. evaluated the efficacy and safety of ursodiol in a small group of patients with PSC.[110] They found significant improvement in serum levels of bilirubin and liver enzymes in the ursodiol-treated group as compared with the placebo group. They also found histopathologic improvement with ursodiol. Further, they showed a marked reduction in expression of HLA class I molecules after ursodiol treatment, thus suggesting the beneficial effect of ursodiol in reducing disease activity.

Bile Acids

Fasting serum bile acid levels are significantly elevated in PSC (approximately 20 ± 5.5 μmol/L vs. 3.6 μmol/L in healthy controls),[108] and ursodiol administration further increases the total serum bile acid concentrations in these patients.[108, 112] Bile acid synthesis does not change, but their pool sizes are reduced, and up to 50% of the total serum bile acid pool becomes ursodiol.[108, 110, 112] This suggests that ursodiol does not replace toxic endogenous bile acids in PSC. Similarly, the elevated urinary excretion of endogenous bile acids remains unchanged after ursodiol administration,[108] and excreted ursodiol accounts for the increase in urinary bile acid output after administration. It is thought that, as in PBC, the increased hydrophilicity of the bile acid pool may contribute to the beneficial effect of ursodiol; even though the pool sizes of the endogenous hydrophobic bile acids CDCA and deoxycholic acid are not reduced,[75, 112] overall hydrophilicity may increase after ursodiol administration and ursodiol may protect against toxicity to the hepatocyte caused by the hydrophobic or other toxic bile acids.[74, 113, 114] On the other hand, an immune mechanism may be possible since the immunoregulating properties of ursodiol in PBC have been observed in PSC also.[75]

Ulcerative Colitis and Primary Sclerosing Cholangitis

The association between PSC and ulcerative colitis has been long recognized, and as many as 80% of patients with PSC have ulcerative colitis.[88, 115, 116] Primary sclerosing cholangitis seems to cause a variety of clinical abnormalities ranging from nonprogressive, small bile duct disease to inflammatory disease of the larger intrahepatic and extrahepatic bile ducts that can lead to cirrhosis and bile duct or gallbladder carcinoma.[117, 118] Approximately 5% of patients with ulcerative colitis have associated PSC,[119] and patients with prolonged ulcerative colitis are at increased risk of colorectal cancer[120, 121] even after liver transplantation.[122] The cause of neoplastic progression in ulcerative colitis is not known. However, alterations of fatty acids or bile acids, which act as tumor promoters, may cause carcinogenesis.[123–125]

BILE ACIDS AND COLON CANCER

Although the etiology of colorectal cancer is complex and includes both environmental and genetic components, bile acids have often been implicated as either causative or contributory agents. Because they are the major human fecal bile acids, most studies have focused on deoxycholic acid and lithocholic acid, which are made by bacterial 7-dehydroxylation of cholic acid and CDCA, respectively. More than 50 years ago Cook et al. reported that deoxycholic acid could produce sarcomas in mice at the site of injection.[126] Aries, Hill, and their colleagues 30 years later[127, 128] proposed that fecal bacteria are capable of creating carcinogens by converting bile acids to polycyclic aromatic hydrocarbons, and several investigators[129, 130] have demonstrated that both deoxycholic acid and lithocholic acid potentiate the activity of known carcinogens.[125, 131–133] Dietary fat and increased serum cholesterol levels are positively correlated with a risk of colorectal adenomas,[123, 124, 134, 135] and a recent study suggests that obese men between the ages of 50.5 and 68.1 are also at high risk of the development of colorectal adenomas.[136] It is thought that excess dietary fat causes an in-crease in biliary secretion of the bile acids necessary for fat absorption. This results in increased amounts of secondary bile acids in the colon formed via bacterial 7α-dehydroxylation of primary bile acids, and early epidemiologic studies[137] have suggested that populations consuming low-fat, low–animal protein diets with concomitantly reduced fecal bile acid concentrations and reduced bacterial transformation of steroids have a much lower incidence of colon cancer. More recent reports have shown that cholic acid (the precursor of deoxycholic acid), when added to the diet of rats, induces proliferation of the colonic epithelium[132] and increases the incidence of tumors.[138, 139] The implication of the above, that high concentrations of deoxycholic acid are toxic to the colonic mucosa, is further bolstered by other studies that have demonstrated that deoxycholic acid is toxic to other tissues such as the liver.[140] Correlations between body pools of deoxycholic acid and colorectal cancer have been demonstrated in human subjects by van der Werf et al., who reported that the deoxycholic acid pool is 55% larger and the input rate of deoxycholic acid is 25% greater in patients with adenomatous polyps.[141] Also, Bayerdorffer et al.[133] found that serum levels of deoxycholic acid were elevated significantly (1.16 ± 0.39 vs. 1.70 ± 0.59 μmol/L, $P < .001$) in men with colorectal adenomas as compared with normal controls.

Although cholic acid in vitro is reported to accelerate the uptake of methylcholanthrene by fibroblasts,[142] in vivo studies of the carcinogenic potential of other bile acids are difficult to interpret because colonic bacteria efficiently and rapidly 7-dehydroxylate most bile acids. Studies in germ-free animals would probably be needed to establish a link between other bile acids and the formation of colonic tumors. Such studies, however, may not be so essential since most bile acids in the large bowel are either deoxycholic or lithocholic acid.

Although humans have been living successfully with bile acids, intestinal bacteria, and colons for a very long time, our recently increased life expectancy and high-fat diet may be partly responsible for an increased incidence of colorectal cancer in Western society. Because both adenomatous polyps and colon cancer correlate well with elevated concentrations of the hydrophobic bile acid deoxycholic acid, perhaps we should be considering hydrophilic bile acids as a protective factor for the intestine. Ursodiol appears to be a prime candidate (see above) because it is well known as a cytoprotective agent when added to hydrophobic cytotoxic bile acids.[27, 34, 35, 74]

URSODIOL AND ORGAN TRANSPLANTATION

Ursodiol appears to be a very useful adjunctive therapy in organ transplantation. The liver transplant unit at the University of Gothenburg now treats all liver transplant recipients with 10 mg/kg/day of ursodiol because they have found that untreated subjects have 4.4 times more rejection episodes than treated patients.[143] This same group also found[144] that ursodiol increased transplant tolerance and graft survival in rats with experimental heart transplants. In addition, Fried et al.[145] observed that ursodiol markedly reduces the signs of cholestatic liver injury in patients after bone marrow transplantation in whom chronic graft-vs.-host disease develops. The mechanism for many of these results probably relates to the protection of the hepatocyte during cholestasis caused by immunosuppressive drugs. The reason for the protection of heart allografts is not at all obvious and likely does not involve a direct immunosuppressive effect. Although ursodiol suppresses the expression of HLA class I antigens,[85-87, 146] which are hepatocyte membrane specific and which may be important for the genesis of PBC, it does not appear to suppress HLA class II antigens[85] or lymphocyte response and proliferation in general.[147]

URSODIOL AND CYSTIC FIBROSIS

Ursodiol, 10 to 20 mg/day, administered to patients with chronic cholestatic liver disease accompanying cystic fibrosis, leads to marked and significant reductions in abnormal liver function test values[148-154] and increased weight gain.[148] Colombo et al.[154] recently have demonstrated, for the first time, that 1 year of 10 to 15 mg/kg/day of ursodiol leads to a significant improvement in biliary function, including reduced ductular dilation and increased bile acid secretion. The positive response of patients with cystic fibrosis to ursodiol is dose dependent.[153] Enrichment of the bile acid pool increases, and abnormal liver function test values decrease steadily with increasing doses of ursodiol between 5 and 20 mg/kg/day.

URSODIOL AND OTHER CHOLESTATIC LIVER DISEASES

Cholestasis of pregnancy is a disease of unknown origin that affects women in the second and third trimesters. It is characterized by elevated liver function test values, cholestasis, and pruritus and can have very serious consequences for both the mother and child.[155] Recently, Palma et al.[156] administered ursodiol, 1,000 mg/day for 20 days, to five women with cholestasis of pregnancy. Pruritus and serum GPT concentrations improved markedly. Three other women were treated for two 3-week intervals separated by a 2-week washout period. Serum GPT levels and pruritus, which were reduced by the first ursodiol therapy, worsened considerably during the 2 weeks without treatment and then ameliorated once ursodiol treatment was resumed.

Alcoholic cirrhosis is one of the most common cholestatic liver diseases. Plevris et al.[157] recently carried out a placebo-controlled crossover trial of ursodiol, 15 mg/kg/day, in 12 patients with biopsy-proven alcoholic cirrhosis. Interestingly, all patients were asked to continue to drink during the study, and blood levels were monitored. After 4 weeks of ursodiol bilirubin, γ-glutamyltranspeptidase and alanine aminotransferase (ALT) levels were all significantly reduced.

BILIARY LITHOTRIPSY

Although extracorporeal shock wave lithotripsy of the gallbladder can be an effective treatment for gallstones in selected patients,[158, 159] unless it is combined with oral dissolution therapy the results are quite poor.[160, 161] Six months after lithotripsy 0%[161] and 9%[160] of subjects with no oral litholytic therapy were stone free. In contrast, 50%[161] and 21%[160] of lithotripsy patients receiving either ursodiol or an ursodiol/CDCA combination were free of gallstones. The question of whether lithotripsy plus ursodiol is more efficacious than ursodiol alone for patients with one or two 10- to 30-mm radiolucent gallstones has been answered in favor of the combination therapy.[159, 162] After comparable treatment periods, 22%[159] and 14%[162] of subjects treated with ursodiol alone were stone free vs. 45% and 48%, respectively, of patients receiving lithotripsy plus ursodiol. Ursodiol appears to have another advantage when used in conjunction with biliary lithotripsy. When gallstone patients are pretreated with ursodiol for a month or more, fragmentation is made easier and the ultimate efficacy increased significantly.[159]

SUMMARY

There is thus ample evidence to believe that ursodiol is the drug of choice in cholestatic liver diseases. It is possible that ursodiol has to be administered for prolonged periods to see appreciable reversal in liver damage. Nevertheless, the amelioration of symptoms and improvement in nutrition of patients are equally important. Disabling symptoms like pruritus are often brought under control, and quality of life improves. Clearly the goal for ursodiol therapy is to slow the rate of disease progression, lessen the mortality risk, and improve the quality of life in patients. It is possible that combination therapy will be more beneficial than ursodiol alone, although the initial results of administering ursodiol with colchicine have shown no improvement in liver histology. However, the administration of ursodiol together with a strong anti-inflammatory drug may be helpful in halting the immune destruction of liver cells.

REFERENCES

1. James SP, et al: Primary biliary cirrhosis: A model autoimmune disease. *Ann Intern Med* 1983; 99:500–512.

2. Goldman MA, et al: Bile acid metabolism in health and disease. *Prog Liver Dis* 1979; 6:225–241.

3. Summerfield JA, et al: Evidence for renal control of urinary excretion of bile acids and bile acid sulfates in the cholestatic syndrome. *Clin Sci Mol Med* 1977; 52:51–65.

4. Vlahcevic ZR, et al: Disturbances of bile acid metabolism in parenchymal liver cell disease. *Clin Gastroenterol* 1977; 6:25–43.

5. Akashi Y, et al: Bile acid metabolism in cirrhotic liver tissue—altered synthesis and impaired hepatic secretion. *Clin Chim Acta* 1987; 168:199–206.

6. Christensen E, et al: Beneficial effect of azathioprine and prediction of prognosis in primary biliary cirrhosis. Final results of an international trial. *Gastroenterology* 1985; 89:1084–1091.

7. Heathcote J, et al: A prospective controlled trial of azathioprine in primary biliary cirrhosis. *Gastroenterology* 1976; 70:656–660.

8. Mitchison HC, et al: Controlled trial of prednisolone for primary biliary cirrhosis: Good for the liver, bad for the bones. *Hepatology* 1986; 6:1211.

9. Matloff DS, et al: A prospective trial of D-penicillamine in primary biliary cirrhosis. *N Engl J Med* 1982; 306:319–326.

10. Neuberger J, et al: Double-blind controlled trial of D-penicillamine in patients with primary biliary cirrhosis. *Gut* 1985; 26:114–119.

11. Hoofnagle JH, et al: Randomized trial of chlorambucil for primary biliary cirrhosis. *Gastroenterology* 1986; 91:1327–1334.

12. Stellaard F, et al: Phenobarbital in treatment of primary biliary cirrhosis. *J Lab Clin Med* 1979; 94:853–861.

13. Ghent CN, et al: Treatment of pruritus in primary biliary cirrhosis with rifampicin. Results of a double-blind crossover randomized trial. *Gastroenterology* 1988; 94:488–493.

14. Minuk GY, et al: Pilot study of cyclosporine A in patients with symptomatic primary biliary cirrhosis. *Gastroenterology* 1988; 95:1356–1363.

15. Wiesner RH, et al: A controlled trial of cyclosporine in the treatment of primary biliary cirrhosis. *N Engl J Med* 1990; 322:1419–1424.

16. Bodenheimer H, et al: Evaluation of colchicine therapy in primary biliary cirrhosis. *Gastroenterology* 1988; 95:124–129.

17. Kaplan MM, et al: A prospective trial of colchicine for primary biliary cirrhosis. *N Engl J Med* 1986; 315:1448–1454.

18. Kaplan MM, et al: Primary biliary cirrhosis treated with low dose oral pulse methotrexate: Resolution of symptoms with improvement in biochemical tests of liver function. *Ann Intern Med* 1988; 109:429–431.

19. Kaplan MM, et al: Treatment of primary biliary cirrhosis with low-dose weekly methotrexate. *Gastroenterology* 1991; 101:1332–1338.

20. Zifroni A, et al: Long-term follow-up of patients with primary biliary cirrhosis on colchicine therapy. *Hepatology* 1991; 14:990–993.

21. Markus BH, et al: Efficacy of liver transplantation in patients with primary biliary cirrhosis. *N Engl J Med* 1989; 320:1709–1713.

22. Greenberg BD, et al: Intrahepatic cholestasis, bile excretory function and hyperbilirubinemia, in Gitnick G (ed): *Current Hepatology,* vol 10. St Louis, Mosby–Year Book, 1989, pp 177–203.

23. Sallie R, et al: Transplantation in primary biliary cirrhosis. *J Gastroenterol Hepatol* 1991; 6:558–562.

24. Polson RJ, et al: Evidence for disease recurrence after liver transplantation for primary biliary cirrhosis. Clinical and histological follow-up studies. *Gastroenterology* 1989; 97:715–725.

25. Rydning A, et al: Factors of prognostic importance of primary biliary cirrhosis. *Scand J Gastroenterol* 1990; 25:119–126.

26. Roll J, et al: The prognostic importance of clinical and histologic features in asymptomatic and symptomatic primary biliary cirrhosis. *N Engl J Med* 1983; 308:1–7.

27. Sasaki H, et al: Primary biliary cirrhosis in Japan: National survey by the Subcommittee on Autoimmune Hepatitis. *Gastroenterol Jpn* 1985; 20:476–485.

28. Goudie BM, et al: Risk factors and prognosis in primary biliary cirrhosis. *Am J Gastroenterol* 1989; 84:713–716.

29. Dickson ER, et al: Prognosis in primary biliary cirrhosis: Model for decision making. *Hepatology* 1989; 10:1–7.

30. Klion FM, et al: Prediction of survival of patients with primary biliary cirrhosis. Examination of the Mayo Clinic Model on a group of patients with known endpoint. *Gastroenterology* 1992; 102:310–313.

31. Hertz R, et al: Inhibition of bile formation by high doses of taurocholate in the perfused rat liver. *Scand J Gastroenterol* 1976; 11:741–746.

32. Palmer RH: Bile acids, liver injury, and liver disease. *Arch Intern Med* 1972; 130:606–617.

33. Fisher RL, et al: A prospective morphologic evaluation of hepatic toxicity of chenodeoxycholic acid in patients with cholelithiasis: The National Cooperative Gallstone Study. *Hepatology* 1982; 2:187–201.

34. Kitani K, et al: Tauroursodeoxycholate prevents biliary excretion of proteins induced by taurocholate and taurochenodeoxycholate in the rat. *Hepatology* 1983; 3:810.

35. Kanai S, et al: Glycoursodeoxycholate is as effective as tauroursodeoxycholate in preventing the taurocholate induced cholestasis in the rat. *Hepatology* 1983; 3:811.

36. Poupon R, et al: Is ursodeoxycholic acid an effective treatment of primary biliary cirrhosis? *Lancet* 1987; 1:834–836.

37. Leuschner U, et al: Ursodeoxycholic acid in primary biliary cirrhosis: Results of a controlled double blind trial. *Gastroenterology* 1989; 97:1268–1274.

38. Batta AK, et al: Effect of ursodeoxycholic acid on bile acid metabolism in primary biliary cirrhosis. *Hepatology* 1989; 10:414–419.

39. Batta AK, et al: Characterization of serum and urinary bile acids in patients with primary biliary cirrhosis by gas-liquid chromatography–mass spectrometery: Effect of ursodeoxycholic acid treatment. *J Lipid Res* 1989; 30:1953–1962.

40. Stiehl A, et al: Ursodeoxycholic acid–induced changes of plasma and urinary bile acids in patients with primary biliary cirrhosis. *Hepatology* 1990; 12:492–497.

41. Oka H, et al: A multi-center double-blind controlled trial of ursodeoxycholic acid for primary biliary cirrhosis. *Jpn Soc Gastroenterol* 1990; 25:774–780.

42. Poupon RE, et al: A multi-center controlled trial of ursodiol for the treatment of primary biliary cirrhosis. *N Engl J Med* 1991; 324:1548–1554.

43. Friman S, et al: Adjuvant treatment with ursodeoxycholic acid reduces acute rejection after liver transplantation. *Transplant Int* 1992; 5(suppl):187–189.

44. Schoenfield LJ, et al: Bile acids on the skin of patients with pruritic hepatobiliary disease. *Nature* 1967; 213:93–94.

45. Stiehl A: Bile acids and bile acid sulfates in the skin of patients with cholestasis and pruritus. *Z Gastroenterol* 1974; 12:121–124.

46. Kirby J, et al: Pruritic effect of bilesalts. *BMJ* 1974; 4:693–695.

47. Jones EA, et al: The pruritus of cholestasis: From bile acids to opiate agonists. *Hepatology* 1990; 11:884–887.

48. Bergasa NV, et al: A controlled trial of naloxone infusions for the pruritus of chronic cholestasis. *Gastroenterology* 1992; 102:544–549.

49. Bachs L, et al: Comparison of rifampicin with phenobarbitone for treatment of pruritus in biliary cirrhosis. *Lancet* 1989; 1:574–576.

50. Bachs L, et al: Effects of long-term rifampicin administration in primary biliary cirrhosis. *Gastroenterology* 1992; 102:2077–2080.

51. Datta DV, et al: Cholestyramine for long-term relief of the pruritus complicating intrahepatic cholestasis. *Gastroenterology* 1966; 50:323–332.

52. Bloomer JR, et al: Phenobarbital effects in cholestatic liver disease. *Ann Intern Med* 1975; 82:310–317.

53. Walt RP, et al: Effect of stanozolol on iching in primary biliary cirrhosis. *BMJ* 1988; 296:607.

54. Borgeat A, et al: Subhypnotic doses of propofol relieve pruritus associated with liver disease. *Gastroenterology* 1993; 104:244–247.

55. Huet PM, et al: Effect of ursodeoxycholic acid (UDCA) on hepatic function and portal hypertension in primary biliary cirrhosis (PBC) (abstract). *Hepatology* 1990; 12:907.

56. Myszor M, et al: No symptomatic or histological benefit from ursodeoxycholic acid treatment in PBC after 1 year controlled pilot study (abstract). *Hepatology* 1990; 12:415.

57. Hadziyannis SJ, et al: A randomized controlled trial of ursodeoxycholic acid (UDCA) in primary biliary cirrhosis (PBC) (abstract). *Hepatology* 1989; 10:580.

58. Vogel W, et al: Deterioration of primary biliary cirrhosis during treatment with ursodeoxycholic acid (letter). *Lancet* 1988; 1:1163.

59. Perdigoto R, et al: Progression of primary biliary cirrhosis with ursodeoxycholic acid therapy. *Gastroenterology* 1992; 102:1389–1391.

60. Cotting J, et al: Biliary obstruction dissipates bioelectrical sinusoidal-cannalicular barrier without altering taurocholate uptake. *Am J Physiol* 1989; 256:312–318.

61. Williams CN, et al: Primary bile acid kinetics in patients with primary biliary cirrhosis and in normal subjects. *Clin Invest Med* 1979; 2:29–40.

62. Batta AK, et al: Effect of long-term treatment with ursodiol on clinical and biochemical symptoms and biliary bile acid metabolism in patients with primary biliary cirrhosis. *Am J Gastroenterol* 1992, in press.

63. Batta AK, et al: Effect of ursodiol on bile acid conjugation in patients with primary biliary cirrhosis. *Gastroenterology* 1991; 100:

64. Tint GS, et al: Ursodeoxycholic acid: A clinical trial of a safe and effective agent for dissolving cholesterol gallstones. *Ann Intern Med* 1982; 97:351–356.

65. Crosignani A, et al: Biliary secretion of unconjugated bile acids in patients with primary biliary cirrhosis before and following ursodeoxycholic acid administration. *Gastroenterology* 1990; 98:A578.

66. Crosignani A, et al: Changes in bile acid composition in patients with primary biliary cirrhosis induced by ursodeoxycholic acid administration. *Hepatology* 1991; 14:1000–1007.

67. Gurantz D, et al: Hypercholeresis induced by unconjugated bile acid infusion correlates with recovery in bile of unconjugated bile acids. *Hepatology* 1991; 13:540–550.

68. Salen G, et al: Familial diseases with storage of sterols other than cholesterol (cerebrotendinous xanthomatosis and sitosterolemia with xanthomatosis), in Stanbury JB, et al (eds): *The Metabolic Basis of Inherited Diseases,* ed 5. New York, McGraw-Hill, 1983, pp 713–730.

69. Huijghebaert SW, et al: Increased urinary excretion of bile alcohol glucuronides in patients with primary biliary cirrhosis. *J Lipid Res* 1989; 30:1673–1679.

70. Karlaganis G, et al: Urinary excretion of bile alcohols in normal children and patients with α_1-antitrypsin deficiency during development of liver disease. *Eur J Clin Invest* 1982; 12:399–405.

71. Karlaganis G, et al: Identification of 27-nor-5β-cholestane-3α,7α,12α,24,25,26-hexol and partial characterization of the bile alcohol profile in urine. *J Lipid Res* 1984; 25:693–702.

72. Ludwig-Kohn H, et al: The identification of urinary bile alcohols by gas chromatography–mass spectrometry in patients with liver disease and in healthy individuals. *Eur J Clin Invest* 1983; 13:91–98.

73. Batta AK, et al: Unpublished results.

74. Heuman DM, et al: Conjugates of ursodeoxycholate protect against cholestasis and hepatocellular necrosis caused by more hydrophobic bile salts. In vivo studies in the rat. *Gastroenterology* 1991; 100:203–211.

75. Beuers U, et al: Effect of ursodeoxycholic acid on the kinetics of the major hydrophobic bile acids in health and in chronic cholestatic liver disease. *Hepatology* 1992; 15:603–608.

76. Poda M, et al: Ursodeoxycholic acid for chronic liver disease. *J Clin Gastroenterol* 1988; 10(suppl):25–31.

77. Katagiri K, et al: Tauro-β-muricholate preserves choleresis and prevents taurocholate-induced cholestasis in colchicine rat liver. *Gastroenterology* 1992; 102:1660–1667.

78. Kanai S, et al: Tauroβ-muricholate is as effective as tauroursodeoxycholate in preventing taurochenodeoxycholate-induced liver damage in the rat. *Life Sci* 1991; 47:2421–2428.

79. Zuin M, et al: Ursocholic acid: A new litholytic agent (abstract). *Hepatology* 1984; 4:1060.

80. Howard PJ, et al: Ursocholic acid: Bile acid and bile lipid response and clinical studies in patients with gallstones. *Gut* 1989; 30:97–103.

81. Loria P, et al: Effect of ursocholic acid on bile lipid secretion and composition. *Gastroenterology* 1986; 90:865–874.

82. Batta AK, et al: Unpublished results.

83. Tint GS, et al: Metabolism of ursocholic acid in humans: Conversion of ursocholic acid to deoxycholic acid. *Hepatology* 1992; 15:645–650.

84. Batta AK, et al: Urinary excretion of bile acids in man. Presented at a Federation meeting, June, 1986.

85. Calmus Y, et al: Hepatic expression of class I and class II major histocompatibility complex molecules in primary biliary cirrhosis: Effect of ursodeoxycholic acid. *Hepatology* 1990; 11:12–15.

86. Calmus Y, et al: Ursodeoxycholic acid (UDCA) in the treatment of chronic cholestatic diseases. *Biochimie* 1991; 73:1335–1338.

87. Yoshikawa M, et al: Immunomodulatory effects of ursodeoxycholic acid on immune responses. *Hepatology* 1992; 16:358–364.

88. LaRusso NF, et al: Current concepts: Primary sclerosing cholangitis. *N Engl J Med* 1984; 301:899–903.

89. Lebovics E, et al: Outcome of primary sclerosing cholangitis: Analysis of long-term observation of 38 patients. *Arch Intern Med* 1987; 147:729–731.

90. McFarlane IG, et al: Leukocyte migration inhibition in response to biliary antigens in primary biliary cirrhosis, sclerosing cholangitis, and other chronic liver diseases. *Gastroenterology* 1979; 76:1333–1340.

91. Bodenheimer HC, et al: Elevated circulating immune complexes in primary sclerosing cholangitis. *Hepatology* 1983; 3:150–154.

92. Minuk GY, et al: Abnormal clearance of immune complexes from the circulation of patients with primary sclerosing cholangitis. *Gastroenterology* 1985; 88:166–170.

93. Whiteside TL, et al: Immunologic analysis of mononuclear cells in liver tissues and blood of patients with primary sclerosing cholangitis. *Hepatology* 1985; 5:468–474.

94. Lindor KD, et al: Enhanced autoreactivity of T-lymphocytes in primary sclerosing cholangitis. *Hepatology* 1987; 7:884–888.

95. Marsh JW, et al: Orthotopic liver transplantation for primary sclerosing cholangitis. *Ann Surg* 1988; 207:21–25.

96. Langnas AN, et al: Primary sclerosing cholangitis. The emerging role for liver transplantation. *Am J Gastroenterol* 1989; 84:1203.

97. Higashi H, et al: Development of colon cancer after liver transplantation for primary sclerosing cholangitis associated with ulcerative colitis. *Hepatology* 1990; 11:477–480.

98. Polter DE, et al: Beneficial effect of cholestyramine in sclerosing cholangitis. *Gastroenterology* 1980; 79:326–333.

99. Myers RN, et al: Primary sclerosing cholangitis: Complete gross and histologic reversal after long-term steroid therapy. *Am J Gastroenterol* 1970; 53:527–538.

100. LaRusso NF, et al: Prospective trial of penicillamine in primary sclerosing cholangitis. *Gastroenterology* 1988; 95:1036–1042.

101. Lindor KD, et al: Prednisone and colchicine are not of benefit after two years in patients with primary sclerosing cholangitis. *Hepatology* 1989; 10:638.

102. Kaplan MM, et al: Primary sclerosing cholangitis and low-dose oral pulse methotrexate therapy. *Ann Intern Med* 1987; 106:231–235.

103. Knox TA, et al: Primary sclerosing cholangitis—improvement with methotrexate treatment. *Hepatology* 1989; 10:688.

104. Kaplan MM: Medical approaches to primary sclerosing cholangitis. *Semin Liver Dis* 1991; 11:56–63.

105. Stiehl A, et al: The effect of ursodeoxycholic acid (UDCA) in primary sclerosing cholangitis (abstract). *Gastroenterology* 1989; 96:664.

106. Chagouilleres O, et al: Ursodeoxycholic acid for primary sclerosing cholangitis. *J Hepatol* 1990; 11:120–123.

107. Hayashi H, et al: Asymptomatic primary sclerosing cholangitis treated with ursodeoxycholic acid. *Gastroenterology* 1990; 99:533–535.

108. O'Brien CB, et al: Ursodeoxycholic acid for the treatment of primary sclerosing cholangitis: A 30-month pilot study. *Hepatology* 1991; 14:838–847.

109. Stiehl L, et al: Effect of ursodeoxycholic acid in patients with primary sclerosing cholangitis, in Paumgertner G, Stiehl A, Gerok W (eds): *Bile Acids as Therapeutic Agents*. Dordrecht, The Netherlands, Kluwer Academic Publishers, 1990, pp 305–307.

110. Beuers U, et al: Ursodeoxycholic acid for treatment of primary sclerosing cholangitis: A placebo-controlled trial. *Hepatology* 1992; 16:707–714.

111. Lebovics E, et al: Resolution of radiographic abnormalities with ursodeoxycholic acid therapy of primary sclerosing cholangitis. *Gastroenterology* 1992; 102:2143–2147.

112. Rudolph G, et al: Effect of ursodeoxycholic acid on the kinetics of cholic acid and chenodeoxycholic acid in patients with primary sclerosing cholangitis. *Hepatology* 1993; 17:1028–1032.

113. Kitani K: Hepatoprotective effect of ursodeoxycholate in experimental animals, in Paumgertner G, et al (eds): *Strategies for the Treatment of Hepatobiliary Diseases*. Dordrecht, The Netherlands, Kluwer Academic Publishers, 1990, pp 43–56.

114. Galle PR, et al: Ursodeoxycholate reduces hepatotoxicity of bile acids in primary human hepatocytes. *Hepatology* 1990; 12:486–491.

115. Wiesner RH, et al: Clinicopathologic features of the syndrome of primary sclerosing cholangitis. *Gastroenterology* 1980; 79:200–206.

116. Thompson HH, et al: Primary sclerosing cholangitis: A heterogeneous disease. *Ann Surg* 1982; 196:127–136.

117. Wee A, et al: Pericholangitis in chronic ulcerative colitis: Primary sclerosing cholangitis of the small bile ducts? *Ann Intern Med* 1985; 102:581–587.

118. Mir-Madjlessi SH, et al: Bile duct carcinoma in patients with ulcerative colitis. Relationship to sclerosing cholangitis: Report of six cases and review of the literature. *Dig Dis Sci* 1987; 32:145–154.

119. Ohlsson R, et al: Prevalence of primary sclerosing cholangitis in ulcerative colitis. *Gastroenterology* 1991; 101:1319–1323.

120. Collins RH Jr, et al: Colon cancer, dysplasia, and surveillance in patients with ulcerative colitis: A critical review. *N Engl J Med* 1987; 316:1654–1658.

121. Gyde S: Screening for colorectal cancer in ulcerative colitis: Dubious benefits and high costs. *Gut* 1990; 31:1089–1092.

122. Higashi H, et al: Development of colon cancer after liver transplantation for primary sclerosing cholangitis associated with ulcerative colitis. *Hepatology* 1990; 11:477–480.

123. Potter JD, et al: Diet and cancer of the colon and rectum. A case control study. *J Natl Cancer Inst* 1986; 76:557–569.

124. Reddy BS: Dietary fat and its relationship to large bowel cancer. *Cancer Res* 1981; 41:3700–3705.

125. Reddy BS, et al: Promoting effect of sodium deoxycholate on colonic adenocarcinomas in germ-free rats. *Natl Cancer Res* 1976; 56:441–442.

126. Cook JW, et al: Production of tumors in mice by deoxycholic acid. *Nature* 1940; 145:627.

127. Aries V, et al: Bacteria and the aetiology of cancer of the large bowel. *Gut* 1969; 10:334–335.

128. Hill MJ: The role of colon anaerobes in the metabolism of bile acids and steroids and its relation to colon cancer. *Cancer* 1975; 36:2387–2400.

129. Narisawa T, et al: Promoting effect of bile acids on colon carcinogenesis after intrarectal instillation of *N*-methyl-*N'*-nitro-*N*-nitrosoguanidine in rats. *J Natl Cancer Inst* 1974; 53:1093–1097.

130. Reddy BS: Role of bile acids in colon carcinogenesis. *Cancer* 1975; 36:2401–2406.

131. Goerg KJ, et al: Effect of deoxycholate on the perfused rat colon. *Digestion* 1982; 25:145–154.

132. Deschner EE, et al: Acute and chronic effect of dietary cholic acid on colonic epithelial cell proliferation. *Digestion* 1981; 21:290–296.

133. Bayerdorffer E, et al: Increased serum deoxycholic acid levels in men with colorectal adenomas. *Gastroenterology* 1993; 104:145–151.

134. Wynder EL, et al: Metabolic epidemiology of colorectal cancer. *Cancer* 1974; 34:801–806.

135. Wynder EL: The epidemiology of large bowel cancer. *Cancer Res* 1975; 35:3388–3394.

136. Bayerdorffer E, et al: Increased risk of "high-risk" colorectal adenomas in overweight men. *Gastroenterology* 1993; 104:137–144.

137. Hill MJ, et al: Faecal steroid composition and its relationship to cancer of the large bowel. *J Pathol* 1971; 104:129–139.

138. Galloway DJ, et al: Experimental colorectal cancer: The relationship of diet and faecal bile acids concentration to tumor induction. *Br J Surg* 1986; 73:233–237.

139. McSherry CK, et al: Effects of calcium and bile acid feeding on colon tumors in the rat. *Cancer Res* 1989; 49:6039–6043.

140. Delzenne NM, et al: Comparative hepatotoxicity of cholic acid, deoxycholic acid and lithocholic acid in the rat: In vivo and in vitro studies. *Toxicol Lett* 1992; 61:291–304.

141. van der Werf SDJ, et al: Colonic absorption of secondary bile-acids in patients with adenomatous polyps and in matched controls. *Lancet* 1982; 1:759–761.

142. Sugezawa A, et al: Possible mechanism for the cocarcinogenic effect of bile acids: Increased intracellular uptake of methylcholanthrene by C3H/10T1/2 fibroblasts in vitro. *Oncology* 1991; 48:138–143.

143. Friman S, et al: Adjuvant treatment with ursodeoxycholic acid reduces acute rejection after liver transplant. *Transplant Int* 1992; 5(suppl 1):187–189.

144. Olausson M, et al: Adjuvant treatment with ursodeoxycholic acid prevents acute rejection in rats receiving heart allografts. *Transplant Int* 1992; 5(suppl 1):539–541.

145. Fried RH, et al: Ursodeoxycholic acid treatment of refractory chronic graft-versus-host disease of the liver. *Ann Intern Med* 1992; 116:624–629.

146. Terasaki S, et al: Hepatocellular and biliary expression of HLA antigens in primary biliary cirrhosis before and after ursodeoxycholic acid therapy. *Am J Gastroenterol* 1991; 86: 1194–1199.

147. Calmus Y, et al: Immunosuppressive properties of chenodeoxycholic and ursodeoxycholic acids in the mouse. *Gastroenterology* 1992; 103:617–621.

148. Cotting J, et al: Effects of ursodeoxycholic acid treatment on nutrition and liver function in patients with cystic fibrosis and longstanding cholestasis. *Gut* 1990; 31:918–921.

149. Colombo C, et al: Effects of ursodeoxycholic acid therapy for liver disease associated with cystic fibrosis. *J Pediatr* 1990; 117:482–489.

150. Nakagawa M, et al: Comprehensive study of the biliary bile acid composition of patients with cystic fibrosis and associated liver disease before and after UDCA administration. *Hepatology* 1990; 12:322–334.

151. Galabert C, et al: Utilisation de l'acids ursodesoxycholique dans le traitment des complications hepatobiliares de la mucoviscidose. *Pathol Biol* 1991; 39:625–628.

152. Galabert C, et al: Effects of ursodeoxycholic acid on liver function in patients with cystic fibrosis and chronic cholestasis. *J Pediatr* 1992; 121:138–141.

153. Colombo C, et al: Ursodeoxycholic acid therapy in cystic fibrosis–associated liver disease: A dose response study. *Hepatology* 1992; 16:924–930.

154. Colombo C, et al: Scintigraphic documentation of an improvement in hepatobiliary excretory function after treatment with ursodeoxycholic acid in patients with cystic fibrosis and associated liver disease. *Hepatology* 1992; 15:677–684.

155. Svanborg A: A study of recurrent jaundice in pregnancy. *Acta Obstet Gynecol Scand* 1954; 33:434–444.

156. Palma J, et al: Effects of ursodeoxycholic acid in patients with intrahepatic cholestasis of pregnancy. *Hepatology* 1992; 15:1043–1047.

157. Plevris JN, et al: Ursodeoxycholic acid in the treatment of alcoholic liver disease. *Eur J Gastroenterol Hepatol* 1991; 3:653–656.

158. Sackmann M, et al: The Munich Gallbladder Lithotripsy Study. Results of the first 5 years with 711 patients. *Ann Intern Med* 1991; 114:290–296.

159. Tint GS, et al: Lithotripsy plus ursodiol is superior to ursodiol alone for cholesterol gallstones. *Gastroenterology* 1992; 102:2042–2049.

160. Schoenfield LJ, the Investigators of the Dornier National Biliary Lithotripsy Study: The effect of ursodiol on the safety and efficacy of extracorporeal shock-wave lithotripsy of gallstones. The Dornier National Biliary Lithotripsy Study. *N Engl J Med* 1990; 323:1239–1245.

161. Darzi A, et al: Gallstone clearance: A randomised study of extracorporeal shockwave lithotripsy and chemical dissolution. *Br J Surg* 1990; 77:1265–1267.

162. Ertan A, et al: Extracorporeal shock-wave lithotripsy versus ursodiol alone in the treatment of gallstones. *Gastroenterology* 1992; 103:311–316.

CHAPTER 10

Liver Transplantation

Jorge Rakela, M.D.

Professor of Medicine, Mayo Medical School; Consultant, Mayo Clinic, Rochester, Minnesota

Jeffrey S. Weinstein, M.D.

Clinical Gastroenterology Fellow, Mayo Clinic, Rochester, Minnesota

Ruud A. F. Krom, M.D.

Professor of Surgery, Mayo Medical School; Consultant in General Surgery and Transplantation, Methodist Hospital, Rochester, Minnesota

PREDICTION OF SURVIVAL AND THE TIMING OF LIVER TRANSPLANTATION

The search for objective predictors that may help in the selection and timing of liver transplantation (LT) continues to be a priority in this arena. Oellerich and colleagues[1] studied predictors of 1-year pretransplant survival in 101 patients with histologically proven cirrhosis. They studied indocyanine green (ICG) half-life, monoethylglycine exylidide (MEGX) formation from lidocaine, serum bilirubin, serum albumin, serum cholinesterase, serum alkaline phosphatase, prothrombin time, development of ascites and encephalopathy, and Child-Pugh's score. After their analysis, Child-Pugh's score, MEGX testing, and ICG half-life were the only independent variables that were related significantly to 1-year survival. The combination of Child-Pugh's score and ICG testing for MEGX had the best specificity as a predictor of 1-year transplant survival. The authors are in the process of evaluating static and dynamic liver function tests in a prospective, multicenter study as predictors of survival before and after LT.

INDICATIONS

Urea Cycle Enzyme Deficiency

There are six hepatic enzymes responsible for the biosynthesis of urea from ammonium and glutamine. A deficiency of one of these enzymes leads to elevated plasma ammonium and glutamine levels, which may be associated with cerebral edema and encephalopathy. LT has been used as a method of enzyme replacement therapy in two patients: a 2-week-old infant with carbamoyl phosphate synthetase-I deficiency and a 35-year-old man with argininosuccinic acid synthetase deficiency.[2] Both patients were comatose before surgery and were doing well at 34 and 40 months, respectively, after transplantation. These two patients can be added to the other seven patients who have undergone transplantation for the same indications (six with ornithine-transcarbamylase deficiency and one with carbamoyl phosphate synthetase-I deficiency). Recent advances in somatic gene therapy hopefully will provide an efficacious therapeutic alternative to LT among patients with a urea cycle enzyme deficiency in the near future.

Primary Hepatic Cancer

The recent trend is to consider LT for hepatocellular carcinoma or cholangiocarcinoma in association with another therapeutic modality (i.e., chemotherapy, radiation therapy). Some patients, however, may be cured with LT alone. Haug and associates,[3] representing the Boston Center for Liver Transplantation, recently have reported their results in 24 patients with hepatocellular carcinoma and 9 patients with cholangiocarcinoma; the actuarial survival rates of the two groups at 3 years were 42% and 59%, respectively. The recurrence rate for cholangiocarcinoma was 56% and that for hepatocellular carcinoma was 25% among those who survived for longer than 3 months. In spite of the fact that no adjuvant therapy was provided, more than 50% of the patients with primary hepatic cancer were considered to be "cured" after LT.

Alcoholic Liver Disease

The University of Michigan Liver Transplantation Program has reported its experience with 99 alcoholic patients who were evaluated for LT.[4] Forty-five patients undergoing this procedure had an actuarial survival rate at 24 months of 73%; this was no different than that of nonalcoholic allograft recipients in the same program. Return to alcohol drinking was documented in 5 patients (11%). Fifty-four patients were not selected for transplantation; 17 were considered to be "too well"; however, their actuarial survival rate at 24 months was only 59%. Nineteen patients were considered to be "too sick": 12 were thought to present a poor operative risk, 5 had hepatoma, 1 had aplastic anemia, and 1 had carcinoma of the lung. The survival rate of this group at 12 months was 0%. Finally, 17 patients were not selected on the basis of "poor prognosis for future sobriety," and their actuarial survival rate was 43% at 18 months, significantly less than that of patients who underwent LT. Sorrell and coworkers[5] in an accompanying editorial, emphasized the need for the authors to provide more data on the value of their approach in predicting sobriety. Their recidivism rate of 11% probably reflects careful patient selection and may not be indicative of the rate that would be observed if alcoholic patients underwent transplantation indiscriminately.

Individuals with end-stage alcoholic liver disease form the largest category of patients with chronic liver disease. They account for a growing percentage of patients undergoing LT in almost every transplant center. The selection process for appropriate surgical candidates continues to be marred with personal biases of members of transplant teams and is perceived unfavorably by the community at large. Efforts to identify appropriate transplant candidates who have the lowest chance of recidivism should be continued.

VIRAL HEPATITIS

Hepatitis B Virus

A high proportion of patients infected with hepatitis B virus (HBV) will have recurrence of this infection in the posttransplant period. A condition defined as fibrosing cholestatic hepatitis is accompanied by increased intrahepatic expression of HBV antigens, suggesting a direct cytopathic effect of the virus.[6] Lau and colleagues[7] have studied the effect of prednisolone, methylprednisolone, azathioprine, and cyclosporine in hepatocyte culture systems using hepatocytes isolated from patients with chronic HBV infection. The authors observed an increase in intracellular HBsAg and HBcAg production with prednisolone and methylprednisolone, but not with azathioprine or cyclosporine. Interestingly, HBsAg secretion was unaffected. This preliminary observation suggests that these patients may not benefit from the use of corticosteroids. This is a hypothesis worthy of further investigation.

Fibrosing cholestatic hepatitis is a distinct clinical entity that occurs in association with HBV infection of hepatic allografts. This condition is characterized by a rapidly progressive clinical course leading to liver failure and a high mortality rate. Histologically, there is extensive periportal fibrosis, canalicular and cellular cholestasis, mild inflammatory changes, and prominent expression of HBV antigens. HBsAg and HBcAg have been measured in liver tissue and found to be at significantly greater concentrations in transplant recipients with fibrosing cholestatic hepatitis than in those without this syndrome or in other patients with chronic HBV infection.[8] Pre-S1 and pre-S2 also were expressed intracellularly. The authors propose that the enhanced expression of viral proteins and the lack of prominent inflammatory changes favor a direct cytopathic effect of these proteins.

Passive Immunoprophylaxis

Liver transplantation among patients with HBV infection is followed almost uniformly by recurrence of the viral infection. Various attempts at preventing this recurrence, such as the use of hyperimmune gamma globulin B, vaccination, and interferon-α, have resulted in either complete failure or controversial protection. An initially promising approach was the use of anti-HBV monoclonal antibody to reduce the risk of HBV infection of donor livers. McMahon and coworkers[9] reported the use of a monoclonal preparation in six patients with HBV infection who were undergoing LT; three of these individuals had recurrence of HBsAg positivity in spite of adequate levels of antibody to HBsAg (anti-HBs). The authors were able to define a genetic variation located in the highly conserved region of the S gene implicated in antiviral binding and neutralizing antibody epitopes. Furthermore, they injected a chimpanzee with two of these variants obtained from one of the patients and were able to observe active immunization by the rising antibody to HBcAg (anti-HBc) and anti-HBs titers; liver biopsies obtained at 6 and 8 weeks showed HBV-DNA by polymerase chain reaction (PCR). Neither elevation of serum aminotransferase levels nor serum HBsAg positivity developed in the chimpanzee during the time of observation; however. This work clearly demonstrates that treatment with human anti-HBs monoclonal antibody is associated with the development of escape mutants of HBV-DNA that lead to amino acid modifications of a viral surface protein determinant that is essential for antibody binding. The clinical implications of this observation remain unclear.

Hepatitis D Virus

Ottobrelli and coworkers[10] prospectively studied 27 patients undergoing liver transplantation for end-stage liver disease associated with HBV and hepatitis D virus (HDV) infection. Thirteen patients had replicating HBV, and HBV was spread along with HDV to the transplanted liver in each case. There were 5 patients among 21 long-term survivors in whom HDV was transmitted to the donor graft in spite of the apparent absence of replicating HBV in either the native or the transplanted liver. This observation may indicate that HDV is able to sustain a chronic infection without HBV. The authors also were able to detect intermittent HDV viremia in the apparent absence of HBV infection; no further data were provided regarding the surface protein of these delta particles that is provided under normal circumstances by HBV. Finally, an intriguing observation was the lack of significant liver disease in patients with delta infection alone; these findings raised the possibility that delta would not be a pathogenic virus unless HBV infection occurred at the same time. Mason and Taylor provided a lucid discussion of the pathogenic implications of these observations in an accompanying editorial[11] and cautioned against accepting these observations fully without further analysis of additional cases.

Hepatitis C Virus

It has become evident that detection of hepatitis C virus (HCV) infection by immunoassay is underestimated in immunosuppressed patients. Shah and associates[12] studied 317 liver transplant donor-recipient pairs and found the prevalence of anti-HCV positivity among recipients to be 13.6% and the seroconversion rate to be 9.2%. The prevalence of presumed chronic non-A, non-B viral hepatitis was 13.8% and that of chronic active hepatitis was very low at 1.6%. A different picture was described by Wright and colleagues[13]; in almost all patients infected before LT, there was recurrence of HCV. Thirty-five percent of patients without a pretransplant HCV infection became infected during the posttransplant period. Furthermore, 96% of patients who had hepatitis were infected with HCV. The clinical spectrum of patients with chronic hepatitis C included 11 patients with chronic active hepatitis, 3 of whom had severe disease. The apparent discrepancy between these studies can be attributed to the use of immunoassays to define HCV infection in one[12] and reverse transcription and PCR for the detection of HCV-RNA in the other.[13]

Feray and associates cloned and sequenced segments of HCV-RNA in patients with HCV infection after LT and demonstrated that the same strain that was infecting the graft was present before transplantation.[14] This observation indicated that, in most patients who have chronic HCV infection before transplantation, the graft becomes infected by the same viral strain. The increasing application of techniques of molecular epidemiology probably will help to define better the mechanism and frequency of transmission of viruses in general in patients undergoing LT.

MEDICAL AND SURGICAL COMPLICATIONS

Bone disease is a frequent complication among patients with end-stage chronic liver disease and, in particular, among those with chronic cholestatic liver disorders. The most frequently described condition is osteoporosis, and the advent of LT has provided the opportunity for further definition of the mechanism of this complication and assessment of the potential therapeutic effect of liver transplantation. McDonald and colleagues[15] studied spinal bone mineral density in 35 adult patients before and after LT. They found a significant decrease in bone mass among men and women with primary biliary cirrhosis. The abnormalities consisted of decreases in the osteoblastic surface, tetracycline surface, and bone formation rate, with a normal reabsorbing surface. The bone loss occurred almost exclusively during the first 3 months after LT and was of 25% with respect to pre-LT levels. Five of the patients sustained vertebral fractures during the first 6 months after LT; 1 patient had a fractured wrist and 3 had osteonecrosis of the hip (2 patients) or knee (1 patient). The authors also were able to demonstrate an increased osteoblastic surface, increased bone formation in men, and elevation of serum osteocalcin levels 3 months after LT. Surprisingly, they found a strong correlation only between the length of hospitalization and bone loss. These findings led to consideration of the possibility of treating this bone loss during the initial period after LT, and they felt that calcitonin and diphosphonates were promising therapeutic agents.

An important and useful publication on first allograft failure has come from the transplant program at the University of Pittsburgh.[16] The authors studied 177 patients who underwent LT for a second time between January 1984 and December 1988. Sixty-eight percent of the grafts failed during the first month after LT, and only 6% failed after 12 months. The leading causes of early graft failure were primary nonfunctioning graft, ischemic graft injury, acute rejection, and vascular complications. The causes of late graft failure included chronic rejection and recurrence of primary disease.

The 6-month survival rate after a second LT was 46.3%, which is worse than after the initial procedure. This observation probably reflects the deteriorating condition of the patient before the second transplantation. This was particularly evident among patients with graft failure resulting from ischemic injury and disease recurrence (associated mainly with HBV disease).

Liver transplant recipients undergo a liver biopsy procedure usually several times during their posttransplant course. This procedure can be associated with morbidity and mortality. Bubak and coworkers[17] reported the incidence and types of liver biopsy complications in their first 160 consecutive LTs. They defined a significant complication as one that required therapeutic intervention. These authors observed a significant complication in 17 of 950 liver biopsies (1.8%), the complications occurring among 13 patients (9.6%). Eleven patients had bleeding complications and 6 had serious infections. The most frequent bleeding complication was hemothorax. An interesting observation was the high incidence of infectious complications among patients who underwent choledochojejunostomy (12.5%) compared with those who had a duct-to-duct biliary anastomosis (1%); this difference was statistically significant ($P < .01$). The most common infections were cholangitis and infected hematomas both of which were associated with bacteremia. The authors concluded that antibiotic prophylaxis probably is appropriate in patients who are at high risk for infection. No patient died in spite of the high frequency of biopsies per patient (6.9 biopsies per graft; range, 1 to 29 biopsies).

Auxiliary heterotropic LT for chronic liver disease has been proposed as an alternative to orthotopic LT by the group in Rotterdam.[6] Their preliminary reports have been encouraging. A potential problem that may arise when the original liver is left in place is functional competition between the two livers.[18] The Rotterdam group has studied this problem in six consecutive patients undergoing auxiliary heterotropic LT. They calculated the sizes of the graft and host livers by planimetry using two-dimensional D-isopropyl iminodiacetic acid scintigrams. They observed that the graft increased from 12.2 cm^2 on day 3 to a maximum of 14.8 cm^2 on day 21, then remained unchanged thereafter. The host liver decreased from 9.6 cm^2 on day 3 to 3.9 cm^2 at 6 months. The investigators stressed that a similar study should be done in patients undergoing this procedure for acute liver failure to determine whether the phenomenon of functional competition occurs in settings other than chronic liver disease. The factors that determine graft growth remain to be determined, but the authors suggest that it probably results from a combination of liver cell proliferation and hypertrophy. Another interesting phenomenon was the rapidity of graft regeneration; it occurred in 3 weeks compared to the 3 to 6 months that regeneration of human liver usually takes after partial hepatectomy.

Autoimmune hepatitis is a frequent indication for LT, in spite of the existence of effective treatment. The Mayo Clinic group has reported prognostic features in 111 patients with autoimmune hepatitis and correlated their findings with those of 24 patients with autoimmune hepatitis who were undergoing LT.[19] No individual features predicted outcome after conventional treatment; those who failed were younger (32 ± 3 years vs. 43 ± 2 years, $P < .02$), required a longer duration of treatment, had ascites more frequently, and were positive for HLA A1, B8 more commonly.

The patients undergoing LT were not different than those who had a poor response to corticosteroid treatment except in their mortality rate, which was 8% vs. 56%, respectively ($P < .01$). Antinuclear antibody and SMA titers decreased after LT and the majority of patients became seronegative 1 year after the procedure. None of the transplant recipients had shown evidence of disease recurrence by the time of this publication.

A different picture is provided by Wright and associates.[20] They found histologic evidence of recurrent disease in 11 of 43 cases (25.6%). The rejection rate was 55.8% and this did not differ from that observed in other conditions. Autoimmune hepatitis was more likely to recur in HLA-DR3–positive recipients of HLA-DR3–negative grafts; recurrence was not seen among patients with HLA-DR3–positive grafts. Surprisingly, HLA-B8 status did not influence the rate of either disease recurrence or rejection.

In 1953, Kowalski and Abelman described several hemodynamic abnormalities in patients with end-stage chronic liver disease, including high cardiac output, low total systemic vascular resistance, tachycardia, decreased mean arterial blood pressure, and increased blood volume. Henderson and colleagues[21] studied cardiac output before and 1 or 2 years after LT in 23 patients. They confirmed the presence of an elevated cardiac output before transplantation and observed that it persisted at 1 and 2 years after LT. The cause of a persistently high cardiac output is unclear so far and the condition does not seem to require treatment; it may contribute to systemic hypertension, however, which is found frequently in patients receiving cyclosporine as part of their immunosuppressive program.

Since the 1983 National Institutes of Health Consensus Conference on Liver Transplantation, this surgical procedure has been considered an essential component of the therapeutic armamentarium for fulminant hepatic failure. Several recent series have demonstrated a survival rate between 50% and 60% in this condition, much better than the 15% to 20% survival rate that was observed before the use of LT. A frequent and potentially lethal complication of transplantation among patients with fulminant hepatic failure is the development of cerebral edema and intracranial hypertension. This complication may lead to brain stem herniation and death. Intracranial pressure monitoring has been proposed as a method of diagnosing and treating this condition, and, more recently, of aiding in the selection of suitable candidates for LT by identifying those patients who already may have sustained irreversible neurologic injury.

Lidofsky and coworkers[22] reported their results with intracranial pressure monitoring in 20 adults and 3 children. Ten patients were treated before LT with mannitol or barbiturates for an intracranial pressure of more than 25 mm Hg. Six of these patients did not respond to therapy; they were removed from the study and subsequently died with brain stem herniation. Twelve of the remaining 17 patients underwent LT; 11 of them required intraoperative treatment of bouts of intracranial hypertension. All the patients who underwent transplantation recovered well and were dismissed from the hospital. Their survival rate after transplantation was 92%. Three other patients died awaiting LT and 2 patients recovered spontaneously.

This study demonstrated the usefulness of intracranial pressure monitoring in the diagnosis and treatment of cerebral edema and suggested that it could be a powerful tool to aid in the selection of suitable candidates for LT. This invasive monitoring procedure can be associated with significant morbidity and mortality, however. In Lidofsky's series, 5 patients had intracranial bleeding; this complication led to death in 2 of them. Two adults had small intraventricular bleeds, but the bleeding was serious in 3 children. One of the children required drainage of an epidural hematoma and the other 2 died of resultant brain stem herniation.

An intriguing biliary complication has been described recently that is characterized by nonanastomotic bile duct strictures and dilatations involving the biliary tree. These can occur at single or multiple sites and may be associated with intrahepatic bile leakage. They tend to appear between 1 and 3 months after transplantation. This condition has been described in association with arteriopathy of chronic ductopenic rejection, ABO incompatibility, and hepatic artery thrombosis.

The Mayo Clinic transplant group has reported a strong association between prolonged cold ischemia time and the development of biliary strictures with both Euro-Collins and the University of Wisconsin solution.[23] The authors also have observed that the incidence of this complication can be decreased significantly by restricting ischemia time to less than 13 hours. If this observation is confirmed in a larger number of patients and by other groups, the current trend toward more prolonged ischemia times using the University of Wisconsin solution may be reexamined. We already have changed our policy at Mayo Clinic and prefer to restrict cold ischemia time to less than 11 hours. Since the implementation of this procedural change, we have observed a sharp decrease in the incidence of biliary strictures.

Neurologic complications may develop in LT recipients during the postoperative period, including alterations in mental status, seizures, and focal-motor deficits. The underlying pathology may include intracranial bleeding, cerebral infarction, central pontine myelinolysis, and central nervous system infection. Cyclosporine and FK-506 also may lead to neurologic syndromes. Lopez and coworkers[24] studied 185 patients who underwent two or more LT procedures. They found alterations in mental status in 84%, seizures in 33%, and focal-motor deficits in 15%. These three complications were more prevalent after the second and third LTs. They also observed that those patients who had a neurologic complication were more likely to die.

Encephalopathy and coma in the posttransplant period were associated with infections, electrolyte abnormalities, and the use of neurotoxic drugs. Seizures were found to be associated with metabolic abnormalities and structural lesions; a high cyclosporine level was noted in 15 of 54 patients with this complication, particularly in those who received the drug intravenously. The causes of motor deficits included cerebral infarcts, intracranial bleeding, and infection.

Large amounts of blood and blood products may be required during LT. Enhanced fibrinolytic activity has been identified as a cause of bleeding, especially during the anhepatic and early postreperfusion phases. Alternatively, this increased fibrinolysis can be attributed to the surgical procedure itself. Bakker and associates[25] studied the fibrinolytic system in 10 patients undergoing orthotopic LT, 18 patients undergoing heterotopic LT, and 10 patients undergoing partial hepatic resection. They found that plasma degradation products of fibrin and fibrinogen increased significantly during the anhepatic phase in patients undergoing orthotopic LT. This was not the case among patients undergoing heterotopic LT or partial resection. They concluded that the lack of hepatic clearance during the anhepatic phase was responsible for the increased amount of tissue type plasminogen activator activity that was observed in this subset of patients.

Significant hypotension may develop during reperfusion and the exact cause of this phenomenon has not been well defined. Khoury and colleagues[26] studied the potential role of prostacyclin, a biologically active prostanoid. They studied 12 patients and found that, in 8 of them, there was a decrease in the systolic blood pressure from 98 ± 5 mm Hg to 61 ± 4 mm Hg, with a rise in cardiac output from 6.9 ± 0.7 l/min to 9.9 ± 1.05 L/min. This coincided with a rise in the prostacyclin level from 524 ± 134 pg/mL to 1,132 ± 264 pg/mL. The hemodynamic measurements were obtained 1 minute before and 3 minutes after reperfusion. These findings suggest that prostacyclin could be a factor in this syndrome.

Graft vs. host disease is a rare complication in LT recipients. Collins and coworkers[27] and Roberts and associates[28] have reported a total of five cases. Skin biopsies and circulating lymphocytes had an HLA phenotype corresponding to that of the respective donor, substantiating the diagnosis in each of the patients. In spite of aggressive immunosuppression, this condition was uniformly fatal. The authors advised that this diagnosis be considered in patients who have undergone LT and have fever, rash, pancytopenia, and diarrhea. Liver allograft recipients with this condition differ from those undergoing bone marrow transplantation in that the liver is not involved because sensitized lymphocytes originate from the donor liver.

ORGAN RETRIEVAL AND PRESERVATION

Hepatic Reperfusion Injury

An excellent review on the mechanisms of preservation and reperfusion injuries in liver allografts has been provided by Clavien and coworkers.[29] A primary non-functioning graft usually haunts transplant surgeons during the postoperative period. This complication may occur in 2% to 15% of all transplant recipients. The mechanism leading to this condition remains obscure and intense research continues. One group of investigators has proposed that a certain type of reperfusion injury may lead in certain patients to alterations in the hepatic microcirculation and subsequently to alterations in hepatic oxygenation.[30] This group studied hepatic oxygenation after ischemia and reflow in a rat model in which the left pedicles were ligated for either 30 or 60 minutes. The group undergoing 60 minutes of ischemia had decreased survival, lower blood oxygenation and blood volume indexes, higher serum alanine aminotransferase levels, and significant hepatocellular degeneration. The authors proposed that the measurement of hepatic tissue oxygenation immediately after reflow with reflectance spectrophotometry, a noninvasive technique, can help to predict liver injury in the posttransplant phase.

Koo and coworkers[31] reported evidence for the role of superoxide anion in the no-reflow phenomenon that is associated with hepatic injury after ischemia-reperfusion. They observed a protective effect of a long-acting form of superoxide dismutase given intravenously. This preparation was able to reduce the hepatocellular necrosis and microcirculatory stasis in liver sinusoids that is associated with reperfusion injury. The relevance of these observations to primary nonfunctioning grafts in humans will have to be defined.

Goto and colleagues[32] approached the study of primary nonfunctioning grafts after LT from a different perspective. They found that endotoxin production, which may stimulate the release of tumor necrosis factor, may be the pathogenic sequence leading to this complication. They studied, in a rat orthotopic LT model, the consequences of storing livers from Lewis rats for either 1 or 4 hours in ice-cold Euro-Collins solution. They found that the group receiving a liver stored for 4 hours had substantial hepatocellular degeneration and higher serum alanine aminotransferase levels 24 hours after surgery. This correlated very closely with elevated serum endotoxin and tumor necrosis factor levels. They also observed that these changes were attenuated effectively by anti–tumor necrosis factor antibody treatment. These observations could have important therapeutic implications if they are confirmed in humans undergoing LT.

The transplanted graft may display variable degrees of functional impairment. A graft may not work at all, a condition known as primary nonfunction, or a gradient of graft dysfunction may be observed. Grande and associates[33] described their experience with poorly functioning grafts among 128 LTs. Fourteen patients (11%) had an alanine aminotransferase level greater than 2,500 units/L, a bile output of less than 40 mL/day, and a prothrombin activity of less than 60% in spite of plasma administration. Two patients underwent a second LT procedure on days 3 and 4, respectively, and hemorrhagic necrosis was found in both grafts. The other 12 patients had slow improvement in liver test results starting on day 3 after transplantation; only 1 of these patients died, as a result of bacterial sepsis and multiorgan failure. Therefore, only 2 of 14 patients (14%) required retransplantation. The authors concluded that most grafts with initially poor function recover and that a decision can be made regarding the need for retransplantation by 3 days postoperatively.

"Marginal donors"have been studied by Mor and colleagues[34] with respect to graft outcome. They found donor body weight exceeding 100 kg to be the only variable associated with increased graft loss and early hepatocellular damage. They suggested that overweight donors should undergo liver biopsy and that their livers should not be used if severe fatty infiltration is found.

REJECTION

Hepatic allograft rejection traditionally has been classified as either "acute" or "chronic." The term "hyperacute" rejection is reserved for the rare condition that is associated with preformed cytotoxic antibodies.[6]

Wiesner and associates[35] proposed an alternate classification of cellular rejection (Table 1). The traditional classification, although it defined rejection temporally, also implied certain specific histologic features. Acute rejection was thought to be reversible and to involve portal or periportal hepatitis, destructive or nondestructive nonsuppurative cholangitis, and endotheliitis or phlebitis of portal or hepatic venules. The newly proposed term is "cellular" rejection. This term is strictly descriptive and has no implications regarding time of occurrence or reversibility.

The term "chronic" rejection has been used to describe a relentless clinical course leading to graft failure. The histologic hallmarks have been damage or progressive loss of small bile ducts, cholestasis, and foam cell arteritis or arteriopathy, the latter being noted rarely. This condition also has been described as vanishing bile duct syndrome. The new term for this state "ductopenic rejection"; this emphasizes the essential pathologic lesion of the diagnosis and does not have any tem-

TABLE 1.
Terminology of Allograft Rejection*

Classification	Present Acute	Proposed Cellular	Present Chronic	Proposed Ductopenic
Morphologic findings	Portal hepatitis, nonsuppurative cholangitis, and endotheliitis	Portal hepatitis, nonsuppurative cholangitis, and endotheliitis	Duct loss ± arteriopathy	Duct loss ± arteriopathy
Time after transplant	Short duration	Independent	Long duration	Independent
Reversibility	Reversible	Independent	Irreversible	Potentially reversible
Additional immuno-suppression	Responsive	Independent	Unresponsive	Independent

*Adapted from Wiesner RH, Ludwig J, Van Hoek B, et al: *Hepatology* 1991; 14:721–729. Used by permission.

poral connotations. This diagnosis is made histologically when bile ducts are not present in more than 50% of the portal tracts. When foam cell arteriopathy or arteritis is present, some investigators make the diagnosis of "vascular" rejection. This lesion is considered to form part of the spectrum of lesions in ductopenic rejection under the proposed new terminology. Ductopenic rejection has a poorer prognosis in terms of graft survival. The prevalence has been described to be between 2% and 17% of patients who have undergone LT (Table 2). It may occur at any time after LT and usually begins as cellular rejection that is refractory to increased immunosuppressive therapy with the subsequent evolution of ductopenic rejection. This type of rejection seems to be more common among patients with

TABLE 2.
Incidence of Chronic Rejection Resulting in Graft Failure*

Transplant Program	Number of First Hepatic Allografts	Incidence of Chronic Rejection (%)
University of Minnesota	47	3(6.3)
Baylor-Dallas	104	8(7.7)
Cambridge/Kings	101	17(16.8)
Birmingham	189	19(10.0)
University of California, Los Angeles	83	3(3.6)
Groningen	83	9(10.8)
Hannover	81	9(11.1)
Pittsburgh	394	22(5.6)
Sydney	28	3(10.7)
Mayo Clinic	164	15(9.1)
University of Wisconsin	127	3(2.4)
Total	1,401	111(7.9)

*Adapted from Wiesner RH, Ludwig J, VanHoek B, et al: *Hepatology* 1991; 14:721–729. Used by permission.

primary sclerosing cholangitis, raising the possibility that it may represent the recurrence of this disorder. HLA-DR matching of donor-recipient pairs and cytomegalovirus infection also were suggested to be associated with this condition; however, Paya and coworkers[36] did not confirm this observation. The presence of a positive lymphocytotoxic crossmatch and the absence of azathioprine as part of the immunosuppressive program have been described as risk factors for ductopenic rejection.

In a minority of patients, this condition is reversible, with clinical, biochemical, and histologic normalization, occasionally occurring spontaneously.

The treatment for progressive ductopenic rejection is retransplantation; unfortunately, this is followed by the recurrence of ductopenic rejection in a large proportion of more than 50% of patients.

Pathologists from five LT centers (Baylor University Medical Center, Mayo Clinic, University of Pittsburgh, University of Minnesota, and University of California, Los Angeles) studied intraobserver variation in the histopathologic diagnosis of allograft rejection.[37] They found the diagnosis of acute cellular rejection to be highly reproducible. It was more difficult to obtain agreement on the diagnosis of chronic rejection. There was excellent agreement in defining portal tract inflammation, subendothelial inflammation, and bile duct damage as the elements necessary for establishing the diagnosis of acute rejection.

A surprising finding was the better agreement on the final diagnosis based on the histologic variables that formed part of the final diagnosis.

Most immunosuppressive programs use prednisone, cyclosporin A, and azathioprine. The latter two medications may cause hepatotoxicity and establishing this diagnosis in an LT recipient who may have multiple causes of hepatic dysfunction is a frequent clinical dilemma. Azathioprine hepatotoxicity is not well defined and its clinical spectrum includes asymptomatic aminotransferase level elevation, cholestasis, veno-occlusive disease with portal hypertension, peliosis hepatitis, and nodular regenerative hyperplasia. Sterneck and coworkers[38] described two patients with azathioprine hepatotoxicity after LT. These individuals had jaundice, elevated serum aminotransferase levels, and sinusoidal congestion with centrilobular hepatocellular degeneration 17 and 61 days, respectively, after LT. Both patients experienced clinical improvement when azathioprine was withdrawn. One of the two patients had a recurrence after rechallenge with the drug. The authors proposed the following sequence of events: The drug initially causes cholestasis and endothelial cell damage manifested as sinusoidal dilatations. The disruption of microvascular hepatic blood flow leads to hepatocyte necrosis in zone III of the hepatic acinus and, if the drug is not withdrawn, hepatic necrosis is followed by regeneration and the development of nodular regenerative hyperplasia. They also emphasized the importance of early drug withdrawal to avoid progression to an irreversible stage.

Hepatic allograft rejection is mainly a T lymphocyte–driven process, expressed and modulated by a multitude of cytokines. Basista and associates[39] evaluated the production of procoagulant activity by Kupffer cells and plasma levels of tumor necrosis factor in a rat allograft rejection model. Procoagulant activity is expressed by monocytes/macrophages and tumor necrosis factor is secreted mainly by macrophages; these cytokines mediate immune cell adherence, vascular thrombosis, and delayed-type hypersensitivity. The researchers found that Kupffer cell procoagulant activity was elevated by day 3 posttransplantation and plasma tumor necrosis factor was elevated by day 1. These observations support a protagonist role for procoagulant activity and tumor necrosis factor in hepatic allograft rejection and raise the possibility of using therapies designed to neutralize their effects as part of the treatment of rejection.

Rapamycin has been described as a potent immunosuppressive substance that is related chemically to FK-506. Cyclosporine and FK-506 inhibit the transcription of early T cell activation genes; rapamycin blocks downstream events derived from T cell activation. Another difference is that cyclosporine and FK-506 have a stimulating effect on liver regeneration; rapamycin has been found to have antiproliferative properties in the liver. Francavilla and coworkers[40] studied the effects of rapamycin on a hepatocyte culture system. They were able to confirm its antiproliferative effect and found it to be dose-dependent and long-lasting after a brief exposure. They also found there to be profound inhibition in the expression of transforming growth factor-β in association with the antiproliferative effect of rapamycin.

Patient monitoring in current cyclosporine-based immunosuppressive programs require the measurement of cyclosporine blood levels. Sandborn and coworkers[41] made an interesting observation in a small group of patients with acute cellular rejection in comparison with a group without rejection. They found that hepatic tissue cyclosporine concentrations were significantly lower in patients with rejection (1,879 ± 998 ng/g vs. 3,493 ± 936 ng/g, $P < .01$); however, they noted no difference in cyclosporine blood levels. They calculated that a hepatic tissue cyclosporine concentration less than 2,500 ng/g was 75% sensitive and 89% specific for predicting cellular rejection. Further studies are needed to define the meaning of this observation because it could be the consequence of the rejection phenomenon itself and not its cause.

The role of cytomegalovirus infection in the vanishing bile duct syndrome continues to be controversial. Proponents of a role for such infection in this condition studied serial biopsies in 12 patients and found cytomegalovirus DNA in the hepatocytes of 10 cases.[42] They observed that cytomegalovirus DNA remained detectable until death or retransplantation among patients with vanishing bile duct syndrome; however, they found cystomegalovirus DNA only in hepatocytes and not in bile duct epithelial cells, the presumed target for injury. Wright[43] pinpointed the weak points of the proposed connection between cytomegalovirus and the vanishing bile duct syndrome and proposed that further work in mice with severe combined immunodeficiency that have been infected with murine cytomegalovirus may help to settle this controversy.

An intriguing finding has been the possible usefulness of bile cytology in the diagnosis of hepatic allograft rejection.[44] Cytologic examination was performed on

128 bile specimens obtained from 12 LT recipients with functioning T tubes. Ten milliliters of bile was collected and a Cytospin preparation was performed. Two types of cells were found: bile duct or epithelial cells and inflammatory cells consisting of polymorphonuclear cells, lymphocytes, and monocytes. The highest specificity for rejection was provided by the presence of lymphoblastic cells and inflammatory cells in bile after the early posttransplant ischemic injury period. This is an interesting observation with potential diagnostic implications.

Hepatic allografts have been considered to be more resistant than other allografts to humoral rejection, and the existence and diagnosis of "hyperacute" liver rejection have been difficult to define. Demetris and associates[45] reported their findings in 26 adult patients with preformed IgG donor lymphocytotoxic antibodies who underwent LT under FK-506 immunosuppression. They found that the crossmatch-positive patients had prolonged early graft dysfunction, a higher incidence of cellular rejection, and a higher incidence of graft failure in the first 180 days. Histologically, these patients had platelet margination in the central veins and sinusoids 60 to 90 minutes after graft revascularization; later on, the biopsies showed neutrophilic portal venulitis, acute cholangitis, cholangiolar proliferation, and centrilobular hepatocyte swelling. None of the patients had hyperacute rejection as such. Primary graft and patient survival rates were diminished significantly among crossmatch-positive patients (56% and 68%, respectively).

Cytokines are soluble glycoproteins that seem to play a central role in the inflammatory reaction that is associated with allograft rejection. Previous publications suggested the potential role of tumor necrosis factor-α, interleukin-1-β, interleukin-6, and interleukin-2 by detecting elevated circulating levels during rejection. Martinez and coworkers[46] took their approach to this problem one step further; they studied the intragraft cytokine profile in liver biopsy specimens taking during rejection. Interleukin-5 gene expression was present predominantly during rejection; interleukin-2, interleukin-4, interleukin-1-β, tumor necrosis factor-α, and interleukin-6 were detected with similar frequency in rejecting allografts and in those without rejection. Interleukin-5 is a cytokine involved in B cell growth and differentiation, the promotion of cytotoxic T lymphocytes and interleukin-2–mediated natural killer cell activity, and the stimulation of eosinophil activation and differentiation.

FK-506, a new immunosuppressant, has been studied in 96 patients who were receiving a cyclosporine-based immunosuppressive program and in whom graft dysfunction or cyclosporine toxicity was developing.[47] The clinical reasons for conversion included rejection in 76 patients, cyclosporine-steroid toxicity in 14 patients, and hepatitis in 6 patients. The latter group was difficult to classify as having either ongoing, refractory rejection or chronic hepatitis. They observed that patients with acute rejection or early chronic rejection benefited the most from switching to FK-506. There was no significant worsening in the mean serum creatinine level after 180 days of FK-506 therapy. These preliminary observations suggest that FK-506 may be a good alternative in the treatment of patients who are receiving cyclosporine and have a rejection episode that is refractory to high-dose steroids or OKT-3. There is an urgent need for more data to define better the position of FK-506 in the immunosuppressive armamentarium.

INFECTIOUS COMPLICATIONS

Cytomegalovirus infection is a major source of morbidity and may contribute to mortality in the posttransplant period. Special attention has been given to cytomegalovirus involvement of the liver, lungs, and retina. Cytomegalovirus enteritis is another complication of cytomegalovirus infection that has been largely ignored. Sakr and colleagues[48] examined 140 LT recipients for the presence of cytomegalovirus enteritis. The incidence was 27.7% in the cyclosporine-treated group and 20% in the FK-506–treated group. The authors found that cytomegalovirus enteritis tended to occur after the first month in the FK-506 group and appeared to be of lesser severity. The stomach and duodenum were involved predominantly. The infection was associated with varying degrees of nausea, vomiting, and abdominal pain. There were no deaths resulting from cytomegalovirus enteritis. The same group demonstrated gastric cytomegalovirus infection to be associated with a significant delay in gastric emptying that led to gastric retention.[49]

The high prevalence of cytomegalovirus infection after LT and its associated morbidity and mortality has stimulated interest in preventive therapy as an approach to improving outcome.[50] The Royal Free Hospital group studied prospectively 46 patients undergoing LT, paying special attention to risk factors for cytomegalovirus infection and disease. Risk factors included donor cytomegalovirus seropositivity, increased volume of pretransplant whole blood transfusion, and high-dose steroids for the treatment of rejection episodes. They also found that a positive blood culture or liver biopsy result was associated significantly with cytomegalovirus disease. They proposed a protocol in which ganciclovir could be tested (vs. placebo) as preventive therapy when a blood or liver biopsy result becomes positive for cytomegalovirus.

IgA deficiency present before LT has been found to be a risk factor for infection and is associated with decreased patient and graft survival.[51] The authors identified 43 adult patients with IgG, IgM, or IgA deficiency, and found that patients who were IgA-deficient had decreased survival at 1 year (50%) and at 2 years (32%). Eight of the 14 patients with IgA deficiency died of bacterial sepsis during the first 3 months, all of them succumbing to an enteric organism. This subset of patients may benefit from selective bowel decontamination and could be ideal candidates for IgA replacement therapy when this becomes available.

PEDIATRIC TRANSPLANTATION

Cohort studies in adult renal and cardiac transplant recipients have revealed increased morbidity and mortality associated with hyperlipidemia. McDiarmid and associates[52] measured serum cholesterol and triglyceride levels in 102 pediatric patients surviving more than 6 months after LT. They found that 50% of the children had a mean cholesterol level greater than 170 mg/dL, and that 56% had a mean triglyceride level greater than 140 mg/dL. These findings raised the concern that a significant proportion of pediatric LT recipients have hyperlipidemia and may be at risk for the development of atherosclerotic disease later in life. The authors were unable to find helpful predictors for the development of hyperlipidemia in this patient population.

The waiting list mortality rate for pediatric patients is about 10%. Several strategies have been designed to increase the donor pool, including living related donors, reduced-size liver allografts, split-liver allografts, and ABO-incompatible LTs. A recent publication[53] reported the use of prophylactic antilymphoblast globulin, plasmapheresis, and splenectomy in seven children undergoing ABO-incompatible LT. The rate of graft survival with this program was 60% and the incidence of rejection was 60%. The authors concluded that this approach should be considered only in emergency situations.

The Liver Transplant group from the University of Nebraska reported their results with 29 patients undergoing transplantation with 30 reduced-size livers.[54] The split-liver technique was used in 10 patients. The 1-year actuarial patient and graft survival rates were 68% and 65%, respectively, with a mean follow-up of 10.6 months. These investigators calculated that the percentage of children who die while awaiting LT has decreased from 13% to 2.6% in association with the introduction of reduced-size techniques to their program. The introduction of reduced-size liver techniques to LT has had a major impact in the pediatric programs in which they are used. They have expanded the donor pool with a consequent decrease in mortality among children awaiting LT. The survival rates have been comparable to those of whole liver transplantation.

There has been concern that reduced-size liver transplantation techniques may be accompanied by a higher incidence of biliary complications. The University of Chicago group, which has pioneered this approach, recently reported their rate of biliary complications among patients with reduced-size liver transplants and compared it to that of patients with full-size grafts.[55] The rate was 11.5% for whole graft recipients vs. 16% for reduced-size graft recipients. The actuarial survival rate was 70% for reduced-size graft recipients compared to 73% for whole-size graft recipients. They concluded that both approaches have comparable results.

The other dreaded complication of these novel techniques has been hepatic artery thrombosis. The University of Chicago group also reported the prevalence of this complication in whole livers, reduced-size grafts, and grafts from living related donors.[56] They found that hepatic artery thrombosis occurred in 25%, 15%, and 23% of patients undergoing the respective procedures. They also observed that the use of a cadaveric left lobe or left lateral segment graft, or an aortic-arterial anastomosis was associated with a lower risk of hepatic artery thrombosis in recipients less than 2 years ago. These results reflect steady progress with the new techniques. Currently, in experienced hands, the results with reduced-size LT are not dissimilar from those obtained with classic whole liver orthotopic LT.

QUALITY OF LIFE

LT is an accepted therapeutic modality for end-stage chronic or acute liver disease and has been shown to improve survival for several diseases when compared with the natural history of disease. A recent publication by Bonsel and colleagues[57] reported a careful analysis of quality of life in 46 adult patients and demonstrated a significant improvement in almost every aspect analyzed. Transplant recipients were better able to perform most of their daily activities and psychiatric morbidity occurred infrequently.

SUMMARY

The selection of patients with end-stage alcoholic liver disease for LT is receiving close scrutiny and better selection criteria should be available in the near future. This etiologic category is growing steadily as an indication for LT. Similar close scrutiny is being given to hepatocellular carcinoma and cholangiocarcinoma.

The use of long-term immunoprophylaxis among patients undergoing LT for end-stage HBV-associated liver disease shows some promise. The lack of an intravenous preparation of hyperimmune B immune globulin in the United States has hindered the evaluation of this approach in American programs, although the European experience is promising. Two clinical pictures of recurrent HBV infection are intriguing: a fulminating course of recurrent HBV infection with fibrosing cholestatic hepatitis has been characterized and found to be almost uniformly fatal; the development of recurrent delta infection without apparent concomitant HBV infection has been observed, defying our conventional dogma regarding delta infection.

Several reports have indicated a high recurrence rate of HCV infection after LT for HCV-associated liver disease and a high prevalence of HCV infection among patients with posttransplant chronic hepatitis. These studies report a rather benign clinical course in association with this infection: however, most of them have had rather short follow-up periods. No successful prophylactic strategies for HCV recurrence have been reported thus far.

An association between the development of nonanastomotic biliary strictures and prolonged ischemia time has been shown. If this observation is confirmed, it may lead to reconsideration of the current trend toward more prolonged ischemia times with the use of the University of Wisconsin solution.

It is anticipated that the role of FK-506– vs. cyclosporin A–based immunosuppression will be resolved in the near future when several ongoing randomized trials are reported.

Finally, this year has brought expansion in the use of reduced-size liver and split-liver techniques as alternatives in the pediatric population, with comparable results to those of whole liver transplantation being demonstrated.

REFERENCES

1. Oellerich M, et al: Predictors of one-year pre-transplant survival in patients with cirrhosis. *Hepatology* 1992; 14:1029–1034.

2. Todo S, et al: Orthotopic liver transplantation for urea cycle enzyme deficiency. *Hepatology* 1992; 15:419–422.

3. Haug CE, et al: Liver transplantation for primary hepatic cancer. *Transplantation* 1992; 53:377–382.

4. Lucey MR, et al: Selection for an outcome of liver transplantation in alcoholic liver disease. *Gastroenterology* 1992; 102:1736–1741.

5. Sorrell MF, Donovan JP, Shaw BW Jr: Transplantation in the alcoholic: A stalking horse for a larger problem (editorial). *Gastroenterology* 1992; 102:1806–1808.

6. Rakela J, et al: Liver transplantation, in Gitnick G (ed): *Current Hepatology,* vol 13. St. Louis, Mosby, 1992, p 293–312.

7. Lau JYN, et al: Modulation of hepatitis B viral antigens expression by immunosuppressive drugs in primary hepatocyte culture. *Hepatology* 1992; 53:894–898.

8. Lau JYN, et al: High-level expression of hepatitis B viral antigens in fibrosing cholestatic hepatitis. *Gastroenterology* 1992; 102:956–962.

9. McMahon G, et al: Genetic alterations in the gene encoding the major HBsAg: DNA and immunological analysis of recurrent HBsAg derived from monoclonal antibody-treated liver transplant patients. *Hepatology* 1992; 15:757–766.

10. Ottobrelli A, et al: Patterns of hepatitis delta virus reinfection and disease in liver transplantation. *Gastroenterology* 1991; 101:1649–1655.

11. Mason WS, et al: Liver transplantation: A model for the transmission of hepatitis delta viris (editorial). *Gastroenterology* 1991; 101:1741–1743.

12. Shah G, et al: Incidence, prevalence, and clinical course of hepatitis C following liver transplantation. *Gastroenterology* 1992; 103:323–329.

13. Wright TL, et al: Recurrent and acquired hepatitis C viral infection in liver transplant recipients. *Gastroenterology* 1992; 103:317–322.

14. Feray C, et al: Reinfection of liver graft by hepatitis C virus after liver transplantation. *J Clin Invest* 1992; 89:1361–1365.

15. McDonald JA, et al: Bone loss after liver transplantation. *Hepatology* 1991; 14:613–619.

16. Quiroga J, et al: Cause and timing of first allograft failure in orthotopic liver transplantation: A study of 177 consecutive patients. *Hepatology* 1992; 14:1054–1062.

17. Bubak M, et al: Complications of liver biopsy in liver transplant patients: Increased sepsis associated with choledochojejunostomy. *Hepatology* 1992; 14:1063–1065.

18. Willemse PJA, et al: Graft regeneration and host liver atrophy after auxiliary heterotopic liver transplantation for chronic liver failure. *Hepatology* 1992; 15:54–57.

19. Sanchez-Urdazpal L, et al: Prognostic features and role of liver transplantation in severe corticosteroid-treated autoimmune chronic active hepatitis. *Hepatology* 1992; 15:215–221.

20. Wright HL, et al: Disease recurrence and rejection following liver transplantation for autoimmune chronic active liver disease. *Transplantation* 1992; 53:136–139.

21. Henderson JM, et al: High cardiac output of advanced liver disease persists after orthotopic liver transplantation. *Hepatology* 1992; 15:258–262.

22. Lidofsky SD, et al: Intracranial pressure monitoring and liver transplantation for fulminant hepatic failure. *Hepatology* 1992; 16:1–7.

23. Sanchez-Urdazpal L, et al: Ischemic-type biliary complications after orthotopic liver transplantation. *Hepatology* 1992; 16:49–53.

24. Lopez OL, et al: Neurological complications after retransplantation. *Hepatology* 1992; 16:162–166.

25. Bakker CM, et al: Increased tissue-type plasminogen activator activity in orthotopic but not heterotopic liver transplantation: The role of the anhepatic period. *Hepatology* 1992; 16:404–408.

26. Khoury GF, et al: Prostacyclia accumulation during orthotopic liver transplantation in man. *Transplantation* 1992; 53:1266–1268.

27. Collins RH Jr, et al: Graft-versus-host disease in a liver transplant recipient. *Ann Intern Med* 1992; 116:391–392.

28. Roberts JP, et al: Graft-versus-host disease after liver transplantation in humans: A report of four cases. *Hepatology* 1991; 14:274–281.

29. Clavien PA, et al: Preservation and reperfusion injuries in liver allografts. *Transplantation* 1992; 53:957–978.

30. Goto M, et al: Hepatic tissue oxygenation as a predictive indicator of ischemia-reperfusion liver injury. *Hepatology* 1992; 15:432–437.

31. Koo A, et al: Contribution of no-reflow phenomenon to hepatic injury after ischemia-reperfusion: Evidence for a role for superoxide anion. *Hepatology* 1992; 15:507–514.

32. Goto M, et al: Tumor necrosis factor and endotoxin in the pathogenesis of liver and pulmonary injuries after orthotopic liver transplantation in the rat. *Hepatology* 1992; 16:487–493.

33. Grande L, et al: Recovery of liver graft after initial poor function. *Transplantation* 1992; 53:228–230.

34. Mor E, et al: The use of marginal donors for liver transplantation. *Transplantation* 1992; 53:383–386.

35. Wiesner RH, et al: Current concepts in cell-mediated hepatic allograft rejection leading to ductopenia and liver failure. *Hepatology* 1991; 14:721–729.

36. Paya CV, et al: Lack of association between cytomegalovirus infection, HLA matching and the vanishing bile duct syndrome after liver transplantation. *Hepatology* 1992; 16:66–70.

37. Demetris AJ, et al: Liver Transplantation Database (LTD) Investigators: *Hepatology* 1991; 14:751–755.

38. Sterneck M, et al: Azathioprine hepatotoxicity after liver transplantation. *Hepatology* 1991; 14:806–810.

39. Basista MH, et al: Procoagulant activity and tumor necrosis factor in rat hepatic allograft rejection. *Hepatology* 1991; 14:883–887.

40. Francavilla A, et al: Effects of rapamycin on cultured hepatocyte proliferation and gene expression. *Hepatology* 1992; 15:871–877.

41. Sandborn WJ, et al: Hepatic allograft cyclosporine concentration is independent of the route of cyclosporine administration and correlates with occurrence of early cellular rejection. *Hepatology* 1992; 15:1086–1091.

42. Arnold JC, et al: Cytomeglovirus infection persists in the liver graft in the vanishing bile duct syndrome. *Hepatology* 1992; 16:285–292.

43. Wright T: Cytomegalovirus infection and vanishing bile duct syndrome: Culprit or innocent by-stander? (editorial) *Hepatology* 1992; 16:494–496.

44. Roberti I, et al: Evidence that the systematic analysis of the bile cytology permits monitoring of hepatic allograft rejection. *Transplantation* 1992; 54:471–474.

45. Demetris AJ, et al: A clinicopathological study of human liver allograft recipients harboring per-formed IgG lymphocytotoxic antibodies. *Hepatology* 1992; 16:671–681.

46. Martinez OM, et al: Intragraft cytokine profile during human liver allograft rejection. *Transplantation* 1992; 53:449–456.

47. Demetris AJ, et al: Conversion of liver allograft recipients from cyclosporine to FK-506 immuno-suppressive therapy—a clinicopathologic study of 96 patients. *Transplantation* 1992; 53:1056–1062.

48. Sakr M, et al: Cytomegalovirus infection of the upper gastrointestinal tract following liver trans-plantation—incidence, location, and severity in cyclosporine- and FK-506-treated patients. *Transplantation* 1992; 53:786–791.

49. VanThiel DH, et al: Cytomegalovirus infection and gastric emptying. *Transplantation* 1992; 54:70–73.

50. Pillay D, et al: Surveillance for CMV infection in orthotopic liver transplant recipients. *Transplantation* 1992; 53:1261–1265.

51. VanThiel DH, et al: The association of IgA deficiency but not IgG or IgM deficiency with a re-duced patient and graft survival following liver transplantation. *Transplantation* 1992; 53:269–273.

52. McDiarmid SV, et al: Serum lipid abnormalities in pediatric liver transplant patients. *Transplantation* 1992; 53:109–115.

53. Renard TH, et al: An approach to ABO-incompatible liver transplantation in children. *Transplantation* 1992; 53:116–121.

54. Langnas AN, et al: The results of reduced-size liver transplantation, including split livers, in pa-tients with end-stage liver disease. *Transplantation* 1992; 53:387–391.

55. Heffron TG, et al: Biliary complications in pediatric liver transplantation. *Transplantation* 1992; 53:391–395.

56. Stevens LH, et al: Hepatic artery thrombosis in infants. *Transplantation* 1992; 53:396–399.

57. Bonsel GJ, et al: Assessment of the quality of life before and following liver transplantation. *Transplantation* 1992; 53:796–800.

CHAPTER 11

Hepatic and Biliary Tract Imaging

Joseph Yee, M.D.

Associate Professor of Radiology, New York University Medical Center, New York, New York

Brian Ginzburg, M.D.

Clinical Instructor of Radiology, University of California, Los Angeles Medical Center, Los Angeles, California

Nagesh Ragavendra, M.D.

Professor of Radiology, University of California, Los Angeles Medical Center, Los Angeles, California

The introduction of contrast agents has boosted magnetic resonance imaging (MRI) into a leadership role in the evaluation of focal liver diseases. Along with advances in MRI technology, the last few years have seen the emergence of a number of innovative interventional procedures designed for both the diagnosis and the treatment of biliary tract diseases. In the following pages, we review the most recent and salient advances in the field of liver and biliary tract imaging by MRI, computed tomography (CT), gray-scale and color Doppler ultrasound, and nuclear medicine techniques.

MALIGNANT DISEASE—HEPATOCELLULAR CARCINOMA

Ultrasonography is an effective imaging modality for screening patients who are at risk for hepatomas. This technique can provide information about the tumor's size, its growth pattern, and the invasion of adjacent vascular structures (e.g., the portal vein). In a view by Bolondi and colleagues,[1] hepatomas were found to have a variable sonographic appearance depending on the size of the tumor. They categorized the tumors by appearance into nodular, massive, and diffuse varieties. The echo pattern also changed as the tumor grew from the nodular variety to diffuse types. Color and duplex Doppler ultrasound gave further insights into the nature of vascular alterations within this tumor. The most common finding was portal vein invasion. An example of the value of ultrasound for depicting hepatoma and tumor thrombus in the portal vein is shown in Figure 1. A study by Imari and associates[2] revealed the usefulness of contrast-enhanced ultrasound. The authors infused carbon dioxide via the hepatic artery to demonstrate lesions that had not been visible by non–contrast-enhanced ultrasound. Among 22 patients with hepatomas, seven additional nodules were found with contrast-enhanced ultrasonography that were not evident on standard scans. The contrast enhancement lasted 15 to 60 minutes. In another study by Dalla Palma and Pozzi-Mucelli[3] using MRI, CT, and ultrasound, the usefulness of ultrasound in the evaluation of hepatocellular carcinoma, as well as its role in guiding percutaneous biopsy was stressed. The authors also concluded that CT and MRI have a supplementary role in the imaging of hepatomas. In a report by Shimamoto and coworkers,[4] intratumoral blood flow was assessed using color Doppler ultrasound and MRI in 15 patients with hepatomas. Doppler signals with shift frequencies ranging from 0.22 to 3.48/kHz were obtained from 14 of the patients. The resistive index became progressively lower as the vessels approached the tumor center, indicating greater neovascularity in the central portion of the tumor. It also was noted that tumors that were hyperintense on MRI with gradient-recalled acquisition in the steady state imaging transmitted Doppler signals of higher amplitude compared with isointense lesions.

Honda and colleagues[5] examined the ability of imaging modalities to visualize the capsule of the tumors. In a study involving 30 patients with histologically proven hepatomas, fibrous capsules were confirmed pathologically in 20 patients. The accuracy of the various techniques in detecting the fibrous capsule was 71% for ultrasound, 82% for CT, and 92% for MRI. Even greater accuracy was obtained when MRI was performed with gadolinium contrast enhancement. In a separate study by Lalonde and coworkers,[6] late-enhanced CT studies (more than 5 minutes after dynamic CT) compared favorably with MRI in demonstrating the fibrous capsule. Both groups of investigators also discussed the mosaic pattern of hepatomas, which is another characteristic feature of these tumors. Other distinctive MRI features included fatty degeneration, daughter nodules, and tumor venous thrombi, as reported by Singcharoen and associates.[7]

The MRI appearance of hepatomas is variable. Kadoya and colleagues[8] correlated MRI findings with histopathology in 72 nodular hepatomas using the

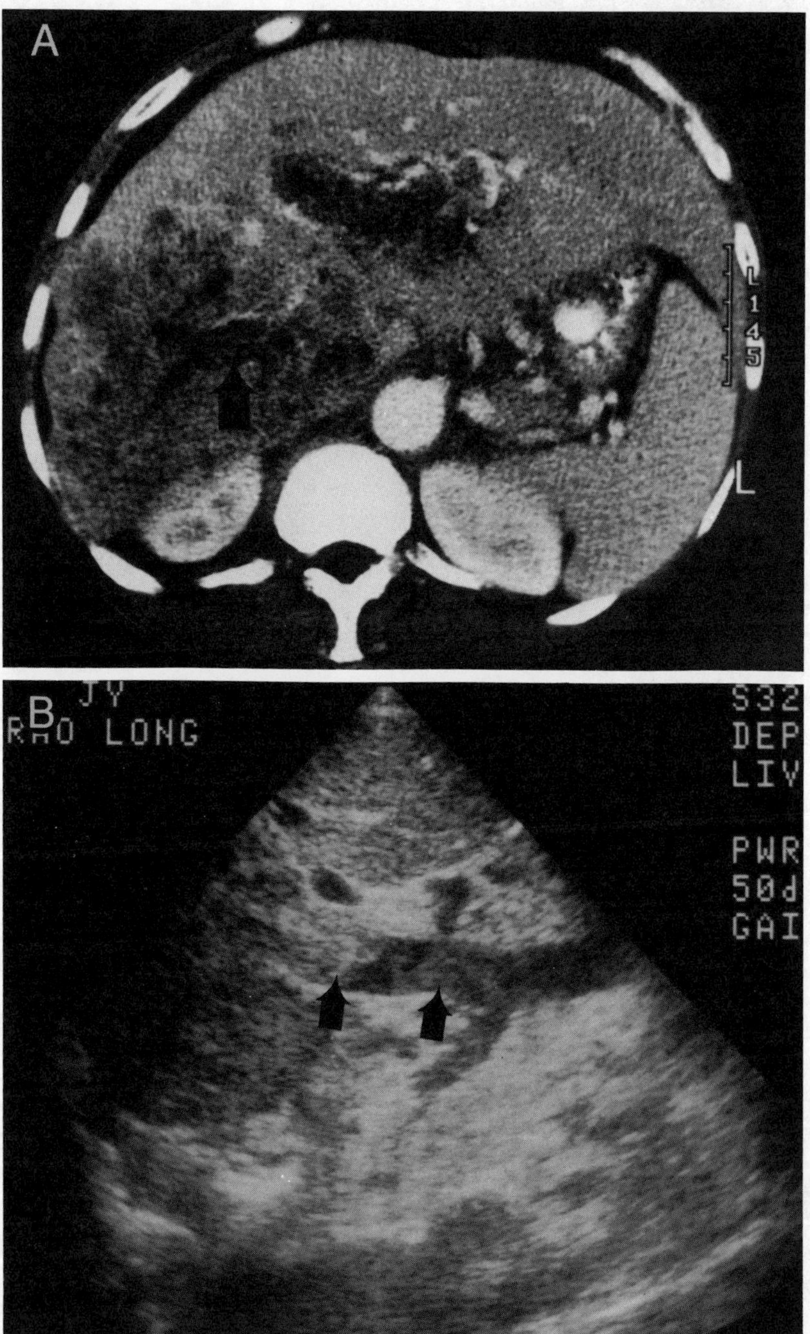

FIG 1.
A 59-year-old man with hepatocellular carcinoma and tumor thrombus in the portal vein. **A,** contrast-enhanced CT of the liver showing thrombus in the portal vein *(arrow)* and an extensive mass in the right and left lobes. **B,** longitudinal sonogram of the portal vein showing extensive thrombus *(arrows)*.

1.5-tesla magnet. Histologic grade I tumors were more likely to be hyperintense on T1-weighted images and isointense on T2-weighted images. Grade II and III lesions had variable intensities on T1-weighted images and most were hyperintense on T2-weighted images. Whenever focal hyperintensity was noted on T2-weighted images, dilated intratumoral sinusoids were identified histologically.

Contrast agents provide important information regarding the vascularity of hepatic masses studied by MRI. Using inversion recovery, fast, low angle shot MRI, hepatomas show total enhancement in the early phase and are isointense in the late phase. On the other hand, hemangiomas demonstrate peripheral and, rarely, total enhancement in the early phase. The majority of hemangiomas show high-intensity uptake in the late phase. In a study by Murakami and associates,[9] 90% of hepatomas and 82% of hemangiomas had these characteristic enhancement patterns. Similar results were reported by Abbas and colleagues[10] regarding the usefulness of dynamic MRI in differentiating hepatomas from hemangiomas. They emphasized the high signal intensities of hemangiomas on delayed spin echo scans.

MALIGNANT DISEASE—OTHER NEOPLASMS

The role of imaging studies in the detection of liver metastases has been the subject of several recent publications. Soyer and associates,[11] studied 28 patients with colorectal cancer metastatic to the liver. They compared intraoperative ultrasound with CT-portography in the detection of liver metastases. Although there were no statistically significant differences in the sensitivity of these two techniques, they concluded that the techniques were complementary. On CT-portography, the hepatic tumors are identified as perfusion defects because they receive most of their blood supply from the hepatic artery and not from the portal vein. A CT portogram is obtained by injecting iodinated contrast medium into the superior mesenteric artery, which in turn opacifies the portal vein.[13] Figure 2 illustrated the usefulness of CT-portography in depicting the morphology of a proven hepatocellular carcinoma.

The use of radioimmunoscintigraphy for the detection of metastatic disease to the liver using 99mTc-anti-carcinoembryonic antigen monoclonal antibodies has been described by Mux'l and coworkers[14] in a study of 64 patients. The specificity of the technique for liver metastases was 100%, but its sensitivity was only 50% and its accuracy 85%. Bock and colleagues[15] in their study of 17 patients with 43 metastatic lesions, noted a sensitivity and accuracy of 21% for all liver lesions. They concluded that the poor sensitivity of the radioimmunoscintigraphic technique for the detection of liver metastases was related to the poor tumor:background ratio caused by nonspecific uptake by the reticuloendothelial system of the liver.

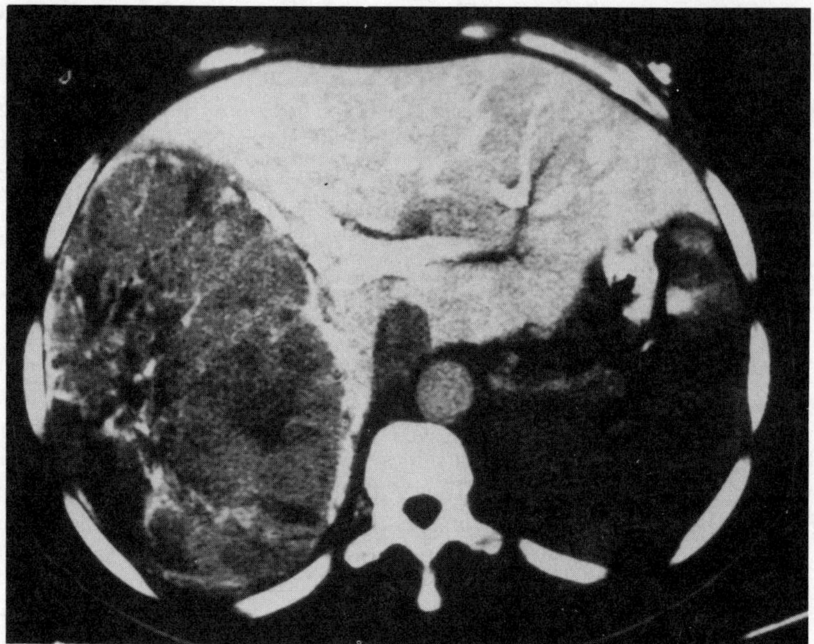

FIG 2.
A 34-year-old women with hepatocellular carcinoma demonstrated by CT arterial portography. Injection via the superior mesenteric artery shows good opacification of the hepatic parenchyma in contrast to the defect produced by the tumor in the right lobe of the liver. (Courtesy of Dr. Richard Gordon, Department of Radiology, Manhattan Veterans Hospital, New York, New York.)

Five patients with hepatic epithelioid hemangioendotheliomas have been characterized by MRI, as reported by Van Beers and associates.[16] Two of these lesions appeared as multiple nodules in a peripheral location; three tumors had macroscopic invasion of portal or hepatic veins. The internal architecture of the tumors was displayed best on T2-weighted images and correlated well with the histopathology.

The use of MRI in two unusual primary hepatic tumors, hepatic carcinoids[17] and malignant mesenchymal hepatic tumors,[18] has been reported in the recent literature. Both these primary tumors are hypointense on T1-weighted MRI sequences and hyperintense on T2-weighted imaging.

BENIGN DISEASE—DIFFUSE CHANGES

The detection of iron overload in the liver continues to be a challenging proposition for CT and MRI. In a study by Harada and colleagues,[19] ten patients with serum ferritin levels greater than 500 ng/mL underwent both MRI and CT. MRI showed decreased signal intensity in the liver when the ferritin level was more than 2,000 ng/mL and was normal in four of six patients at lower levels. CT demonstrated increased density of the liver parenchyma in five of seven patients with high ferritin levels. One patient with hepatic steatosis had normal CT findings with high serum ferritin levels. Liver biopsy, however, detected iron deposits in nine of ten patients and, therefore, was the most accurate technique for the detection of iron in the liver. In another study, Guyader and associates[20] showed decreased MRI signal intensity in the liver of patients with genetic hemochromatosis. Villari and coworkers[21] used MRI in 12 patients with transfusion-dependent thalassemia and found it to be useful in predicting iron overload. In a group of patients with cirrhosis, Murakami and colleagues[22] found MRI to be a more sensitive technique in depicting iron deposits in cirrhotic nodules than was CT.

Kreft and associates[23] studied fatty livers by MRI in rat models. Quantitative analysis of conventional and chemical shift images were correlated with the chemically determined fat content of the liver. Although both techniques showed good correlation between signal intensity and the degree of fatty infiltration, the authors concluded that only chemical shift imaging was reliable for the detection of fat in the liver.

MRI has been used in patients with hepatitis. Itoh and coworkers[24] noted periportal high signal intensity in 50% of patients (n = 32) with acute viral hepatitis on T2-weighted images when the serum glutamic-oxaloacetic transaminase (SGOT) levels were greater than 500 IU. The authors concluded that the degree of increase in MRI signal intensity is directly proportional to the severity of the illness. Yankelevitz and associates[25] noted MRI signal changes in patients with Hodgkin's disease and radiation hepatitis. Increased signal intensities on T2-weighted images were noted by 4 weeks after therapeutic irradiation and returned to normal by 8 weeks.

BENIGN DISEASE—FOCAL CHANGES

Blood pool single photon emission CT (SPECT) imaging is a very accurate technique for the detection of hemangiomas.[26] The sensitivity of this method, however, is dependent on the size of the hemangioma. A detection rate of 83% for lesions 2 to 3.5 cm in diameter falls to 51% for lesions 2 cm or less in diameter.

Focal nodular hyperplasia (FNH) was the subject of two recent publications on MRI. Haggar and Bree[27] reported ten cases of FNH in which the most common finding was isointensity of the lesion on all pulse sequences. In this small series of patients, a central scar, which was hyperintense on the T2-weighted sequence, was seen in only one patient. Based on this series and a review of the literature, FNH seems to have a variable appearance on MRI and no single characteristic MRI feature can be identified. Vilgrain and colleagues[28] came to a similar conclusion when they studied 37 patients with FNH and found the typical MRI findings to be present in only 43%; in the remainder, the findings were atypical.

Liver abscess and hydatid disease have been the subject of two recent papers. Barreda and coworkers[29] reviewed their experience with 100 patients with liver abscesses derived from two separate geographic locations (Mexico and Florida). They described characteristic imaging features of pyogenic, amebic, and fungal abscesses. This paper should be reviewed for further information. El-Tahir and associates[30] reported CT and ultrasound findings in 41 patients with hydatid disease. CT detected the lesions in all cases, whereas ultrasound was nondiagnostic in two cases because of heavy calcification of the wall and the presence of intracavitary air.

Last, there have been a number of unusual case reports of focal lesions of the liver. Hainaux and colleagues[31] reported the case of a 3½-year-old girl with Gaucher's disease and extensive hepatic necrosis who had involvement of the lungs and bone detected by plain radiography, MRI, CT, and ultrasound. Focal lesions were reported in two patients with sarcoidosis using multiple imaging modalities.[32] A macronodular tuberculoma was reported using CT and MRI.[33] A cyst of the falciform ligament was found to be the cause of an unusual case of right upper quadrant pain in a patient described by Bryan and Pillarisetty.[34] Castleman's disease (giant lymph node hyperplasia) presenting as a hypervascular mass in the porta hepatis mimicking hepatic tumor was described by Rahmouni and colleagues.[35]

NEW HORIZONS

Among recent innovations in imaging technology is the sonolaparoscope. With an increasing number of laparoscopic procedures being performed for both diagnosis and treatment, it would be advantageous to be able to evaluate the solid or cystic organs of the abdomen beyond simple visual inspection. A preliminary report from Fukuda and coworkers[36] described the use of a mechanical radial ultrasound scanner in conjunction with the surgical laparoscope. These researchers found the sonolaparoscope to be useful in the detection of occult liver cysts, tumors, and granulomas.

Less spectacular, but worthy of mention, is a study by Suzuki and associates[37] using radionuclide SPECT imaging with 99mTc macro aggregated albumin (MAA) for the evaluation of perfusion patterns of the liver during chemotherapy for metastases. Three-dimensional reconstruction of the perfusion patterns then was performed.

Recent technical advances also have enabled the nonsurgical creation of a portosystemic shunt using the transjugular approach and a balloon-expandable stent. This new procedure, called the transjugular intrahepatic porta caval shunt, is described by Zemel and colleagues and by Richter and associates.[38, 39]

New MRI contrast agents have been introduced recently to increase the specificity and sensitivity of MRI. Gadobenate dimeglumine (Gd-BOPTA) was developed as a paramagnetic contrast agent that has both biliary and renal properties.[40] Rofsky and Weinreb[41] reported the use of manganese-DPDP (N.N' Dipyridoxylethylenediamine-N,N'-diacetate 5, 5'-Bis phosphate) as a more specific hepatocellular agent with greater affinity for hepatomas. Figure 3 illustrates the superior definition of hepatomas that can be obtained using this currently investigative paramagnetic MRI contrast agent. Violante and coworkers[42] have introduced microparticles (nanoparticles) for diagnostic use with CT, ultrasound, and MRI.

INTERVENTIONAL SONOGRAPHY OF THE GALLBLADDER

vanSonnenberg and colleagues[43] and Ascher and coworkers[44] used a new catheter-based ultrasound technique to visualize the gallbladder and bile duct. vanSonnenberg's group introduced a miniature ultrasound transducer into the gallbladder percutaneously in 22 patients and via the laparoscope in 4 patients. This new technique facilitated the differentiation of intraluminal filling defects, the examination of areas inaccessible to conventional imaging, and observations about the walls of the ducts and gallbladder. Ascher and coworkers used this modality as an adjunct to laparoscopic cholecystectomy in 20 patients. In this technique, the ultrasound catheter is introduced alongside the laparoscope. The common hepatic duct and common duct were visualized in all patients. The integrity of the cystic duct and presence of any retained stones was assessed after cholecystectomy. In another, related study, Mosnier and associates[45] used conventional ultrasound intraoperatively before and after operative cholecystectomy. They concluded that sonography is a simple, efficient technique that provides good detection of biliary stones and observed that operative cholangiography is required only in instances in which the sonographic visualization of bile ducts is incomplete.

INTERVENTIONAL DIAGNOSTIC AND THERAPEUTIC PROCEDURES

Three areas have been particularly topical within the interventional arena: intraoperative procedures, endoscopic and endoluminal procedures, and percutaneous procedures, including biopsy techniques.

The use of intraoperative ultrasonography for the detection of primary and secondary hepatic tumors was examined in a prospective study of 82 operations.[46] This modality was shown to have had a major impact on the course of the operation, leading to a strategic change of procedure in 22% of cases. Intraoperative sonography supplied additional information over the preoperative workup, which included ultrasound, CT, and MRI, in 38% of cases. The particular clinical advan-

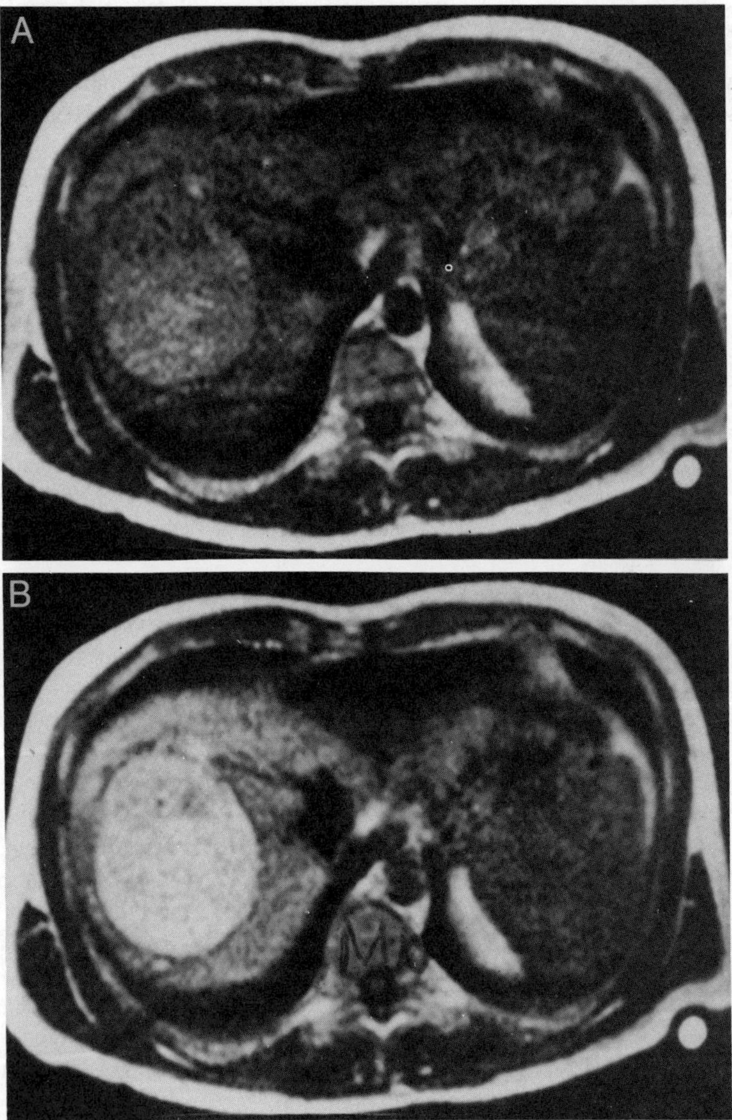

FIG 3.
A 41-year-old man with hepatocellular carcinoma in the right lobe of the liver on T1-weighted spin-echo MRI. **A,** before contrast enhancement. **B,** after contrast (Mn II DPDP) enhancement. (From Rofsky N, Weinreb J: *Magn Reson Q* 1992; 8:156–168. Used by permission.)

tages of intraoperative ultrasound are an increased tumor detection rate, better discrimination between solid and cystic lesions, and identification of the tumor location with respect to the vascular anatomy. It also has the financial advantage of being more cost-effective than is an extensive preoperative workup.

A multicenter prospective study showed that the use of ultrasonic surgical dissectors reduced the amount of blood loss incurred during surgical resection of benign and malignant hepatic lesions.[47] The ultrasonic surgical dissectors did not decrease the length of the operation, but did decrease the amount of blood loss by facilitating access to intrahepatic and extrahepatic arterial and venous tributaries, particular the hepatic veins. Overall, the technique was considered helpful or very helpful in 75% of the resections, with the greatest benefit occurring in the resection of hydatid cysts.

Another study of the use of intraoperative ultrasound demonstrated its accuracy and usefulness in diagnosing the extent of spread of gastric carcinoma with respect to stomach wall invasion, para-aortic lymph node metastases, and hepatic metastases.[48] The accuracy rates were 81% for depth of stomach wall invasion and 93% for para-aortic lymphadenopathy, and were significantly better than those of preoperative studies. In 10% of operations (3 of 30), operative sonography identified hepatic metastases that were not recognized during preoperative investigation.

Several recent studies have concentrated on endoscopic and endoluminal ultrasonography. Two of these studies have examined the use of intraductal sonography to visualize the pancreatic and biliary ducts. Very–high-frequency (30-MHz) transducers produce high-resolution cross-sectional images of the main pancreatic duct and the bile duct. One study attempted to establish baseline normal criteria for the anatomy of these ducts by in vitro scanning of 15 patients at the time of autopsy.[49] The images revealed three distinct layers with a fine reticular pattern in the pancreas. In attempting to determine the clinical usefulness of this procedure, the authors scanned four live patients in vivo and were able to insert the transducer into the major papilla without sphincterotomy being necessary. The other study used intraductal radial sonography to investigate 11 cases of bile duct carcinoma and 5 cases of pancreatic carcinoma.[50] Two approaches were used: percutaneous insertion via a transhepatic biliary fistula established for cholangioscopy and transpapillary insertion via the duodenoscope. The common bile duct wall, pancreatic head, adjacent major blood vessels, and extent of carcinomatous involvement could be demonstrated clearly, raising the hopes that this method will become routine or staging of biliopancreatic malignancy.

Endoluminal ultrasound also can facilitate the treatment of extrahepatic bile duct tumors. Intraluminal brachytherapy with tritium-192 can be used for biliary neoplasms. The treatment is administered through a biliary duct drainage tube. The endoluminal ultrasound transducer is small enough to be inserted into the biliary drainage tube and thereby provide accurate tumor volume determinations to assess response to treatment. A case of recurrent islet cell carcinoma treated and assessed in this way has been used to illustrate this concept.[51]

Endoscopic ultrasound also has the ability to display much of the portal venous system, including the splenic, mesenteric, and portal veins, as well as the azygos vein. In a study of 40 patients with portal hypertension and 48 control patients, esophageal and gastric varices, periesophageal and perigastric collateral veins, and submucosal gastric venules were seen only in the patients with portal hypertension.[52] Endoscopic ultrasound was inferior to endoscopy for the detection and grading of esophageal varices, but superior for the detection of gastric fundal varices. In fact, endoscopic ultrasound, with an overall sensitivity of only 50%, is not a reliable method for studying esophageal varices and does not permit flow measurements or assessment of bleeding risk. On the other hand, endoscopic sonography can detect portal hypertensive gastropathy, distinguishing it from inflammatory gastritis, thereby influencing therapeutic decisions.

The range of topical percutaneous procedures varies from diagnostic fine-needle aspirations to new techniques in performing core biopsies to therapeutic interventions in the treatment of hepatocellular carcinoma and portal hypertension. A review of 142 ultrasound-guided, fine-needle (22-gauge) aspirations of suspected malignant hepatic lesions found that the overall diagnostic accuracy was 89.4%.[53] The technique failed to demonstrate malignancy in 13.1% of malignant tumors (13 patients). All the benign lesions were shown correctly to be benign by fine-needle aspiration. The sensitivity, specificity, and positive and negative predictive values were 86.5%, 100%, 100%, and 76.9% respectively. Fatal complications are rare, but there was one death related to the procedure in a patient with incipient chronic disseminated intravascular coagulation who sustained an intraperitoneal hemorrhage.

A comparative randomized study of two biopsy techniques in 200 cases of chronic liver disease was performed.[54] A large-bore, ultrasound-guided liver biopsy technique using a cutting needle via an anterior subcostal route proved to be able to provide better diagnostic samples with fewer complications than could the conventional intercostal Menghini technique of core liver biopsy. Adding a second pass to this anterior subcostal technique increased the diagnostic specificity, as demonstrated by three cases in which the diagnoses were changed from chronic active hepatitis to active cirrhosis by the second-pass biopsy.

Another study of 203 hepatic biopsies in diffusing liver disease used a spring-propelled 18-gauge cutting needle and ultrasound guidance.[55] The biopsy specimen was adequate for histologic diagnosis in 97% of cases (197 biopsies). Only four complications requiring treatment occurred. These included one vasovagal reaction and three bleeding episodes. Significant bleeding occurred only in patients with preexisting coagulopathy. There was no difference in efficacy between biopsies of native or transplanted livers and no difference between biopsies of the right and left lobes, except for more frequent pain with right-lobe biopsies. The described technique was shown to be safe and efficacious in the diagnosis of diffuse liver disease.

Transjugular biopsy of the liver is an accepted technique in patients with coagulation disorders. An alternative procedure in these higher-risk patients is ultrasound-guided percutaneous liver biopsy with plugging of the needle track. Seventy-eight percutaneous biopsies were performed in 72 patients with abnormal coagulation status of varying severity.[56] Embolization of the biopsy track was accomplished with gelatin particles and thrombin. Only two serious bleeding complications occurred, and these were in patients with severe coagulation disorders. This technique is a feasible alternative to transjugular liver biopsy.

Percutaneous ethanol injection of hepatocellular carcinoma under ultrasound guidance is a new therapeutic technique used in cirrhotic patients with small hepatomas. In one study, no serious complications occurred in 70 patients as a consequence of this procedure.[57] The 1-, 2-, and 3-year survival rates were 94%, 84%, and 72%, respectively, for solitary tumors smaller than 5 cm. Multiple lesions treated similarly had 94%, 84%, and 25% survival rates over 1, 2, and 3 years, respectively. The authors believe that percutaneous ethanol injection of single lesions smaller than 5 cm may be indicated if there is a contraindication to surgical resection.

The percutaneous placement of intrahepatic portosystemic shunts between the portal and hepatic veins is becoming a more frequently used method of decompressing the portal venous system in portal hypertension. The actual placement procedure requires access to the portal system via a transjugular approach. Color Doppler is a highly effective means of graphically demonstrating the portal veins and thereby directing the transhepatic portal puncture. This was shown to facilitate a quick and safe puncture under real-time monitoring in a study of four patients.[58]

VASCULAR ABNORMALITIES AND DOPPLER IMAGING

The liver is an organ particularly well suited to investigation by duplex and color Doppler imaging. These modalities can be applied to studying the unique dual blood supply of the liver by the hepatic artery and the portal vein, and the drainage by the hepatic veins and the inferior vena cava. The hemodynamics of these vessels are intricate both in the normal state and in the many diseases that alter the flow patterns in complex ways. Duplex and color Doppler imaging can distinguish readily portal from systemic vessels and can provide rapid assessment of low direction and velocity in each vessel. Collateral vessels are appreciated easily with color imaging.

Color Doppler is a valuable modality in the initial diagnosis of Budd-Chiari syndrome. To assess this technique, five patients were studied with the following hemodynamic findings: absent hepatic venous flow (one patient), reversal of hepatic venous flow (two patients), and narrowing of the hepatic veins (three patients).[59] Collateral vessels, which were undetectable by other imaging modalities, were seen with color Doppler. These collaterals included hepatic vein to hepatic vein (four patients), hepatic veins to subcapsular systemic veins (two patients), and portosystemic collaterals (three patients). Color Doppler imaging also improved the identification of structural anatomic changes such as irregularity or compression of the hepatic veins in three patients. Spectral Doppler of the hepatic veins produced flat, aphasic waveforms indicative of distal hepatic venous compression.

MRI also can be used in the investigation of Budd-Chiari syndrome. MRI was performed on nine patients with membranous obstruction of the inferior vena cava.[60] The morphologic findings were a curvilinear soft-tissue membrane (five cases) or an obliterated lumen of a hepatic segment of the inferior vena cava (four cases). Inferior to the obstruction, MRI demonstrated a flow-related signal in seven cases, an intraluminal thrombus in one case, and thrombotic occlusion in one case. MRI showed narrowing and disorientation of the hepatic veins with loss of their usual connection to the inferior vena cava. MRI also was able to demonstrate the ancillary findings of hepatosplenomegaly, caudate lobe enlargement, cirrhosis, hepatoma, and collaterals.

Duplex sonography can be used in many ways in the evaluation of cirrhosis and portal hypertension. One hundred and eighteen patients with proven portal hypertension were studied with duplex sonography to find a sensitive sonographic sign of portal hypertension.[61] A patent paraumbilical vein was present in 85.6% of patients overall and in 82.5% of patients with varices, indicating a relatively high sensitivity. Varices were found in 73.3% of patients overall and in 100% of patients with a patent paraumbilical vein combined with ascites. Other parameters, such as an enlarged portal venous caliber, thrombosed portal vein, reversed portal venous flow, abnormal portal velocities, and splenomegaly, were shown to have very low sensitivity in the diagnosis of portal hypertension. The authors concluded that a patent paraumbilical vein is a practical, useful, and sensitive ultrasound sign of portal hypertension.

Doppler flowmetry can be used to monitor acute changes in flow in portal hypertension. A study showed that, in cirrhotic patients, the portal venous velocity increased significantly after a standardized meal and decreased significantly after the administration of propranolol.[62] The cross-sectional area of the portal vein did not change significantly with either of these interventions. Therefore, the use of blood velocity alone is suggested to monitor acute changes in flow in patients with portal hypertension.

Another study showed that portal venous flow velocity, as measured by duplex sonography, is of use in differentiating compensated cirrhosis (i.e., no ascites, encephalopathy, jaundice, or hematemesis) from other chronic compensated liver diseases.[63] Patients with biopsy-proven, noncirrhotic chronic liver disease (e.g., steatosis, chronic hepatitis) had maximum portal venous flow velocities similar to those of normal individuals. Cirrhotic (biopsy-proven) patients had significantly lower maximum portal velocities. Therefore, a low maximum portal flow velocity is a reliable indication of liver cirrhosis as opposed to other forms of chronic liver disease.

Color Doppler imaging can detect intrahepatic aneurysms, which may appear merely as cysts on gray-scale ultrasonography. Thirteen cases of cystic liver lesions that were suspected to communicate with vessels on ordinary sonography were examined by color Doppler.[64] Blood flow was detected in 5 of these and the communication to a vessel was confirmed. Color imaging also was able to define the hemodynamics of these lesions. Two of the lesions were shown to be aneurysmal portahepatic venous fistulas, two others were portal venous aneurysms, and one was a hepatic venous aneurysm.

BILIARY TRACT IMAGING

In these days of expanding options in imaging, it is important to know which diagnostic tests are suited best to the clinical problem. A prospective comparison was performed between endoscopic retrograde cholangiopancreatography (ERCP), CT, and fat-suppression MRI in the evaluation of bile duct disease.[65] Eleven patients with malignant disease and 17 patients with benign disease were studied by all three modalities and the results were interpreted blindly. ERCP allowed the correct diagnosis of all the malignant cases by revealing the presence of a narrowed bile duct with irregular margins. CT and MRI enabled the detection of all the malignant cases, but allowed the characterization of only 9 as definitely malignant, as demonstrated by wall thickening greater than 5 mm or enhancing periportal tissue on MRI. Benign disease was diagnosed correctly using ERCP in 16 cases, as shown by smooth, tapered ductal narrowing. CT and MRI allowed the correct diagnosis of only 13 cases as benign, as revealed by mild to moderate intrahepatic biliary dilatation and wall thickness of less than 5 mm. Overall, ERCP allowed the correct characterization of 27 cases as benign or malignant, whereas CT and MRI both allowed the correct characterization of 22 cases. Therefore, ERCP was thought to be superior to CT and MRI in characterizing bile duct disease.

The search for more noninvasive methods of investigation will continue and research into different MRI sequencing techniques appears promising. Three-dimensional MRI has been evaluated as an alternative to cholangiography in 12 patients with malignancy-related obstructive jaundice.[66] Dilatation and obstruction of the bile ducts was well documented in all cases. There was good correlation with percutaneous transhepatic biliary drainage performed some time after the MRI.

One of the potential problems of MRI is the presence of metallic objects within the body. The concerns are twofold: (1) the metal may move in response to the strong magnetic field, causing tissue damage, and (2) the metal may cause image artifact, degrading the diagnostic quality of the scan. These concerns were evaluated in vitro and in eight patients with the most commonly used metallic biliary prosthesis (the Wallstent endoprosthesis).[67] In vitro, the stent produced no tip deflection at 0.6- or 1.5-tesla magnetic field strengths. Trace magnetic susceptibility artifact, similar to that from an air column, paralleled the stent. In patients, there was only minimal image degradation with conventional pulse sequences. Middle field strength spin-echo images produced minimal artifacts indistinguishable from those seen with pneumobilia.

The combination of noninvasive imaging, percutaneous transhepatic cholangiography (PTC), and percutaneous biliary drainage (PBD) was examined in the context of the respective roles of the individual techniques in the diagnosis and treatment of choledochal cysts.[68] Thirteen patients with choledochal cysts were investigated: 6 had CT scans, 2 had sonograms; PTC was performed in all 13 patients and 16 PBD procedures were performed. PTC was the important diagnostic imaging modality because of its superior ability to define the anatomy of the cysts, to show the site of origin from the bile ducts, and to delineate associated biliary abnormalities such as strictures and calculi. PBD was valuable in preoperative intervention, as an aid to surgical reconstruction, and in postoperative care.

Nuclear medicine imaging is a relatively noninvasive method of assessing the biliary tract. Twenty-two patients infected with the human immunodeficiency virus (HIV) who had right upper quadrant pain, and in whom sclerosing cholangitis related to the acquired immunodeficiency syndrome was suspected, were studied with biliary scintigraphy.[69] Fourteen abnormal scan results were obtained and ascending cholangitis was confirmed in 10 of these patients by liver biopsy, ERCP, or postmortem examination. One patient with mild ascending cholangitis on ERCP had normal results on scintigraphic scanning. Biliary scintigraphy appears to be a useful noninvasive screening test in HIV-positive patients with right upper quadrant pain and may help in the selection of those patients who should proceed to the more invasive ERCP.

In summary, technical advances and improvements in contrast agents have led the way in the design and implementation of a wide variety of new diagnostic methods and treatment options for biliary tract diseases that were nonexistent only a few years ago. The major emphasis of many of the papers reviewed for this chapter was on interventional procedures, and this trend is likely to continue.

REFERENCES

1. Bolondi L, et al: Ultrasonography and guided biopsy in the diagnosis of hepatocellular carcinoma. *Ital J Gastroenterol* 1992; 24:46–49.

2. Imari Y, et al: Hepatocellular carcinoma not detected with plain US: Treatment with percutaneous ethanol injection under guidance with enhanced US. *Radiology* 1992; 185:497–500.

3. Dalla Palma L, et al: Computed tomography and magnetic resonance imaging in diagnosing hepatocellular carcinoma. *Ital J Gastroenterol* 1992; 24:87–91.

4. Shimamoto K, et al: Hepatocellular carcinoma: Evaluation with color Doppler US and MR imaging. *Radiology* 1992; 182:149–153.

5. Honda H, et al: Characteristic findings of hepatocellular carcinoma: An evaluation with comparative study of US, CT, and MRI. *Gastrointest Radiol* 1992; 17:245–249.

6. Lalonde L, et al: Capsule and mosaic pattern of hepatocellular carcinoma: Correlation between CT and MR imaging. *Gastrointest Radiol* 1992; 17:241–244.

7. Singcharoen T, et al: Hepatocellular carcinoma: MR imaging. *Australas Radiol* 1992; 36:34–36.

8. Kadoya M, et al: Hepatocellular carcinoma: Correlation of MR imaging and histopathologic findings. *Radiology* 1992; 183:819–825.

9. Murakami T, et al: Differentiation between hepatoma and hemangioma with inversion recovery snap-shot FLASH MRI and Gd-DTPA. *J Comput Assist Tomogr* 1992; 16:198–205.

10. Abbas Y, et al: Differential diagnosis of hepatic neoplasms: Spin echo versus Gd-DTPA-enhanced gradient echo imaging. *Magn Reson Q* 1991; 7:275–292.

11. Soyer P, et al: Preoperative assessment of resectability of hepatic metastases from colonic carcinoma: CT portography vs. sonography and dynamic CT. *AJR Am J Roentgenol* 1992; 159:741–744.

12. Soyer P, et al: Detection of liver metastases from colorectal cancer: Comparison of intraoperative US and CT during arterial portography. *Radiology* 1992; 183:541–544.

13. Peterson M, et al: Hepatic parenchymal perfusion defects detected with CTAP: Imaging-pathologic correlation. *Radiology* 1992; 185:149–155.

14. Mux'l A, et al: Radioimmunoscintigraphy of colorectal carcinoma with a 99mTc-labeled anti-CEA monoclonal antibody. *Nucl Med Commun* 1992; 13:261–270.

15. Bock E, et al: Diagnostic accuracy of 99mTc anti-CEA immunoscintigraphy in patients with liver metastases from colorectal carcinoma. *Nuklearmedizin* 1992; 31:80–83.

16. Van Beers B, et al: Epitheliod hemangioendothelioma of the liver: MR and CT findings. *J Comput Assist Tomogr* 1992; 16:420–424.

17. Takayasu K, et al: Findings in primary hepatic carcinoid tumor: US, CT, MRI, and angiography. *J Comput Assist Tomogr* 1992; 16:99–102.

18. Ohtomo K, et al: MR imaging of malignant mesenchymal tumors of the liver. *Gastrointest Radiol* 1992; 17:58–62.

19. Harada M, et al: Comparative study of magnetic resonance imaging, computed tomography and histology in the assessment of liver iron overload. *Intern Med* 1992; 31:180–184.

20. Guyader D, et al: Magnetic resonance imaging and assessment of liver iron content in genetic hemochromatosis. *J Hepatol* 1992; 15:304–308.

21. Villari N, et al: Assessment of liver iron overload in thalassemic patients by MR imaging. *Acta Radiol* 1992; 33:347–350.

22. Murakami T, et al: CT and MRI of siderotic regenerating nodules in hepatic cirrhosis. *J Comput Assist Tomogr* 1992; 16:578–582.

23. Kreft B, et al: Diagnosis of fatty liver with MR imaging. *J Magn Reson Imaging* 1992; 2:463–471.

24. Itoh H, et al: Periportal high intensity on T2-weighted MR images in acute viral hepatitis. *J Comput Assist Tomogr* 1992; 16:564–567.

25. Yankelevitz D, et al: MR appearance of radiation hepatitis. *Clin Imaging* 1992; 16:89–92.

26. Bonanno N, et al: Diagnosis of hepatic hemangiomas with 99mTc-labeled red blood cell scanning: Value of SPECT. *J Nucl Biol Med* 1991; 35:135–140.

27. Haggar A, et al: Hepatic focal nodular hyperplasia: MR imaging at 1.0 and 1.5 T. *J Magn Reson Imaging* 1992; 2:85–88.

28. Vilgrain V, et al: Focal nodular hyperplasia of the liver: MR imaging and pathologic correlation in 37 patients. *Radiology* 1992; 184:699–703.

29. Barreda R, et al: Diagnostic imaging of liver abscess. *Crit Rev Diagn Imaging* 1992; 33:29–58.

30. El-Tahir M, et al: Hydatid disease of the liver. *Br J Radiol* 1992; 65:390–392.

31. Hainaux B, et al: Gaucher's disease. Plain radiography, US, CT and MR diagnosis of lungs, bone and liver lesions. *Pediatr Radiol* 1992; 22:78–79.

32. Panasci D, et al: Sarcoidosis of the liver: Evaluation with multiple imaging modalities. *Comput Med Imaging Graph* 1992; 16:55–58.

33. Kawamori Y, et al: Macronodular tuberculoma of the liver: CT and MR findings. *AJR Am J Roentgenol* 1992; 158:311–313.

34. Bryan D, et al: Cyst of the falciform ligament of the liver: A rare cause of right upper quadrant pain. *Am Surg* 1992; 58:779–781.

35. Rahmouni A, et al: Castleman disease mimicking liver tumor: CT and MR features. *J Comput Assist Tomogr* 1992; 16:699–703.

36. Fukuda M, et al: Preliminary evaluation of sonolaparoscopy in the diagnosis of liver diseases. *Endoscopy* 1992; 24:701–708.

37. Suzuki Y, et al: Application of single photon emission computed tomography (SPECT) with 99mTc-MAA in evaluation of perfusion patterns during hepatic infusion chemotherapy. *Ann Nucl Med* 1991; 5:123–126.

38. Zemel G, et al: Technical advances in transjugular intrahepatic portosystemic shunts. *Radiographics* 1992; 12:615–622.

39. Richter M, et al: Transjugular intrahepatic portacaval stent shunt: Preliminary clinical results. *Radiology* 1990; 174:1027–1030.

40. Vogl T, et al: Gadobenate dimeglumine—a new contrast agent for MR imaging: Preliminary evaluation in healthy volunteers. *AJR Am J Roentgenol* 1992; 158:887–892.

41. Rofsky N, et al: Manganese (II) N,N'-dipyridoxylethylene-diamine-N,N'-diacetate 5,5'-bis (phosphate): Clinical experience with a new contrast agent. *Magn Reson Q* 1992; 8:156–168.

42. Violante M: Potential of microparticles for diagnostic tracer imaging. *Acta Radiol Suppl* 1990; 374:153–156.

43. vanSonnenberg E, et al: Percutaneous intraluminal US in the gallbladder and bile ducts. *Radiology* 1992; 182:693–696.

44. Ascher SM, et al: Intraoperative bile duct sonography during laparoscopic cholecystectomy: Experience with a 12.5 MHz catheter-based US probe. *Radiology* 1992; 185:493–496.

45. Mosnier H, et al: Intraoperative sonography during cholecystectomy for gallstones. *Surg Gynecol Obstet* 1992; 174:469–473.

46. Boutkan H, et al: The impact of intraoperative ultrasonography of the liver on the surgical strategy of patients with gastrointestinal malignancies and hepatic metastases. *Eur J Surg Oncol* 1992; 18:342–346.

47. Millat B, et al: Prospective evaluation of ultrasonic surgical dissectors in hepatic resection: A cooperative multicenter study. *HPB Surg* 1992; 5:135–144.

48. Kodama I, et al: The value of operative ultrasonography in diagnosing tumor extension of carcinoma of the stomach. *Surg Gynecol Obstet* 1992; 174:479–484.

49. Furukawa T, et al: New technique using intraductal ultrasonography for the diagnosis of diseases of the pancreatobiliary system. *J Ultrasound Med* 1992; 11:607–612.

50. Yasuda K, et al: Clinical application of ultrasonic probes in the biliary and pancreatic duct. *Endoscopy* 1992; 24:370–375.

51. Minsky B, et al: Ultrasound directed extrahepatic bile duct intraluminal brachytherapy. *Int J Radiat Oncol Biol Phys* 1992; 23:165–167.

52. Caletti GC, et al: Value of endoscopic ultrasonography in the management of portal hypertension. *Endoscopy* 1992; 24:342–346.

53. Edoute Y, et al: Ultrasonically guided fine-needle aspiration of liver lesions. *Am J Gastroenterol* 1992; 87:1138–1141.

54. Papini E, et al: A randomized trial of ultrasound-guided liver biopsy versus the conventional Menghini technique. *Hepatology* 1991; 13:291–297.

55. Sheets PW, et al: Safety and efficacy of a spring-propelled 18-gauge needle for ultrasound-guided liver biopsy. *J Vasc Interv Radiol* 1991; 2:147–149.

56. Zins M, et al: Ultrasound-guided percutaneous liver biopsy with plugging of the needle track: A prospective study in 72 high-risk patients. *Radiology* 1992; 184:841–843.

57. Livraghi T: Percutaneous ethanol injection of hepatocellular carcinoma: Survival after 3 years in 70 patients. *Ital J Gastroenterol* 1992; 24:72–74.

58. Longo JM, et al: Color Doppler-ultrasound guidance in transjugular placement of intrahepatic portosystemic shunts. *Radiology* 1992; 184:281–284.

59. Ralls PW, et al: Budd-Chiari syndrome: Detection with color Doppler sonography. *AJR Am J Roentgenol* 1992; 159:113–116.

60. Park JH, et al: Membranous obstruction of the inferior vena cava with Budd-Chiari syndrome: MR imaging findings. *J Vasc Interv Radiol* 1991; 2:463–469.

61. Ditchfield MR, et al: Duplex Doppler ultrasound signs of portal hypertension: Relative diagnostic value of examination of paraumbilical vein, portal vein and spleen. *Australas Radiol* 1992; 36:102–105.

62. Sabb'a C, et al: Echo-Doppler evaluation of acute flow changes in portal hypertensive patients: Flow velocity as a reliable parameter. *J Hepatol* 1992; 15:356–360.

63. Cioni G, et al: Duplex-Doppler assessment of cirrhosis in patients with chronic compensated liver disease. *J Gastroenterol Hepatol* 1992; 7:382–384.

64. Tanaka S, et al: Intrahepatic venous and portal venous aneurysms examined by color Doppler flow imaging. *J Clin Ultrasound* 1992; 20:89–98.

65. Semelka RC, et al: Bile duct disease: Prospective comparison of ERCP, CT and fat suppression MRI. *Radiographics* 1992; 12:269–279.

66. Morimoto K, et al: Biliary obstruction: Evaluation with three-dimensional MR cholangiography. *Radiology* 1992; 183:578–580.

67. Girard MJ, et al: Wallstent metallic biliary endoprosthesis: MR imaging characteristics. *Radiology* 1992; 184:874–876.

68. Savader SJ, et al: Choledochal cysts: Role of noninvasive imaging, percutaneous transhepatic cholangiography and percutaneous biliary drainage in diagnosis and treatment. *J Vasc Interv Radiol* 1991; 2:379–385.

69. Buscombe JR, Miller RF, Ell PJ: Hepatobiliary scintigraphy in the diagnosis of AIDS-related sclerosing cholangitis. *Nucl Med Commun* 1992; 13:154–160.

CHAPTER 12

Review of the Japanese Literature

Kunio Okuda, M.D., Ph.D.

Emeritus Professor, Department of Medicine, Chiba University School of Medicine, Chiba, Japan

Mikio Nishioka, M.D.

Professor of Medicine, Kagawa Medical College; Chief of Gastroenterology Service, Third Department of Medicine, Kagawa Medical College Hospital, Mikimachi, Kagawa-ken, Japan

This chapter summarizes the reports that appeared during the past year mainly in *Acta Hepatologica Japonica* and the *Japanese Journal of Gastroenterology*. During this period most reports were concerned with hepatitis C virus (HCV) and HCV-associated liver diseases, thus indicating where the greatest interest currently lies in Japan. For reasons that are unclear, it now seems that Japan ranks first in the world in the endemicity of HCV-associated chronic liver disease. There is a large difference between the United States and Japan in the incidence of HCV-associated hepatocellular carcinoma (HCC). About 30% of chronic hepatitis C progresses to cirrhosis in 10 years and 15% to HCC.[1] One recent multicenter study in the United States demonstrated no difference in long-term mortality between those in whom non-A, non-B hepatitis developed and those in whom it did not after blood transfusion.[2] The difference in the prognosis of non-A, non-B hepatitis between the two countries is striking; in Japan many contract HCC after a long time lapse from posttransfusion non-A, non-B hepatitis,[3] and the yearly incidence of HCC among patients with cirrhosis is 6% to 10% per year.[4] There has been some shift in interest in the study of HCC; there were more papers dealing with treatment in the recent past whereas in the time period this review covers there were fewer such papers and more histopathologic investigations on preneoplastic lesions and early HCC in cirrhotic livers. Japan now leads the world in the study of early HCC appearing in posthepatitic cirrhotic livers in man, but it is not clear whether the same histologic sequence in the evolution of HCC occurs in the liver in Western countries. Recent studies in the United States on cirrhotic livers harvested for transplantation seem to confirm some of the Japanese experience with slight differences,[5] and it is interesting to see how many of the observations made in Japan concerning this particular problem will be confirmed or disproved by similar studies in Western countries.

METABOLISM AND BIOCHEMISTRY

In 1984, Nakamura and associates[6] partially purified and characterized hepatocyte growth factor (HGF) from the sera of 70% hepatectomized rats by using primary liver cell cultures and succeeded in purification and determination of the chemical structure of rat HGF derived from platelets.[7, 8] Their HGF is now widely accepted as the major growth-stimulating factor for the liver. Shortly thereafter, Gohda et al.[9, 10] independently isolated and purified a similar HGF from the sera of patients with fulminant hepatic failure. Andoh et al.[11] used Nakamura's assay system to partially purify and characterize a hepatotrophic factor from the plasma of rats treated with carbon tetrachloride. It was unstable to heat and acid treatment, as is HGF, and behaved much the same as HGF on chromatography. It showed synergistic effects with insulin and epidermal growth factor (EGF) on primary cultured hepatocytes. Thus it was suggested that the HGF plays an important role in the liver cell regeneration that follows liver damage. The same group has already shown that HGF is elaborated by mesenchymal cells, not hepatocytes, in the liver and other organs.[12]

Hepatic triglyceride lipase (HTGL) is an isoenzyme of lipoprotein lipase (LPL) synthesized only by the liver, and plasma levels may reflect liver function or reserve. Determination of these enzymes in serum was difficult because they were not readily separable. In 1989, Ikeda et al. succeeded in purification of LPL and HTGL from human plasma[13] and developed monoclonal antibodies that were then made into enzyme immunoassay (EIA)-sandwich assays.[14] Fujiwara et al.[15] used these assay systems to measure the two enzymes in postheparin plasma from patients with chronic liver disease. They found that the levels of HTGL were 124 ± 120 ng/mL in cirrhosis, 316 ± 193 ng/mL in chronic active hepatitis, 587 ± 432 ng/mL in chronic persistent hepatitis, and 612 ± 354 ng/mL in controls. Hepatic triglyceride lipase levels were also correlated with the results of other liver tests such as the hepaplastin test, albumin, total cholesterol, the cholesterol-ester ratio, and pseudocholine esterase activities. By contrast, no difference in LPL was shown among the four groups of patients and control subjects.

The proposal put forward by Fisher et al.[16] that branched-chain amino acids (BCAAs) are useful in correcting disturbances in the metabolism of amino acids and albumin in patients with cirrhosis and hepatic encephalopathy has not been substantiated in Western countries. By contrast, most Japanese hepatologists favor his recipe.[17, 18] In fact, several preparations of BCAA-enriched amino acid solutions have been commercialized for quite some time in Japan, and more recently an oral preparation was made commercially available. However, little is known about the metabolic effects induced by BCAAs. Kato et al.[19] gave a BCAA-enriched nutrient mixture (17.7 g of BCAAs per day) to five cirrhotic patients with hypoalbuminemia for 8 weeks and studied the metabolic changes induced. The plasma BCAA (valine) level and BCAA/aromatic amino acid molar ratio were significantly elevated. The biological half-life of albumin was significantly shortened, whereas degradation and synthesis rates increased and showed recovery toward the control range. No significant change occurred in body weight, plasma volume, plasma albumin concentration, the intravascular albumin pool, and the total albumin pool. However, there was a shift of albumin from the extravascular to the intravascular pool. They concluded that administration of a BCAA-enriched nutrient mixture is useful in patients with cirrhosis.

Indian childhood cirrhosis, a peculiar malady of unknown etiology, occurs in certain areas of India. Some investigators suspect excess copper intake as a likely cause[20] because sporadic observations of similar cases associated with excess copper intake have been made outside India.[21, 22] Sato et al.[23] studied the relationship between nutrition and copper metabolism from the embryonic stage to 8 weeks postpartum by feeding excess copper in solutions to two groups of rats, one given a normal diet and one given a low-protein diet. Copper content in the liver was determined chemically as well as histologically by atomic absorption flame photometry and copper staining. It was found that in the rats given the normal diet no copper deposition occurred in the liver whereas in the low-protein diet group marked copper deposition was seen in the centrilobular region. Thus this study failed to produce copper deposition in the periportal area as seen in Indian childhood cirrhosis, Wilson's disease, and primary biliary cirrhosis. It was postulated that because hepatocytes are unable to secrete copper into bile during malnutrition, copper accumulates in the centrilobular zone.

Thrombomodulin (TM) is a 105-kd glycoprotein specifically present in the plasma membrane of endothelial cells and has a strong affinity to thrombin. It was first isolated by Esmon and Owen in 1981[24] and subsequently characterized.[25] This protein is released into blood from damaged endothelial cells after degradation by cytoplasmic proteases. It is increased in serum in systemic lupus erythematosus, disseminated intravascular coagulopathy syndrome (DIC), renal failure, diabetes mellitus, and other diseases in which vascular damage occurs. A preliminary study of serum TM and liver disease was reported in 1990,[26] but no detailed study is as yet available. On an assumption that in severe liver disease vascular endothelial cells within the liver are damaged, Mori et al.[27] set out to measure serum TM levels in various liver diseases by using an enzyme-linked immunosorbent assay (ELISA) system in which monoclonal antibody to TM is used. Thrombomodulin levels were markedly elevated in acute hepatic failure (85.6 ± 30.3 ng/mL) when compared with normal controls (13.6 ± 2.6 ng/mL) and patients with other acute and chronic liver diseases (all below 33.8 ng/mL), the differences being significant ($P < .001$). They did not correlate with the thrombin–antithrombin III complex, a marker of DIC. A negative or positive correlation was noted between the serum TM level and platelet count, serum albumin, choline esterase activity, prothrombin time, and indocyanine green (ICG) clearance. In patients with acute and subacute hepatic failure, serum TM levels kept rising as the clinical course worsened, and the suggestion was made that the serum TM concentration would be a good predictor of prognosis in severe hepatitis.

Short-chain (C_2–C_8) fatty acids are physicochemically volatile, produced by bacterial fermentation in the colon, absorbed into portal vein blood, and metabolized in the liver. In hepatic coma, short-chain fatty acid levels increase markedly in peripheral blood, and this is thought to be an important factor contributing to the development of hepatic coma.[28] In the past, measurement was done by a technique that employed steam distillation and gas chromatography. Subsequent studies have improved the quantitation of volatile fatty acids. Hori[29] employed the modified technique of Brazier et al.[30] in which ether extraction and gas chromatography are used. By this method, each fatty acid is quantified in a pure form with a stable and reproducible calibration curve. The total volatile fatty acid concentration in peripheral blood was 110.9 ± 20.1 μmol/L in young control subjects and 250.6 ± 131.7 μmol/L in hepatic failure with marked increases in C_3, C_6, and C_8. Portal blood taken during abdominal surgery showed a level twice that in the peripheral blood. The preoperative and postoperative (hepatic resection) volatile fatty acid levels were similar except for an increase in C_8 shortly after hepatectomy. In rats given carbon tetrachloride, C_3 and C_6 increased as in humans with hepatic failure. The authors postulate that C_3, C_6, and C_8 exert ill effects on energy metabolism within the liver.

Tumor necrosis factor α (TNF-α) was first identified in the sera of mice sensitized with bacille Calmette-Guérin (BCG) and then challenged by endotoxin in 1975.[31] After biochemical characterization and production of pure TNF-α by a recombinant method,[32] physiologic functions of this factor have come to be known. Many recent studies suggest involvement of various cytokines in the development of acute hepatic failure. Kayano et al.[33] measured TNF-α levels in acute liver disease including fulminant hepatic failure and attained values of less than 10 pg/mL for normal controls, 26.8 ± 32.0 pg/mL in acute hepatitis, 50.0 ± 16.2 pg/mL in severe acute hepatitis, 112.0 ± 75.7 pg/mL in patients with fulminant hepatic failure who survived, and 95.8 ± 35.5 pg/mL in those who succumbed. The peak value in fulminant hepatic failure and subacute hepatic failure occurred 8.8 and 34.4 days after onset, respectively. No correlation was demonstrated between TNF-α levels and the degree of histologic hemorrhage in the liver parenchyma. They interpret these data to be suggestive of a role of TNF-α in the induction and development of acute liver injury.

It has been suggested that bacterial endotoxin or lipopolysaccharide has an important role in the pathophysiology of liver cirrhosis and certain other diseases. In the past, the limulus test based on horseshoe crab clotting enzyme was the only method, but the test had many difficulties because gelation was not very quantitative. The test was subsequently improved with the introduction of a chromogenic substrate,[34] and after elucidation of two reaction pathways involved in the test,[35] inhibitory factors, and nonspecific amidase activities, a further improvement was introduced to the limulus test by perchloric acid (PCA) heat precipitation and then redissolution of the precipitate.[36] Narita used this new PCA technique (Endospecy assay), which is much more specific and quantitative than the previous methods, to determine endotoxin levels in the plasma of patients with cirrhosis[37]: 9.8 pg/mL in the controls and 5.7 ± 5.3 pg/mL in the cirrhotics. Plasma endotoxin levels significantly correlated with the severity of liver dysfunction (Child-Turcotte grade), total bilirubin, and ICG clearance and negatively correlated with the prothrombin time and high-density lipoprotein (HDL)-cholesterol. There was no correlation between esophageal varices and plasma endotoxin. Against the previously held notion, the author failed to demonstrate elevated endotoxin levels in cirrhosis, although certain correlations with some liver tests results were shown. It remains to be seen whether his findings disprove the role of endotoxin currently suspected in the pathophysiology of cirrhosis.

It is now known that cirrhosis-associated hypoxemia and digital clubbing improve after liver transplantation,[38] and certain humoral factors are thought to be a cause.[39, 40] Shijo et al.[41] studied four patients with hepatopulmonary syndrome. All patients showed a reduction in arterial oxygen tension in the standing position and diffusion within the lung, but no other pulmonary function impairment was demonstrated. Contrast-enhanced echocardiography showed delayed opacification of the left ventricle, and pulmonary perfusion imaging with ^{99m}Tc-macroaggregated albumin revealed significant uptake in extrapulmonary organs such as the brain, spleen, and kidneys. A discrepancy was also noted between the physiologic shunt ratio and the percentage of right-to-left shunting as estimated by the quantitative radionuclide technique. A postmortem study in two patients confirmed the presence of intrapulmonary vascular dilations. There were no anatomically established arteriovenous anastomoses in the lung. These observations suggest that abnormally dilated alveolar capillaries are a major cause of severe hypoxemia in this syndrome. Furthermore, these observations suggest that some humoral factors such as prostacyclin and/or other vasoactive substances play a role in the development of this syndrome.

HEPATITIS

Hepatitis B

DNA sequence analysis of the hepatitis B virus (HBV) genome identified four open reading frames (ORFs). The smallest of the four ORFs, initially designated as region 5 by Galibert et al.[42] and recently called ORFX,[43] has the potential to encode a 154–amino acid polypeptide. Recently, Moriarty et al.[44] studied X gene products and found circulating antibodies specific for X protein in the sera of patients with HBV infection. Interestingly, the antibodies were detected predominantly in the sera from patients with HCC. Furukata et al.[45] studied localization of the X antigen by indirect immunoperoxidase staining of rabbit antisera to a synthetic X peptide (N-terminal amino acid sequence 116–134) in liver specimens from 36 patients with chronic hepatitis B. It was distributed diffusely in the cytoplasm of hepatocytes as fine granules. Hepatitis B core antigen (HBcAg) was detected in nearly the same area when it was stained by the same method but with anti-HBc antibodies. Hepatitis B x antigen in the liver was found in 4 of 5 (80%) patients with chronic persistent hepatitis, in 14 of 23 (60.8%) with chronic active hepatitis, and in 3 of 8 (37.5%) with chronic active hepatitis and cirrhosis. It is suggested that levels of HBX antigen in the liver decrease as the disease progresses. Its turnover dynamics were studied in connection with interferon (IFN) treatment. After treatment, HBX antigen in the liver disappeared in 4 of 11 patients and decreased in 2. Five of these 11 patients also showed a loss of HBc antigen in the liver, and the seroconversion of hepatitis B e (HBe) antigen to HBe antibody occurred within 6 months of IFN treatment. These observations suggest that HBX antigen is associated with active viral replication and can be used as an additional marker of HBV infection.

Some Japanese hepatologists use corticosteroids before the administration of IFN for the treatment of HBeAg-positive patients with chronic active hepatitis. One group at Toranomon Hospital, Tokyo, advocates steroid withdrawal therapy in which 40 mg of prednisolone per day is given for 1 week, the dose reduced stepwise to 30 mg and 20 mg weekly, and then the medication discontinued. The same group[46] analyzed HBV-DNA in the sera of 15 patients who were followed for more than 5 years after the disappearance of HBeAg by using polymerase chain reaction (PCR) plus ethidium bromide staining (EB) and Southern blotting with digoxigenin-labeled HBV-cDNA.[47] In ten patients alanine aminotransferase (ALT) levels were normalized, PCR + EB became negative, whereas HBV-DNA persisted in the sera of five patients in whom the ALT level remained elevated. When sera were studied by PCR + EB, HBV-DNA was still positive in the majority. Thus, PCR + EB is too sensitive, and PCR + EB negativity seems to be a better predictor of clinical improvement.

Hepatitis C

Progress in the field of hepatology has been most remarkable as regards study of HCV and HCV-induced diseases as discussed in the same chapter in the previous edition of this book.[48] The complete sequence of nucleotides has been deciphered.[49] Hepatitis C virus RNA can now be readily demonstrated by reverse transcription PCR (RT-PCR), and this method is widely used throughout Japan. Quantification of HCV in aliquots has also become possible by competitive PCR,[50–52] and it is becoming common practice in large laboratories. Several groups of investigators in Japan represented by Okamoto,[53] Kato,[54] Takada,[55] Mizogami,[56] and others have been studying the nucleotide sequence of HCV and subtyping HCV according to the heterogeneity of the base sequence. It is known that RNA viruses readily undergo changes in nucleotide sequence, and HCV is no exception. Changes in sequence may be demonstrated in isolates from the serum of the same patient.[57] According to Okamoto et al.,[49] who determined the full-length genome sequence of HCV, there may be four major subtypes (I to IV), the percent difference in nucleotide being 21% between I and II, 32% for I vs. III, 33% for I vs. IV, 32% for II vs. III, 33% for II vs. IV, and 23% for III vs. IV. Shimotono and his group add two more subtypes. There is as yet no international nomenclature for these subtypes. Takada and his group,[58] who use names such as PT (American prototype), K1, K2a, K2b, etc., analyzed 71 Japanese patients with chronic C disease, 13 patients without HCC from Spain, and 22 such patients from China. Of the 58 Japanese patients without HCC, K1 (type II or J) constituted 76.9%; K2a (III), 15.5%; and K2b (IV), 6.9%. Only one patient had the American prototype (I or PT), which was acquired from an American plasma product. Eleven of 13 (84.6%) patients with HCC had K1. Among the Spanish patients, 38.5% had PT (I) and 53.8% had K1 (II). There was no K2 (III and IV). Chinese patients were similar to the Japanese, and none had PT (I). They contend that K1 (II) is the original strain of HCV that evolved into the Western (PT or I) and the Eastern type (K2 or III, IV) and postulate that the differences in clinical features are in part due to different subtypes. The C-100 assay system contains polypeptides derived from the N3/N4 region of the virus genome, which is thought to have a relatively conserved sequence. Hayashi et al.[59] were able to identify Japanese variants from pooled sera with high ALT levels by using mixed primers derived from C5–11 within C-100 and prepared by the technique of Cheng et al.[60] for RT-PCR. The cDNA fragments 93 nucleotides in length showed a 65 to 67% homology at the nucleotide level and an 81% homology at the amino acid level when compared with the American prototype (PT or I) HCV-cDNA.

The epidemiology of hepatitis C somewhat resembles that of hepatitis B, and the clinical course is also similar to that of hepatitis B in that it progresses from chronic persistent hepatitis to chronic active hepatitis and then to cirrhosis. Hepatocellular carcinoma usually evolves on the background of cirrhosis in C disease, but it may develop before the stage of cirrhosis in B disease. One of the major differences between B and C disease is that the quantity of virus in the blood decreases as the disease progresses in the former but the reverse is true in the latter.[51] It was recently found that persons with a history of household or sexual exposure to a person who had hepatitis have a significantly higher positivity rate for anti-HCV. In addition, there are reports showing intrafamilial clusters of HCV infection.[61, 62] According to Michitaka et al.,[63] clustering of anti-HCV–positive persons was observed in 2 of 16 families (12.5%) studied in Japan. Four of 35 family members (11.4%) with no history of blood transfusion were positive for anti-HCV. Two of 17 offsprings (11.8%) of anti-HCV–positive mothers were positive for anti-HCV, whereas 1 of 5 spouses (20%) was positive for anti-HCV. These data suggest that intrafamilial transmission is one of the routes of HCV infection. Mother-to-infant transmission of HCV is still controversial. Both mother and child were positive for anti-HCV in 3 mother-child pairs, as reported by Takahashi et al.,[64] who studied 160 family members of 76 index parents. In 2 pairs, transmission from mother to child after birth was suspected, and in the other pair, perinatal transmission from father to child seemed likely. These three children had progressive chronic liver disease although they were still young, an indication of the development of chronic hepatitis C even in childhood.[65]

There have been more than a dozen small areas in Japan where chronic liver disease and anti-HCV are reported to be very prevalent. The first such study was made in Saga Prefecture by Setoguchi et al. in 1990.[66] In most studies,[67–70] one village has an exceptionally high prevalence rate for HCV infection and is contrasted by neighboring villages where the prevalence rate is far lower than the national average. Suou et al.[70] reported yet another area in Shimane Prefecture where anti-HCV was positive in 16.6% of 459 adults. Within the village, region A of the three regions (A, B, and C) had an anti-HCV rate of 21.2% as contrasted by region C, where it was 5.7%, and the physician frequently consulted in region A was the prime suspect for spread of the virus; other possible etiologic factors showed no difference in frequency among the three regions. A similar observation had already been made by Kiyosawa and Tanaka a year or so earlier[68] in a village in Nagano Prefecture where one particular physician was the most likely source of infection; he often used unsterilized needles for injection. One other possible mode of transmission in this region was a folk remedy in which blood is suctioned from the skin by negative pressure. Tokita et al.[69] tested beside C-100-3 antibody, nucleocapsid polypeptide CP-9[71] and CP-10,[72] and GOR[73] antibodies in 1,062 adults in a village in Gifu Prefecture where non-A, non-B hepatitis had been endemic. The positivity rate for C-100-3 was 15.3%; CP-9, 36.0%; CP-10, 33.3%; and GOR, 22.3%. Of the total of 1,062 examinees, 45.4% tested positive for at least one of the four antibodies. Within the 3 regions (A, B, C) in the village, region A showed the highest prevalence for elevated ALT and HCV antibodies. They were unable to pinpoint any particular factor to explain the high prevalence rate in region A.

A recent interest is HCV superinfection in HBV carriers and vice versa. The frequency of anti-HCV in hepatitis B surface antigen (HBsAg)-positive patients with chronic hepatitis has been found to be slightly higher than in healthy adult controls. Chayama et al.[74] studied the positivity rate for anti–C-100 antibody in patients with chronic hepatitis B and their clinical features. Anti–C-100 was detected in 24 (3.9%) of 613 patients with chronic hepatitis B. In a further analysis of 24 patients with chronic hepatitis B, anti–C-100 was found more frequently in the patients negative for HBeAg than in those positive for HBeAg (22 of 385 vs. 2 of 227; $P < .01$). As detected by reverse transcription and nested PCR, HCV-RNA, was positive in 20 of 22 patients negative for HBeAg, whereas it was detected in only 1 of 2 patients positive for HBeAg, thus suggesting a high prevalence of HCV infection in HBeAg-negative patients with chronic hepatitis. In their follow-up study, a patient had become HCV-RNA positive after seroconversion from HBeAg to anti-HBe in spite of the fact that HCV-RNA was undetectable during the HBeAg-positive phase. These data suggest that HCV infection becomes active after seroconversion from HBeAg to anti-HBe.

Chen et al.[75] also reported a higher anti-HCV prevalence in HBsAg-positive patients with chronic liver diseases as compared with volunteer blood donors. However, among patients with chronic hepatitis, anti-HCV positivity was much higher in HBsAg-negative patients than in HBsAg-positive patients. The positivity rate for anti-HCV became higher with progression in the severity of chronic hepatitis and with progression to cirrhosis and from cirrhosis to HCC in HBsAg-positive patients. It would be interesting to determine whether HCV superinfection accelerates the liver disease in HBsAg carriers, although preexisting chronic or concurrent acute non-A, non-B virus infection has already been found to interfere with HBV replication and to modulate the development of disease related to HBV infection in chimpanzees.[76] The mechanism for this phenomenon remains to be elucidated.

Higuchi[77] studied HCV superinfection in HBV carriers. Hepatitis B virus markers and antibodies to HCV (anti–C-100 and anticore) were tested in 774 nonalcoholic adults in areas of high endemicity of liver disease in northern Japan. Ninety-seven individuals (12.5%) were positive for HBsAg and 94 (12.1%) positive for antibodies to HCV. Ten (10.3%) of those 97 positive for HBsAg were superinfected with HCV. This is a very high prevalence rate for HCV infection because the anti-HCV positivity in healthy adults is 1% to 2% in Japan. The titer of HBsAg, frequency of HBe antigenemia, and level of DNA polymerase were found to be significantly lower in individuals with HCV superinfection than in HBV carriers negative for anti-HCV. Such observations suggest that HCV may reduce the replication of HBV in superinfected livers.

Kobayashi et al.[78] at Toranomon Hospital, Tokyo, tested sera from 1,619 patients with chronic non-A, non-B liver disease for C-100 antibody titers; 73.8% of males and 65.0% of females tested positive. Among the cirrhotic patients, 76.2% of males and 56.0% of females were positive ($P < .05$). The percentage of patients who showed an antibody titer greater than 2^5 was less in females than in males. Among 52 patients who were followed for more than 8 years, 14 turned negative for the antibody. Of these, 12 were cirrhotic from the beginning. Of the 14, 11 were female, and in 4 of these 11 females, serum ALT levels became normal, and as yet no HCC has developed. These observations suggest certain differences between males and females in the clinical course and natural history of HCV-associated liver disease.

The Ministry of Health and Welfare of Japan now permits the administration of IFN to patients with histologically proven chronic active hepatitis C for up to 6 months, and the costs are borne by the health insurance funds. A flux of reports on the clinical experience of IFN treatment is expected in a short while. Hagiwara et al.[79] examined HCV-RNA in sera from 20 patients with chronic hepatitis C during IFN therapy by using RT-PCR; primers were chosen from the NS3 region of the prototype HCV-RNA sequence. In 18 of 20 (90%) patients, HCV-RNA was detected before IFN therapy. However, in patients in whom the serum ALT level improved, HCV-RNA became undetectable at 4 weeks of therapy. Within 4 weeks after therapy HCV-RNA reappeared in those who had a relapse. In the group without response, HCV-RNA did not disappear during the therapy. They concluded that IFN therapy was beneficial for viremia and the detection of HCV-RNA in serum is useful for evaluating the antiviral effect of IFN. Matsumoto et al.[80] studied the effect of IFN therapy on hepatic HCV-RNA in chronic hepatitis C. Levels of HCV-RNA were estimated by RT-PCR with RNA extracted from the liver tissue of 14 patients. It was found that the levels of hepatic HCV-RNA were suppressed after treatment in all patients except for 1. The hepatic HCV-RNA level before therapy was lower ($P < .01$) in the responding group (ALT normalized, 6 cases) than in the nonresponder (ALT remained elevated, 8 cases). They simultaneously measured HCV-RNA in the serum. Serum HCV-RNA in the responder group became undetectable 1 month after therapy. In the nonresponder group, it was detected in 7 of 8 patients 1 month after therapy. It is interesting that patients having small amounts of HCV-RNA in the liver before IFN therapy responded well to the therapy. Interferon therapy has side effects that include chills, fever, myalgia, fatigue, nausea, vomiting, and bone marrow suppression. As reported by Conlon et al.[81] in 1990, exacerbation of autoimmune disease following IFN therapy has been noted. Chikazawa et al.[82] reported psychiatric problems in two patients with chronic active hepatitis C treated with IFN-α. Anxiety, suicidal ideation, and delusions of persecution occurred in one of them. Indeed, the psychiatric side effect of IFN-α is one of the reasons for discontinuation of therapy.

Imaging

Hepatocytes have an asialoglycoprotein (Ashwell) receptor on the plasma membrane that is very specific for the hepatocyte. Vera et al. in 1985 first synthesized ^{99m}Tc-labeled asialoglycoprotein for receptor binding and hence imaging of hepatocytes. They used this system to mathematically analyze hepatocyte mass and liver function.[83] The compound they used was glycosyl-neoglycoalbumin. Subsequently, Kubota et al. of Japan covalently attached a chelating agent, diethylenetriaminepentaacetic acid (DTPA) to galactosyl-albumin (GSA) to stabilize the technetium atom.[84] Kudo et al.[85] assessed this compound as an imaging agent for evaluating liver function in 3 normal subjects and 54 patients with various liver diseases. They set the receptor index as the ratio of radioactivity of the liver to the activity of the liver plus the heart 15 minutes after intravenous injection of 3 mg of ^{99m}Tc GSA. Receptor concentration $[R_O]$ was obtained by kinetic analysis of liver and heart time-activity data and pharmacokinetic nonlinear modeling. Values for the receptor index and $[R_O]$ were significantly different between controls and the patients with liver disease. Good correlations were obtained between the receptor index, $[R_O]$, and conventional liver tests such as Child-Turcotte score, prothrombin time, and ICG test. These parameters could be adequately estimated even in patients with obstructive jaundice or remarkable portacaval shunts. These observations suggest that receptor imaging as well as its parameters receptor index and $[R_O]$ are practical and reliable for estimating the functioning hepatocyte mass and assessing liver function.

There have already been a number of studies on the measurement of portal venous blood flow velocity by Doppler flowmetry outside the liver after the first report by Ohnishi et al. in 1985.[86] However, intrahepatic portal blood flow has not been studied extensively. Furuse et al.[87] studied the hemodynamics of intrahepatic portal flow velocity in the first- to third-order branches in 35 normal subjects and 74 patients with cirrhosis. The flow velocity decreased from the portal trunk to the first-order branch and further from the first-order to the second-order branch in both lobes. The abrupt drop in velocity in the umbilical portion of the left portal branch was the most remarkable finding. The drop in velocity from the second- to the third-order branch was greater than the gradient between the first- and second-order branches in the right lobe, but no such drop was observed in the left lobe in which the velocity in the second- and third-order branches was about the same. Furthermore, velocity in the third-order branch was the same regardless of the lobe. Intrahepatic portal thrombosis was found in a first- or second-order branch in 31 cirrhotic patients with 36 thrombi. Of the 36 thrombi, 25 were in the left lobe; of these 25, 16 (64%) were intraluminal and 9 (36%) were mural. Thus, the slower velocity in the left portal branches seems to predispose to more frequent thrombus formation than in the right lobe.

Urita et al.[88] evaluated the branching structure of hepatic arteries in 14 subjects without liver disease and 16 patients with cirrhosis on the premise that the normal branching structure, namely, the angle and caliber, is optimal so that loss of blood flow energy is kept minimal. Angiograms provide only two-dimensional information. They first analyzed hepatic arteriograms for the measurement of calibers before and after branching and then measured the branching angles by ultrasound. They chose the site where the third-order branches divide from the right anterior hepatic artery. Theoretical equations have been proposed by several investigators, but they used the curve proposed by Zamir and Medeiros.[89] They analyzed the data in points for the degree of scatter in reference to the theoretical curve. The data in control subjects plotted near the theoretical curve, whereas those obtained in cirrhotic patients tended to plot far away from the curve when both the diameter and branching angle were considered. The authors postulate that such deviation seen in cirrhosis is caused by hemodynamic changes resulting from increased intrahepatic shunts and morphologic changes due to fibrosis and/or regenerative nodules in the parenchyma.

Kashiwagi and his group have been studying portal hemodynamics by scintiphotosplenoportography[90] and more recently by less invasive single-photon emission computed tomography (SPECT) with ^{99m}Tc-labeled erythrocytes (blood pool SPECT).[91] They further studied hemodynamic changes after sclerotherapy in 36 patients with cirrhosis by injecting 740 MBq (20 mCi) of ^{99m}Tc-O$_4$$^-$ (in vivo labeling) and using a digital camera attached to a high-resolution collimeter for low energy.[92] Before sclerotherapy, blood pool images of the left gastric vein were obtained in 34 patients. The varix recurrence rate was 11.1% in the group in which the blood pool disappeared after sclerotherapy, whereas it was 90% in patients in whom the pool remained unchanged. These results indicate that abdominal blood pool SPECT is useful for evaluating the therapeutic effects of sclerotherapy and predicting variceal recurrence.

Yoshida[93] combined scintiphotosplenoportography with angiography (postceliac arteriographic splenoportography) and measured the time-activity curve over the area of interest set on the splenic vein and portal trunk by using ^{99m}Tc-O$_4$$^-$ for in vivo labeling and a gamma camera. From the Stewart-Hamilton equation they calculated the relative percentage of splenic vein blood (SV%) within the portal venous flow. The 96 patients they studied consisted of 74 with cirrhosis, 8 with chronic hepatitis, 4 with idiopathic portal hypertension (IPH), and 10 controls who had no liver disease. The percentage of splenic vein blood was significantly lower in patients without liver disease or without collateral veins than in patients with collaterals. Among the latter, patients with IPH showed significantly higher SV%, and in these patients, 74% of portal venous flow was derived from the splenic vein. They interpreted these results as demonstrating a hyperdynamic state in and around the spleen.

Attempts have recently been made to use ultrasound for tissue characterization[94, 95] on the assumption that histologic changes will alter ultrasonic absorption by that particular tissue. The group at the First Department of Medicine, Osaka University Hospital, developed a new system with the Shimazu Laboratories that consists of a 10-MHz A-mode transducer, pulse generator, A/D converter, personal computer, and oscilloscope.[96] The ultrasonic transducer is placed in contact with the liver surface and the frequency-dependent attenuation (FDA) coefficient of the liver is determined in vivo from the ultrasonic signals. They applied this system first to rabbits with fatty livers. The FDA coefficient significantly correlated with the microscopic degree of fatty infiltration and with the content of total lipids and triglycerides in the liver. They also applied this system to patients with liver diseases during peritoneoscopy. There was a significant correlation between the FDA coefficient and the microscopic degree of fatty infiltration in the liver.[97] They claim that the degree of fatty change in the liver can be quantitatively assessed by their ultrasonic system, although it is invasive because laparoscopy is required. The volume of the liver can be quantitatively assessed by slicing the liver by computed tomography (CT) and adding the liver areas. Ibe et al.[98] studied the change in liver volume in one patient with idiopathic acute fatty liver of pregnancy (IAFLP); there have already been several reports on the liver volume in this disease, but the observations vary. In this case report, the volume was rapidly reduced to 703 cm^3 on the second day of illness but climbed to 1,390 cm^{23} in 6 days, thus indicating a very rapid volume alteration in this disease.

IMMUNOLOGY

Primary biliary cirrhosis (PBC) is one of the common forms of nonviral and nonalcoholic chronic liver disease of unknown etiology. It affects all races and socioeconomic classes. The immunogenetic background has been studied for a number of autoimmune diseases by evaluating the association of antigen of the major histocompatibility complex (MHC), but association of PBC with MHC class I or II antigen has not yet been clearly determined. Recent studies revealed an increased frequency of HLA-DRw8 in patients with PBC in the United States[99] and more recently in German patients as well.[100] Maeda et al.[101] studied the possibility of an immunogenetic association in Japanese patients with PBC by examining their HLA class I and II antigens. The HLA antigen typing was carried out with the standard National Institutes of Health (NIH) microdroplet lymphocyte cytotoxicity test. The distribution of its phenotypes in patients with PBC for class I antigens A, B, and C did not differ from that in the control group. A highly significant increase in HLA-DRw8 was found in patients with PBC vs. controls (78% vs. 24.2%; relative risk, 11.978; P [corrected] < .001). Their studies clearly showed a strong immunogenetic background in Japanese patients with PBC as shown by an increased frequency of HLA-DRw8. This may be true for all races because the association of HLA-DRw8 in PBC was found in North America,[99] Europe,[100] and the Far East.[3]

In Japan, PBC was thought to be very rare in the past, but it rapidly increased in frequency after diagnostic criteria were established.[102] Enzan et al.[103] surveyed all autopsied PBC cases in the autopsy registries edited by the Japanese Pathological Society from 1984 to 1987. Fourty-two patients with PBC were autopsied in 1984, 37 in 1985, 38 in 1986, and 49 in 1987. Thus, a total of 166 PBC cases were found to be recorded. Its incidence among total autopsies was 0.10%. This rate is quite high in comparison with the previous analysis that showed a rate of 0.03% from 1958 to 1983. The number of patients with PBC seems to be increasing in Japan as well as in Western countries.[104] The mean age of those patients with PBC at autopsy in the study of Enzan et al. was 57.6 years. There was a female preponderance of 7.3:1. These findings appear to be common worldwide. The majority of patients were in a cirrhotic stage with portal hypertension and jaundice. Interestingly, their analysis revealed 7 patients with HCC out of 166 cases. Hepatocellular carcinoma mainly develops in patients with cirrhosis of viral origin. In recent years, Melia et al.[105] reported the occurrence of HCC in patients with PBC in the United Kingdom, although it had been thought to be extremely rare in patients with PBC.[106, 107] They emphasized that HCC was the cause of death in 33% of the men and 5% of the women who suffered from PBC, thus suggesting that HCC is not less frequent in PBC than other types of cirrhosis.

In a survey carried out by Nakanuma et al.[108] similar to the one just quoted,[103] not even a single case of HCC in PBC was reported up to the end of 1982 in Japan. Hepatocellular carcinoma began to be noticed in patients with PBC in 1983. It seems that HCC complicating PBC is a recent phenomenon.[109] It would be of great interest to know whether patients with PBC in whom HCC developed had HCV infection. More recently, Hata et al.[110] described a 63-year-old woman with HCC complicating PBC. She had received a blood transfusion 32 years earlier and had been followed after PBC was diagnosed. Hepatocellular carcinoma was detected when α-fetoprotein (AFP) levels were continuously elevated. Her liver was Scheuer's stage 4. Hepatitis C virus infection was confirmed by anti-HCV and HCV-RNA. Further epidemiologic observations are necessary for understanding the relationship between the recent rise in HCC incidence in PBC and HCV infection.

The histologic features of autoimmune hepatitis (AIH) are characterized by periportal piecemeal necrosis and have plasma cells infiltration, but they are not specific for AIH. Recently, Dienes et al.[111] reported broad collapsing hepatocellular areas extending from the portal tracts into the parenchyma and encompassing groups of hepatocytes with microacinal transformation as the most conspicuous lesions in AIH when compared with chronic hepatitis B and chronic hepatitis C. Hino[112] also studied the characteristics of hepatocytes with acinar arrangements called rosettes. Rosettes were seen more frequently in AIH than in acute and chronic viral hepatitis. They were divided into two types by electron microscopic analysis: one is the degenerative type which contains many lipofuscin granules and dilated rough endoplasmic reticula (rER) in the cytoplasm, and the other is the regenerative type, which contains abundant glycogen granules and rER with many ribosomes. A number of mononuclear cells and plasma cells were seen in close contact with the rosettes. The phenotypes of the mononuclear cells were mainly those of non-T and non-B cells. This suggests that antibody-dependent cell-mediated cytotoxicity (ADCC) may participate in the hepatocyte destruction seen in AIH, as previously described by Eggink et al.[113] These findings do not, of course, exclude T-cell–mediated cytotoxicity.

It is thought that hepatitis caused by HBV is a host immune response to the virus and that the intensity of the immune response determines the infection patterns,[114] but direct evidence is lacking. Duck hepatitis B virus (DHBV) is one of the hepadnaviruses[115] and may be a useful model of HBV infection for studying host-viral interaction and the immunologic mechanism of viral hepatitis. Fukuda et al.[116] studied the relationship between the host immune state and hepatic inflammation by experimentally transmitting DHBV to 7-day-old ducks that were pretreated with immunoregulatory drugs. Immunosuppressive treatment with cyclophosphamide extended the viremia period without inflammatory changes in the liver. Steroid hormone treatment also extended the period of viremia by increased viral DNA replication. Remarkable infiltration of inflammatory cells in the liver was observed by pretreatment with OK-432, a streptococcal pyrogen preparation that has immunostimulatory effects.[117] To further ascertain the specific immune response of DHBV, Takashita and Fukuda[118] immunized DHBV carrier ducks intraperitoneally or intrahepatically with major polypeptides of DHBV surface antigen (DHBV viral protein)[119] and Freund's Complete Adjuvant (FCA). Histologically, focal necrosis and accumulation of lymphocytes in the portal tract along with destruction of the limiting plate were found in DHBV carrier ducks injected with DHBV viral protein and FCA. These findings are the characteristics of chronic active hepatitis in ducks. By contrast, no significant inflammatory changes were seen in DHBV carrier ducks receiving microsomal proteins of duck liver along with FCA or FCA alone. The severity of hepatitis was closely associated with the amount of DHBV viral proteins injected. Interestingly, the amount of DHBV-DNA was decreased in the DHBV carrier ducks that had severe hepatitis. They hypothesize that viral hepatitis is due to a host immune response against viral protein(s) present on hepatocytes.

Human T-lymphotrophic virus type 1 (HTLV-1) is a virus that causes adult T-cell leukemia (ATL). It is also well known that HTLV-1 causes immunodeficiency. Almost all persons positive for anti–HTLV-1 are considered to be carriers.[120] Carriers are densely distributed in Western Japan, particularly in Kyushu at a frequency of 3.5% of the population as reported by Motoori et al.[121] Nakano et al.[122] studied anti–HTLV-1 in patients with liver disease and in HBsAg carriers in comparison with healthy controls in the same area of Japan as surveyed by Motoori et al. The rate of anti–HTLV-1 carriage in patients with liver disease (8.1%, 14 of 171) was higher than that in healthy controls (3.5%, 7 of 200). In patients with liver disease who had a history of blood transfusion, the positivity rate was 18.4% (7/38). Surprisingly, anti–HTLV-1 was significantly higher in HBsAg carriers (11.3%, 6 of 53). They suggested that the high incidence of anti–HTLV-1 in patients with liver disease was due to transmission of HTLV-1 by the same routes as for HBV infection such as maternal transmission and blood transfusion. They also described a 31-year-old woman who became an HBV carrier after being exposed to both HTLV-1 and HBV simultaneously through blood transfusions. One of the reasons for the high rate of anti–HLTV-1 in HBV carriers, even without a history of transfusion, may be that the state of HTLV-1 carriage permits the persistence of HBV infection.

Liver Cancer

One of the major issues currently discussed in Japan[109] has been the distinction between adenomatous hyperplasia (AH) as a preneoplastic lesion in cirrhotic livers,[123, 124] abnormal AH (AH containing foci of abnormal cells), and early HCC. Differentiation based on conventional histologic features has struck a snag, and other criteria are being sought. Kudo et al. at Kobe City Hospital[125] studied the hemodynamic characteristics of 17 patients with resected early-stage HCCs and 49 patients with resected advanced HCC lesions smaller than 3 cm by using in vivo vascular imaging techniques. They defined early-stage HCC as a nodule uniformly composed of well-differentiated HCC or AH containing well-differentiated HCC foci within the nodule. Imaging techniques were ultrasound angiography with intra-arterial administration of CO_2 microbubbles for the assessment of arterial vasculature and CT during arterial portography (CTAP) for the assessment of portal perfusion within the nodule. Of the 17 early-stage HCC nodules, 5 were hypervascular, 5 were isovascular, 4 were hypovascular, and 3 had vascular spots within a hypovascular pattern, whereas 43 of 49 advanced HCC nodules were hypervascular and 6 were isovascular. Of 14 patients with early-stage HCC, 9 showed perfusion defects on CTAP, and 5 did not, whereas all 37 cases of advanced HCC showed perfusion defects on CTAP. Seven of 17 (41%) patients with early-stage HCCs showed fatty metamorphosis in contrast to only 8% (4/49) of those with advanced HCC. It was concluded that (1) arterial tumor neovascularization is relatively low in early-stage HCC, (2) portal perfusion is present in some cases of early-stage HCC, (3) a hypoperfusion state involving both the arterial and portal supply is present in some cases of early-stage HCC, (4) vascular spots in a hypovascular pattern is a characteristic arterial pattern in AH containing HCC foci, and (5) fatty metamorphosis may be related to hypoperfusion of the nodule in early-stage HCC. The same group[126] used the same techniques to study arterial vascularity (AV) and portal perfusion (PP) in 55 nodular lesions found in cirrhotic livers and resected. They classified tumor hemodynamic patterns into six types: type I, PP(+), AV (hypo); type I', PP(+), AV (iso); type II; PP(+), AV (iso); type III, PP(−), AV (iso); type IV, PP(+), AV (hyper); and type V, PP (practically +), AV (vascular spots in a hypovascular background). Eight benign nodules all exhibited a type I pattern, and all type II lesions and 88% of type III lesions were well-differentiated HCC as contrasted to only 8% being well-differentiated HCC in type IV nodules. Seventy-five percent of type III lesions had fatty changes. They concluded that in the stage of transformation from AH to HCC, a reduction in portal flow occurs in the nodule before tumor begins to form arterial vessels; early-stage HCC exhibits either a hypovascular pattern (types I, II), isovascular pattern (type III), or vascular spots in the background of hypovascularity (type V) as contrasted by typical HCC (type IV). They also suggest that the more mature as a neoplasia the HCC becomes, the greater the number of vessels the tumor would contain and that fatty changes are related to hypoperfusion from the arterial and portal vessels within the nodule.

They further studied[127] the vasculature of small HCC lesions histologically in relation to CO_2 ultrasound angiography in 44 small HCC lesions resected from 39 patients. Of the 44 lesions, 35 were hypervascular, 5 isovascular, 3 with vascular spots in a hypovascular background, and 1 hypovascular. Of 11 HCC lesions of

Edmondson-Steiner grade I, 4 were isovascular, 6 hypervascular and 1 hypovascular. The sensitivity in demonstrating hypervascularity improved to 80% by the use of ultrasound angiography vs. 70% with conventional angiography and 73% with Lipiodol CT. It was concluded that practically all HCC lesions have arterial vascularity, that about half of well-differentiated HCC lesions exhibit an isovascular or hypovascular pattern suggesting immature neovascularization, and that tumors not detectable by angiography or Lipiodol CT are isovascular and unencapsulated or very small. They maintain that ultrasound angiography is sensitive in the detection of arterial vascularity within the HCC nodules and will contribute to the diagnosis of small HCC lesions. These studies of Kudo and his group and other reports from Japan have clearly shown that early HCC lesions often have fatty changes[128] and are seen as hyperechoic lesions. Kanno et al.[129] compared echogenic and nonechogenic HCC lesions smaller than 2 cm for histology and prognosis. They followed 87 such HCC lesions: 32 were diffusely or partially echogenic and 55 were nonechogenic. Histologically, Edmondson-Steiner grade I HCC was more frequent in the former, and the transition of tumor cells from more differentiated to less well differentiated types seems to be slower. The survival rate in the former was 73% at 3 years, 56% at 5 years, and 48% at 7 and 9 years as contrasted by the corresponding figures of 46%, 42%, and 0% in the nonechogenic HCCs. These results suggest that the echogenicity of small HCC lesions is a predictor of relatively benign prognosis.

The diagnosis of a small HCC lesion largely depends on its vascularity as the quoted papers suggest, and many hepatologists are conscious of the importance of vascularity assessment. In this connection, the case report by Shuto et al.[130] may be of interest. During surgery on two patients in whom a small mass lesion was detected by frequent ultrasound follow-up, they injected ICG into the portal vein branch flowing into the particular subsegment that contained the lesions. The dye was not taken up by the tumors, which were found to be unencapsulated well-differentiated HCC lesions each measuring 15 and 20 mm. The two lesions were hyperechoic on ultrasound examination and histologically showed fatty changes, but portal veins were recognized within the nodule. Since cellularity was high, the histologic diagnosis was well-differentiated HCC. They speculate that these lesions did not have enough portal perfusion despite the presence of portal veins and that such discrepancy between portal vasculature and flow may represent a feature of unencapsulated early HCC.

A number of studies have been made in Japan on Doppler signals derived from HCC,[131–133] but analysis and interpretation[134] of the signals were still preliminary, and a critical view has been voiced.[135] It is not yet clear whether Doppler study contributes to the differential diagnosis of early HCC lesions. Tohara[136] analyzed Doppler signals obtained from 42 HCC lesions smaller than 2 cm and 62 HCC lesions larger than 2 cm, 21 metastatic lesions, 21 hemangiomas, and 5 large regenerative nodules. Diagnosis was made by biopsy. Doppler signals were detected in 70% of the HCC lesions, significantly more frequently than in metastatic cancers. Color signals obtained from the tumors were divided into feeding signals, spotty signals, draining signals, and penetrating signals. Feeding signals entering the tumor from the boundary or draining signals flowing out of the tumor were detected only in HCC. Thus, if feeding or draining signals were obtained from the tumor, a diagnosis of HCC was possible. It was suggested that feeding signals are derived from a feeding artery or portal vein and draining signals from the flow draining the tumor. Furthermore, Doppler flowmetry is useful for evaluating the efficacy of transcatheter embolization treatment or percutaneous ethanol injection and for appraising whether or not additional treatment is required, according to the author.

From the above discussion it is clear that tumor vasculature is an important feature that has clinical relevance. The neovasculature of advanced HCC has been extensively studied by Nakashima[137] and his group. Edamitsu[138] carried out a morphologic study on tumor vessels of small HCC lesions less than 5 cm. He histologically classified vessels of small HCC lesions into types A and V; in the former there is a muscular wall resembling ordinary arteries, and the latter lacks the muscular wall and resembles a vein. The number of type A vessels increased along with the increase in tumor size up to 2 cm, but no further increase was recognized after the tumor reached the size of 2 cm. The number of type A vessels was smaller in tumors that did not show a tumor stain upon arteriography as compared with the more frequent type A vessels in tumors that showed stains.

Several techniques are currently available for demonstrating damage to DNA in vitro such as detection of unscheduled DNA synthesis in primary liver cell culture,[139] constant-velocity sedimentation in a sucrose gradient,[140] and alkaline elution.[141] More recently, Nose and Okamoto[142] developed a nick translation method for detecting carcinogen-induced DNA breaks. Tsutsumi et al.[143] used the nick translation technique to evaluate its usefulness in primary cultures of rat hepatocytes. They used dimethylnitrosamine (DMN), aflatoxin B_1 (AFB_1), lysophosphatidylcholine (LPC), phospholipase A_2 (PLA_2), and lithocholic acid (LCA) because the latter three substances are suspected carcinogens for gallbladder carcinoma commonly associated with abnormal pancreaticobiliary ductal union. DNA damage was detected at concentrations higher than 2×10^{-5}M, 1.6×10^{-6}M, and 5×10^{-7}M for DMN, AFB_1, and LCA, but no damage occurred with PLA_2 and LPC. When compared with unscheduled DNA synthesis and alkaline elution methods, this system was far more sensitive and simple. They concluded that this technique can be used to screen the carcinogenicity of many other compounds.

Proteasomes are newly discovered ring-shaped, large protease complexes with multicatalytic activities.[144] Takai et al.[145] determined their levels in sera from patients with liver cirrhosis, metastatic liver cancer, and HCC by sandwich EIA with their monoclonal and polyclonal antibodies. The levels of proteasomes in sera from 50 healthy adults were uniformly low, whereas the levels of proteasomes in sera from patients with metastatic liver carcinoma and HCC were high. When the neoplastic parts of metastatic liver cancer or HCC were removed by hepatectomy, the proteasome levels in sera dropped. Statistical analysis showed no significant correlation between the levels of proteasomes and AFP or carcinoembryonic antigen (CEA). These results suggest that measurement of the levels of proteasomes in sera might be useful for the diagnosis of HCC.

It is now established that abnormal prothrombin, des-γ-carboxy prothrombin or PIVKA-II, increases in the serum of some patients with HCC and is diagnostic.[146] The exact mechanism whereby PIVKA-II increases is not yet known. Aoyagi and his group at Niigata University Hospital have been working with the sugar moiety of AFP in HCC that distinguishes itself from other types of AFP produced in other diseases. The same group studied the biantennary sugar chain of PIVKA-II produced by HCC tissue.[147] Using a column of concanavalin A (Con-A)-Sepharose, they demonstrated a fraction not binding to Con-A in four of eight patients with HCC, but no such fraction was found in patients with other diseases. Although this is a preliminary report requiring confirmation, it may prove diagnostic in distinguishing HCC-specific and HCC-nonspecific increases in PIVKA-II.

Hypercitrullinemia is frequently associated with hepatocarcinogenesis. Japanese reports indicate that HCC developed in 8 of 56 (14%) patients, the ages of these patients ranging from 22 to 44 years, an unusual age distribution for HCC. Nakayama et al. used primary hepatocyte culture to demonstrate that citrulline acts as a growth-promoting factor and can act as a promotor in high concentrations.[148] They extended their study[149] by using rats given diethylnitrosamine (DEN) and acetylaminofluorene (AAF) and then given either citrulline, phenobarbital, or no medication. Hyperplastic nodules developed in 83.3% of the phenobarbital-treated rats, in 100% of the citrulline-treated rats, and in 16.7% of the controls. These investigators suspect that besides being a genetic factor, citrulline may act as a promotor in initiated liver cells in animals.

Because of the established policy of monitoring cirrhotic patients at short intervals with abdominal ultrasound and serum AFP examinations at major gastrointestinal units throughout Japan, most patients are now detected at an early stage of HCC. Recently about 70% of HCC lesions have been smaller than 5 cm at detection, and many are even smaller than 2 cm. The question remains whether such early detection has really increased the number of complete cures or improved prognosis. Since 1965 the Liver Cancer Study Group of Japan has been analyzing records of individual patients seen and compiled by cooperating major hospitals throughout the country with a questionnaire. The data are put into the computer at Kyoto University. The first report was made in 1980.[150] One area of emphasis has been to monitor changes in the survival rate after surgical treatment. Since 1980, data have been analyzed every 2 years.[151–153] The latest, or the ninth report, was published in 1991[154]; 601 institutes participated and a total of 9,564 cases that included 2,982 histologically confirmed cases of HCC were analyzed. The follow-up of patients with HCC and cholangiocarcinoma who were operated on after January 1, 1978, showed a 1-year survival rate of 71.9%, a 2-year survival rate of 56.6%, a 3-year survival rate of 45.6%, and a 5-year survival rate of 30.9%. The survival rate for patients with HCC lesions smaller than 2 cm was

86.9% at 1 year, 81.5% at 2 years, 74.5% at 3 years, and 60.5% at 5 years, significantly better than that in patients with larger HCC lesions. Operative death occurred in 3.1%, which is much lower than 11.9%, the operative mortality in the period 1968 to 1977.[150]

The problem with Japanese investigators in clinical medicine has been the paucity of randomized controlled studies. Many past studies on therapy have been criticized. The autologous lymphokine-activated killer (LAK) cell treatment initiated by Rosenberg et al. in 1985[155] has been applied to the treatment of HCC by several investigators in Japan.[156–159] In some studies, activated killer cells were transferred from the hepatic artery.[147, 148] However, these studies were made in a small number of patients in an uncontrolled fashion. The overall results have been rather disappointing, although serum AFP levels came down in many patients.[160] Wakizaka et al.[161] carried out a randomized clinical trial among 30 patients with HCC after radical resection in order to compare the efficacy of postoperative arterial infusion of doxorubicin (Adriamycin [ADR]), recombinant interleukin-2 (rIL-2), and spleen-derived LAK cells (chemoimmunotherapy) vs. ADR alone (chemotherapy). Twenty-four patients, 12 in each group, were judged to be evaluable. The total number of transferred LAK cells per patient ranged from 3.2 to 18.0 $\times$ 10^9 in the immunochemotherapy group. They were followed for 11 to 29 months. There were no significant differences between the two groups with regard to preoperative conditions. No major adverse side effects were noted with the therapy. The cumulative recurrence rate in the chemoimmunotherapy group was 41.7% (5/12), and that of the chemotherapy group was 58.3% (7/12) 21 months after surgery, the difference being insignificant.

After the intratumor ethanol injection therapy was developed in 1983 at Chiba University Hospital,[162, 163] no exciting novel treatment modality has evolved in this country. The surgical group headed by Nakayama at Kurume started using a microwave coagulator developed in Japan in 1979[164] for the treatment of small HCC lesions located near the liver surface.[165] They modified the microwave coagulator to fit the laparoscope and reported their experience in treating one patient with a small HCC lesion near the surface by laparoscopic coagulation.[166] There was no adverse reaction, and the lesion, which turned to a low-density lesion on CT, was no longer enhanced on hepatic arteriography. The results of long-term follow-up are awaited. Ethanol and the microwave coagulator are similar in a sense that both induce tissue necrosis by coagulation. Several other new coagulating substances or devices are currently being tested in Japan, and the results will soon appear in publications. Seki et al.[167] applied both the microwave coagulator and ethanol coagulation to the treatment of large 5- to 8-cm HCC lesions in 7 patients. The average size reduction was 40%. During heating with the microwave needle placed through the skin, the skin also became heated, and the authors had to keep cooling the needle by applying cold wet gauze around it. The results remain to be objectively evaluated with proper controls in a large number of patients.

SUMMARY

The major defect in this chapter is the lack of studies on liver transplantation in Japan, where only living related donor liver transplantation has been carried out. As stated in the introduction, studies on HCV will gain an impetus in the coming year or two. Routes of infection other than blood transfusion will be made clear, and the question of whether subtypes make any differences in the response to IFN therapy and the frequency of hepatocarcinogenesis will be solved shortly. Another question of whether the close association between chronic HCV infection and HCC is simply through cirrhosis, which in itself is a premalignant state, or through as yet unknown mechanisms induced by this virus has to be resolved. Along with the progress in our understanding of molecular events that underlie the multistep process of carcinogenesis currently investigated by molecular oncologists will come a stage where the sequential events involving oncogene activation/antioncogene suppression that lead to hepatocarcinogenesis are understood, like the Vogelstein model for colon carcinoma. The histologic alterations that occur stepwise in the preneoplastic lesions of the liver will eventually be correlated with the molecular changes. The authors of this chapter expect that discovery of a new hepatitis virus (HFV) is imminent. The preliminary reports in this country suggest that this virus causes a rather severe hepatitis. Next comes the important question of which virus is the main or most frequent cause of subfulminant hepatic failure and whether HCV is its common cause. The data from Japan and Europe are at variance in this regard at the moment. Hepatology will never keep us bored.

REFERENCES

1. Yano M: Natural history of C hepatitis (in Japanese). *Clin Gastroenterol* 1992; 7:1995–2000.

2. Seeff LB, et al: Long-term mortality after transfusion-associated non-A, non-B hepatitis. *N Engl J Med* 1992; 327:1906–1911.

3. Kiyosawa K, et al: Interrelationship of blood transfusion, non-A, non-B hepatitis and hepatocellular carcinoma: Analysis by detection of antibody to hepatitis C virus. *Hepatology* 1990; 12:671–675.

4. Oka H, et al: Prospective study of early detection of hepatocellular carcinoma in patients with cirrhosis. *Hepatology* 1990; 12:680–687.

5. Ferrell L, et al: Incidence and diagnostic features of macroregenerative nodules vs. small hepatocellular carcinoma in cirrhotic livers. *Hepatology* 1992; 16:1372–1381.

6. Nakamura T, et al: Partial purification and characterization of hepatocyte growth factor from serum of hepatectomized rats. *Biochem Biophys Res Commun* 1984; 122:1450–1459.

7. Nakamura T, et al: Purification and characterization of a growth factor from rat platelets for mature parenchymal hepatocytes in primary cultures. *Proc Natl Acad Sci U S A* 1986; 83:6489–6493.

8. Nakamura T, et al: Purification and subunit structure of hepatocyte growth factor from rat platelets. *FEBS Lett* 1987; 224:311–316.

9. Gohda E, et al: Human hepatocyte growth factor in plasma from patients with fulminant hepatic failure. *Exp Cell Res* 1986; 166:139–150.

10. Gohda E, et al: Purification and partial characterization of hepatocyte growth factor from plasma of a patient with fulminant hepatic failure. *J Clin Invest* 1988; 81:414–419.

11. Andoh T, et al: Partial purification and characterization of HGF-like hepatotrophic factor from the plasma of rats treated with carbon tetrachloride. *Acta Hepatol Jpn* 1992; 33:238–245.

12. Kinoshita T, et al: Marked increase of HGF mRNA in nonparenchymal liver cells of rats treated with hepatotoxins. *Biochem Biophys Res Commun* 1985; 133:1042–1050.

13. Ikeda Y, et al: Purification and characterization of lipoprotein lipase and hepatic triglyceride lipase from human postheparin plasma: Production of monospecific antibody to the individual lipase. *Biochim Biophys Acta* 1989; 103:254–269.

14. Ikeda Y, et al: A sandwich-enzyme immunoassay for the quantification of lipoprotein lipase and hepatic triglyceride lipase in human postheparin plasma using monoclonal antibodies to the corresponding enzymes. *J Lipid Res* 1990; 31:1911–1924.

15. Fujiwara S, et al: Enzyme-linked immunoassay of hepatic triglyceride lipase in chronic liver disease. *Acta Hepatol Jpn* 1992; 33:219–224.

16. Fisher JE, et al: The effect of normalization of plasma amino acids on hepatic encephaloopathy in man. *Surgery* 1976; 80:77–91.

17. Yoshimura NN, et al: Protein-sparing effect of intravenously administered branched chain amino acids in adult rats. *JPEN J Parenter Enteral Nutr* 1978; 2:525–531.

18. Muto Y, et al: Effect of oral supplementation with branched-chain amino acid granules on improvement of protein nutrition in decompensated liver cirrhosis: A cross over controlled study, in Ogoshi S, Okada A (eds): *Parenteral and Enteral Hyperalimentation*. Amsterdam, Elsevier, 1984, pp 280–292.

19. Kato M, et al: Effect of branched-chain amino acid (BCAA) enriched-nutrient mixture on albumin metabolism in cirrhotic patients. *Acta Hepatol Jpn* 1991; 32:692–699.

20. Tanner MS, et al: Early introduction of copper-contaminated animal milk feeds as a possible cause of Indian childhood cirrhosis. *Lancet* 1983; 2:992–995.

21. Müller-Hocker J, et al: Copper storage disease of the liver and chronic dietary copper intoxication in two further German infants mimicking Indian childhood cirrhosis. *Pathol Res Pract* 1988; 183:39–45.

22. Lefkowitch JH, et al: Hepatic copper overload and features of Indian childhood cirrhosis in an American sibship. *N Engl J Med* 1982; 307:271–277.

23. Sato M, et al: A study on high copper deposition in rodent liver induced by low-protein diet—an experimental copper administration to SD rats from embryonal to neonatal periods. *Acta Hepatol Jpn* 1991; 32:1017–1026.

24. Esmon CT, et al: Identification of endothelial cell cofactor for thrombin catalyzed activation of protein. *Proc Natl Acad Sci U S A* 1981; 78:2249–2252.

25. Salem HH, et al: Isolation and characterization of thrombomodulin from human placenta. *J Biol Chem* 1984; 259:12246–12251.

26. Iwabuchi S, et al: Plasma thrombomodulin in liver disease. *Gastroenterol Jpn* 1990; 25:661.

27. Mori K, et al: Clinical significance of serum level of thrombomodulin in severe liver diseases: Especially in acute liver failure. *Acta Hepatol Jpn* 1992; 33:147–152.

28. Takahashi Y: Hepatic coma (in Japanese). *Metabolism* 1969; 6:536–544.

29. Hori K: Plasma volatile fatty acids in liver dyfunction, especially after hepatectomy and in surgical liver disorder. *Acta Hepatol Jpn* 1992; 33:152–160.

30. Brazier N, et al: A rapid, simple and sensitive gas chromatographic micromethod for the quantitation of butyric acid and other short-chain fatty acids in serum. *Clin Chim Acta* 1985; 148:261–265.

31. Carswell EA, et al: An endotoxin-induced serum factor that causes necrosis of tumors. *Proc Natl Acad Sci U S A* 1975; 72:3666–3670.

32. Shirai T, et al: Cloning and expression in *Escherichia coli* of the gene for human tumor necrosis factor. *Nature* 1985; 313:803–806.

33. Kayano K, et al: Clinical investigations on the levels of serum TNF-α in the patients with acute liver injury. *Acta Hepatol Jpn* 1992; 33:213–218.

34. Iwanaga S, et al: Chromogenic substrates for horseshoe crab clotting enzyme. Its application for the assay of bacterial endotoxins. *Haemostasis* 1978; 7:183–188.

35. Morita T et al: A new (1–>3)-β-D-glucan–mediated coagulation pathway found in limulus amoebocyte lysate. *FEBS Lett* 1981; 129:318–321.

36. Inada K, et al: Establishment of a new perchloric acid treatment method to allow determination of the total endotoxin content in human plasma by the limulus test and clinical application. *Microbiol Immunol* 1991; 35:303–314.

37. Narita T: Plasma endotoxin measured by the combination of new perchloric acid pretreatment method and endotoxin specific assay in liver cirrhosis. *Jpn J Gastroenterol* 1992; 89:1252–1259.

38. Stoller JK, et al: Reduction of intrapulmonary shunt and resolution of digital clubbing associated with primary biliary cirrhosis after liver transplantation. *Hepatology* 1990; 11:54–58.

39. Krowka MJ: Hepatopulmonary syndrome: An evolving perspective in the era of liver transplantation. *Hepatology* 1990; 11:138–142.

40. Agusti AGN, et al: The lung in patients with cirrhosis. *J Hepatol* 1990; 10:251–257.

41. Shijo H, et al: Marked hypoxemia associated with liver cirrhosis: Clinicopathological study on hepatopulmonary syndrome. *Acta Hepatol Jpn* 1991; 32:817–825.

42. Galibert F, et al: Nucleotide sequence of the hepatitis B virus genome (subtype ayw) cloned in *E. coli. Nature* 1979; 281:646–650.

43. Tiollais P, et al: Biology of hepatitis B virus. *Science* 1981; 213:406–411.

44. Moriarty AM, et al: Antibodies to peptides detect new hepatitis B antigen: Serological correlation with hepatocellular carcinoma. *Science* 1984; 227:429–433.

45. Furukata A, et al: Localization of HBx antigen in the liver tissues from patients with chronic hepatitis. *Acta Hepatol Jpn* 1991; 32:675–682.

46. Arase Y, et al: Changes of HBV DNA after seroconversion from hepatitis B e antigen to anti-HBe after corticosteroid withdrawal therapy. *Acta Hepatol Jpn* 1991; 32:757–761.

47. Matsumoto T, et al: Production of digoxigenin labeled HCV-cDNA probe using PCR and the multiprime technique. *Acta Hepatol Jpn* 1990; 31:1248.

48. Okuda K, et al: Review of the Japanese literature, in Gitnick G (ed): *Current Hepatology*, vol 12. St Louis, Mosby–Year Book, 1992, pp 309–331.

49. Okamoto H, et al: Full-length sequence of a hepatitis C virus genome having poor homology to reported isolates: Comparative study of four distinct genotypes.*Virology* 1992; 188:331–341.

50. Gilliland G, et al: Analysis of cytokine mRNA and DNA: Detection and quantitation by competitive polymerase chain reaction. *Proc Natl Acad Sci U S A* 1990; 87:2725–2729.

51. Kato N, et al: The relationship between the amount of hepatitis C virus quantified by competitive RT-PCR (CRT-PCR) and the effect of interferon treatment. *Acta Hepatol Jpn* 1991; 32:750–751.

52. Chayama K, et al: Quantitation of HCV by competitive PCR using an internal control. *Acta Hepatol Jpn* 1991; 32:754.

53. Okamoto H, et al: Nucleotide sequence of the genomic RNA of hepatitis C virus isolated from a human carrier: Comparison with reported isolates for conserved and divergent regions. *J Gen Virol* 1991; 72:2697–2704.

54. Kato N, et al: Molecular cloning of the human hepatitis C virus genome from Japanese patients with non-A, non-B hepatitis. *Proc Natl Acad Sci U S A* 1990; 87:9524–9528.

55. Takada N, et al: Genotyping of hepatitis C virus and its clinical significance. *Acta Hepatol Jpn* 1992; 33:121–126.

56. Mizokami M, et al: Molecular evolution of HCV and its subtypes (abstract). *Hepatology* 1992; 16:570.

57. Tanaka T, et al: Molecular cloning of hepatitis C virus genome from a single Japanese carrier: Sequence variation within the same individual and among infected individuals. *Virus Res* 1992; 23:39–53.

58. Takada N, et al: Clinical backgrounds of the patients having different types of hepatitis C virus genomes. *J Hepatol* 1992; 14:35–40.

59. Hayashi N, et al: Analysis of HCV variants by RT-PCR using mixed-degenerative primers on C-100 region of HCV. *Acta Hepatol Jpn* 1991; 32:688–691.

60. Cheng CL, et al: Generation of cDNA probes directed by amino acid sequence: Cloning of urate oxidase. *Science* 1988; 239:1288–1291.

61. Kamitsukasa H, et al: Intrafamilial transmission of hepatitis C virus. *Lancet* 1989; 2:987.

62. Ideo G, et al: Intrafamilial transmission of hepatitis C virus. *Lancet* 1990; 335:353.

63. Michitaka K, et al: Intrafamilial transmission of hepatitis C virus in Japan. *Gastoenterol Jpn* 1991; 26:619–622.

64. Takahashi M, et al: Intrafamilial transmission of hepatitis C. *Gastroenterol Jpn* 1991; 26:483–488.

65. Hopf U, et al: Long-term follow-up of post-transfusion and sporadic chronic hepatitis non-A, non-B and frequency of circulating antibodies to hepatitis C virus (HCV). *J Hepatol* 1990; 10:69–76.

66. Setoguchi Y, et al: Prevalence of chronic liver diseases and anti-HCV antibodies in different districts of Saga. *Acta Hepatol Jpn* 1990; 31(suppl):62.

67. Ito S, et al: Massive seroepidemiological survey of hepatitis C virus: Clustering of carriers on the southwest coast of Tsushima, Japan. *Jpn J Cancer Res* 1991; 82:1–3.

68. Kiyosawa K, et al: Route of HCV infection other than blood transfusion. *Acta Hepatol Jpn* 1991; 32:219–221.

69. Tokita H, et al: Seroepidemiological survey of hepatitis C virus related anti C100-3, anti CP-9, anti CP-10 and anti GOR antibodies in an endemic area for non-A, non-B hepatitis. *Acta Hepatol Jpn* 1991; 32:1093–1100.

70. Suou T, et al: Prevalence of HCV antibodies in Yatsuka town of Simane Prefecture, Japan. *Jpn J Gastroenterol* 1992; 89:1173–1178.

71. Okamoto H, et al: Enzyme-linked immunosorbent assay for antibodies against the capsid protein of hepatitis V virus with a synthetic oligopeptide. *Jpn J Exp Med* 1990; 60:223–233.

72. Okamoto H, et al: Antibodies against synthetic oligopeptides deduced from the putative core gene for the diagnosis of hepatitis C virus infection. *Hepatology* 1992; 15:180–186.

73. Misiro S, et al: Non-A, non-B hepatitis specific antibodies directed at host-derived epitope: Implication for an autoimmune process. *Lancet* 1990; 336:1400–1403.

74. Chayama K, et al: Clinical features and viral markers in patients with chronic hepatitis positive for both HBs antigen and anti–C-100 antibody. *Jpn J Gastroenterol* 1991; 88:2113–2118.

75. Chen DS, et al: Hepatitis C virus infection in an area hyperendemic for hepatitis B and chronic liver disease: The Taiwan experience. *J Infect Dis* 1990; 162:817–822.

76. Brotman B, et al: Interference between non-A, non-B and hepatitis B virus infection in chimpanzees. *J Med Virol* 1983; 11:191–205.

77. Higuchi S: Virological studies on the superinfection in hepatitis B virus carriers with hepatitis C virus. *Acta Hepatol Jpn* 1991; 32:1085–1092.

78. Kobayashi M, et al: Positive rate of C-100 antibody and changes of long term follow up cases of chronic liver disease. *Acta Hepatol Jpn* 1991; 32:683–687.

79. Hagiwara H, et al: Detection of hepatitis C virus RNA serum during treatment of chronic hepatitis C with interferon alpha. *Jpn J Gastroenterol* 1991; 88:1420–1425.

80. Matsumoto M, et al: Changes of hepatic and serum HCV RNA level on interferon therapy in patients with chronic hepatitis C. *Acta Hepatol Jpn* 1991; 32:983–989.

81. Conlon KC, et al: Exacerbation of symptoms of autoimmune disease in patients receiving alpha-interferon therapy. *Cancer* 1990; 65:2237–2242.

82. Chikazawa H, et al: Two cases of chronic active hepatitis type C accompanied with psychiatric symptoms during interferon therapy. *Acta Hepatol Jpn* 1992; 33:44–48.

83. Vera DR, et al: Technetium-99m galactosyl-neoglycoalbumin: Preparation and preclinical studies. *J Nucl Med* 1985; 26:1157–1167.

84. Kubota K, et al: New liver function test using a system for asialo asialoglycoprotein receptor system. I. Liver imaging using Tc-99m labeled neoglycoprotein. *Nucl Med* (Japanese) 1986; 23:899–905.

85. Kudo M, et al: Clinical utility of receptor imaging in the assessment of liver function. *Jpn J Gastroenterol* 1992; 89:1349–1359.

86. Ohnishi K, et al: Pulsed Doppler flow as a criterion of portal venous velocity: Comparison with cineangiographic measurements. *Radiology* 1985; 154:495–498.

87. Furuse J, et al: Hemodynamics of intrahepatic portal vein studied in healthy subjects and liver cirrhosis by pulsed Doppler method. *Jpn J Gastronenterol* 1992; 89:1341–1348.

88. Urita Y, et al: Optimal branching of hepatic artery in patients with liver cirrhosis. *Jpn J Gastroenterol* 1992; 89:610–615.

89. Zamir M, et al: Optimal branching of the vascular bifurcations in the human retina. *J Gen Physiol* 1979; 537–548.

90. Kashiwagi T, et al: Dynamic studies on the portal hemodynamics by scintiphotosplenoportography: The visualization of portal venous system using ^{99m}Tc. *Gastroenterology* 1974; 67:668–673.

91. Kashiwagi T, et al: Portosystemic collaterals in portal hypertensino: Visualization by using blood-pool SPECT imaging. *AJR Am J Roentgenol* 1989; 153:281–285.

92. Azuma M, et al: Relationship between recurrence of esophageal varices and changes of portal circulation after endoscopic injection sclerotherapy: Evaluation by single photon emission Ct. *Jpn J Gastroenterol* 1992; 89:498–502.

93. Yoshida H: Splenic venous hemodynamics in portal hypertension. *Jpn J Gastroenterol* 1991; 88:2763–2770.

94. Zimmerman KP, et al: Ultrasound velocity in fixed human liver: Empirical ANOVA and regression modeling on histologically assessed abnormalities. *Ultrason Imaging* 1983; 5:280–294.

95. Ophir J, et al: A narrowband pulse-echo technique for in vivo ultrasonic attenuation estimation. *IEEE Trans Biomed Eng* 1985; 32:205–212.

96. Suzuki K, et al: Ultrasonic tissue characterization of chronic liver disease using cepstral analysis. *Gastroenterology* 1991; 101:1324–1331.

97. Kono M, et al: In vivo ultrasound tissue characterization for the fatty infiltration in the liver using the frequency-dependent attenuation coefficient. *Acta Hepatol Jpn* 1991; 29:919–925.

98. Ibe T, et al: Consecutive follow up of liver volume change measured by computed tomography in a survived case of idiopathic acute fatty liver of pregnancy. *Acta Hepatol Jpn* 1992; 33:174–181.

99. Gores GJ, et al: Primary biliary cirrhosis: Associaton with class II major histocompatibility complex antigen. *Hepatology* 1987; 7:889–892.

100. Manns MP, et al: HLA DRw8 and complement C4 deficiency as risk factors in primary biliary cirrhosis. *Gastroenterology* 1991; 101:1367–1373.

101. Maeda T, et al: Relationship between Japanese primary biliary cirrhosis and HLA DRw8. *Acta Hepatol Jpn* 1992; 33:438.

102. Ichida F: Primary biliary cirrhosis. *Jpan J Gastroenterol* 1975; 72:1428–1430.

103. Enzan H, et al: Autopsy cases of primary biliary cirrhosis in Japan—A statistical study based on

the annuals of the pathological autopsy cases in Japan, from 1984–1987. *Acta Hepatol Jpn* 1991; 32:897–904.

104. Nakamura Y, et al: Pathologic study of primary biliary cirrhosis of early histologic stages presenting cholestatic jaundice. *Liver* 1988; 8:319–324.

105. Melia WM, et al: Hepatocellular carcinoma in primary biliary cirrhosis: Detection by α-fetoprotein. *Gastroenterology* 1984; 87:660–663.

106. Peters RL: Pathology of hepatocellular carcinoma, in Okuda K, Peters RL (eds): *Hepatocellular Carcinoma*. New York, John Wiley & Sons, 1976, pp 107–168.

107. Edmondson HA, et al: Neoplasms of the liver, in Schiff L, Schiff ER (eds): *Diseases of the Liver*, ed 6. Philadelphia, JB Lippincott, 1987, pp 1125.

108. Nakanuma Y, et al: Hepatocellular carcinoma in primary biliary cirrhosis: An autopsy study. *Hepatology* 1990; 11:1010—1016.

109. Okuda K: Hepatocellular carcinoma: Recent progress. *Hepatology* 1992; 15:948–963.

110. Hata K, et al: A case of hepatocellular carcinoma in primary biliary cirrhosis positive for anti-HCV. *Acta Hepatol Jpn* 1992; 33:167–173.

111. Dienes HP, et al: Histologic features in autoimmune hepatitis. *Z Gastroenterol* 1989; 27:325–330.

112. Hino T: Studies on rosette formation in the liver of patients with autoimmune hepatitis. *Acta Hepatol Jpn* 1991; 32:997–1007.

113. Eggink HF, et al: Cellular and hormonal immune reactions in chronic active liver disease. *Clin Exp Immunol* 1982; 50:17–24.

114. Eddleston ALWF, et al: Inadequate antibody response to HBsAg or suppressor T-cell defect in development of active chronic hepatitis. *Lancet* 1974; 2:1543–1545.

115. Mason WS, et al: Virus of Pekin ducks with structural and biological relatedness to human hepatitis B virus. *J Virol* 1980; 36:829–836.

116. Fukuda R, et al: Alteration of infection pattern of duck hepatitis B virus by immunomodulatory drugs. *J Med Virol* 1988; 26:387–396.

117. Hojo H, et al: Cytotoxic cells induced in tumor bearing rats by a streptococcus preparation (OK-432). *Gann* 1981; 72:692–699.

118. Takashita N, et al: Attempt to cause hepatitis in duck hepatitis B virus carrier ducks by immunization with DHBV protein. *Jpn J Gastroenterol* 1992; 89:1242–1251.

119. Marion PL, et al: Major polypeptide of duck hepatitis B virus surface antigen particles. *J Virol* 1983; 48:534–541.

120. Gotoh Y, et al: Healthy carriers of a human retrovirus, adult T-cell leukemia virus (ATLV): Demonstration by clonal culture of ATLV-carrying T-cells from peripheral blood. *Proc Natl Acad Sci U S A* 1982; 79:478–482.

121. Motoori T, et al: Malignant lymphoma in Chikugo district: II) Study on the cell surface markers and the incidence of anti-ATLA antibody. *J Jpn Soc Res* 1984; 24:281–287.

122. Nakano H, et al: Incidence of anti–HTLV-1 antibody in liver disease. *Gastroenterol Jpn* 1992; 27:37–42.

123. Arakawa M, et al: Emergence of malignant lesions within an adenomatous hyperplastic nodule in a cirrhotic liver. Observations in five cases. *Gastroenterology* 1986; 91:198–208.

124. Okuda K: What is the precancerous lesion for hepatocellular carcinoma in man? *J Gastroenterol Hepatol* 1986; 1:79–85.

125. Kudo M, et al Hemodynamic characteristics of early stage hepatocellular carcinoma: In vivo evaluation with vascular imagings. *Acta Hepatol Jpn* 1992; 33:283–291.

126. Kudo M, et al: Tumor hemodynamics in hepatic nodules associated with liver cirrhosis: Relationship between cancer progression and tumor hemodynamics changes. *Jpn J Gastroenterol* 1991; 88:1554–1565.

127. Kudo M, et al: Arterial vascularity within the nodules of small hepatocellular carcinoma: Analy-

sis with ultrasound angiography using intraarterial CO_2 microbubbles and resected specimens. *Acta Hepatol Jpn* 1991; 32:1008–1016.

128. Kojiro M, et al: Pathomorphologic characteristics of early hepatocellular carcinoma, in Okuda K, Tobe T, Kitagawa T (eds): *Early Detection and Treatment of Liver Cancer*, Gann Monogr Cancer Res No 38. Tokyo, Japanese Cancer Association, 1991, pp 29–37.

129. Kanno T, et al: Prognostic significance of echogenic lesion within small hepatocellular carcinoma. *Jpn J Gastroenterol* 1992; 89:55–60.

130. Shuto T, et al: Two cases of well differentiated hepatocellular carcinoma with an unusual supply of portal blood. *Acta Hepatol Jpn* 1992; 33:252–258.

131. Yasuhara K, et al: Pulsed Doppler in the diagnosis of small liver tumors. *Br J Radiol* 1988; 61:898–902.

132. Ohnishi K, et al: Ultrasonic Doppler studies of hepatocellular carcinoma and comparison with other hepatic focal lesions. *Gastroenterology* 1989; 97:1489–1497.

133. Tanaka S, et al: Color Doppler flow imaging of liver tumors. *AJR Am J Roentgenol* 1990; 154:509–514.

134. Taylor KJW, et al: Correlation of Doppler US tumor signals with neovascular morphologic features. *Radiology* 1988; 166:57–66.

135. Gaiani S, et al: Caution in the interpretation of Doppler signals of HCC (letter). *Gastroenterology* 1990; 99:1860.

136. Tohara K: Evaluation of the hemodynamics of liver masses by ultrasonic Doppler method: Usefulness in differential diagnosis of tumor. *Acta Hepatol Jpn* 1991; 32:843–851.

137. Nakashima T: Vascular changes and hemodynamics in hepatocellular carcinoma, in Okuda K, Peters RL (eds): *Hepatocellular Carcinoma*. New York, John Wiley & Sons, 1976; pp 169–203.

138. Edamitsu O: Pathomorphologic study on tumor vessels of hepatocellular carcinoma. *Acta Hepatol Jpn* 1992; 33:15–20.

139. Williams GM: Detection of chemical carcinogens by unscheduled DNA synthesis in rat liver primary cell culture. *Cancer Res* 1977; 37:1845–1851.

140. Noll H: Characterization of macromolecules by constant velocity sedimentation. *Nature* 1967; 215:360–363.

141. Kohn KW, et al: Alkaline elution analysis, a new approach to the study of DNA single-strand interruptions in cells. *Cancer Res* 1973; 33:1849–1853.

142. Nose K, et al: Detection of carcinogen-induced DNA breaks by nick translation in permeable cells. *Biochem Biophys Res Commun* 1983; 111:383–389.

143. Tsutsumi N, et al: Rat hepatocyte in situ nick translation assay as a screening model to detect chemical carcinogens. *Acta Hepatol Jpn* 1992; 33:161–166.

144. Tanaka K, et al: A high molecular weight protease in the cytosol of rat liver. (Purification, enzymological properties and tissue distribution). *J Biol Chem* 1986; 261:15197–15203.

145. Takai S, et al: Abnormal high level of proteasomes in sera from patients with hepatoma. *Acta Hepatol Jpn* 1992; 33:383–389.

146. Okuda H, et al: Vitamin K–dependent proteins and hepatocellular carcinoma. *J Gastroenterol Hepatol* 1991; 6:392–399.

147. Ogura H, et al: Alteration in the sugar chain of PIVKA-II in patients with hepatocellular carcinoma—Con A nonbinding fraction. *Acta Hepatol Jpn* 1991; 32:894.

148. Nakayama M, et al: Promotion effect of citrulline in hepatocarcinogenesis: Possible mechanism in hypercitrullinemia. *Hepatology* 1990; 11:819–823.

149. Nakayama M, et al: Experimental study on hepatocarcinogenesis in hypercitrullinemia—Promoting effect of citrulline. *Acta Hepatol Jpn* 1991; 32:812.

150. Okuda K: Liver Cancer Study Group of Japan: Primary liver cancers in Japan. *Cancer* 1980; 45:2663–2669.

151. The Liver Cancer Study Group of Japan: Primary liver cancer in Japan. Fifth report. *Cancer* 1984; 54:1747–1755.

152. The Liver Cancer Study Group of Japan: Primary liver cancer in Japan. Sixth report. *Cancer* 1987; 60:1400–1411.

153. The Liver Cancer Study Group of Japan: Primary liver cancer in Japan. Clinicalpathological features and results of surgical treatment. *Ann Surg* 1990; 211:277–287.

154. The Liver Cancer Study Group of Japan: Survey and follow-up study of primary liver cancer in Japan. Report 9. *Acta Hepatol Jpn* 1991; 32:1138–1147.

155. Rosenberg SA, et al: Observation on the systemic administration of autologous lymphokine-activated killer cells and recombinant interleukin-2 to patients wth metastatic cancer. *N Engl J Med* 1985; 313:1485–1492.

156. Onishi S, et al: Adoptive immunotherapy with lymphokine-activated killer cells plus recombinant interleukin-2 in patients with unresectable hepatocellular carcinoma. *Hepatology* 1989; 10:349–353.

157. Komatsu T, et al: Transcatheter arterial injection of autologous lymphokine-activated killer (LAK) cells into patients with liver cancers. *J Clin Immunol* 1990; 10:167–174.

158. Okuno K, et al; Treatment for unresectable hepatoma via selective hepatic arterial infusion of lymphokine-activated killer cells generated from autologous spleen cells. *Cancer* 1986; 58:1001–1006.

159. Ishikawa T, et al: Immunotherapy of hepatocellular carcinoma with autologous lymphokine-activated killer cells and/or recombinant interleukin-2. *J Cancer Res Clin Oncol* 1988; 114:283–290.

160. Saibara T, et al: Defective function of lymphokine-activated killer cells and natural killer cells in patients with hepatocellular carcinoma. *Hepatology* 1989; 9:471–476.

161. Wakizaka Y, et al: Postoperative chemoimmunotherapy with autologous spleen-LAK cells to patients wtih resected hepatocellular carcinoma—Prospective randomized study. *Acta Hepatol Jpn* 1992; 33:304–311.

162. Sugiura N, et al: Treatment of small hepatocellular carcinoma by percutaneous injection of ethanol into tumor with real-time ultrasound monitoring. *Acta Hepatol Jpn* 1983; 24:920.

163. Ebara M, et al: Percutaneous ethanol injection for the treatment of small hepatocellular carcinoma. Study of 95 patients. *J Gastroenterol Hepatol* 1990; 5:616–626.

164. Tabuse K: A new operative procedure of hepatic surgery using a microwave tissue coagulator. *Arch Jpn Chir* 1979; 48:160–172.

165. Mada Y, et al: New surgical treatment of small hepatocellular carcinoma—Usefulness of systematic microwave coagulator method. *Acta Hepatol Jpn* 1990; 31:832.

166. Sato H, et al: A case of laparoscopic microwave coagulo-necrotic therapy for small hepatocellular carcinoma. *Acta Hepatol Jpn* 1992; 33:478–483.

167. Seki T, et al: Local treatment for large hepatocellular carcinoma—Combination therapy with percutaneous microwave coagulation therapy and percutaneous ethanol injection therapy. *Acta Hepatol Jpn* 1992; 33:466–472.

Index

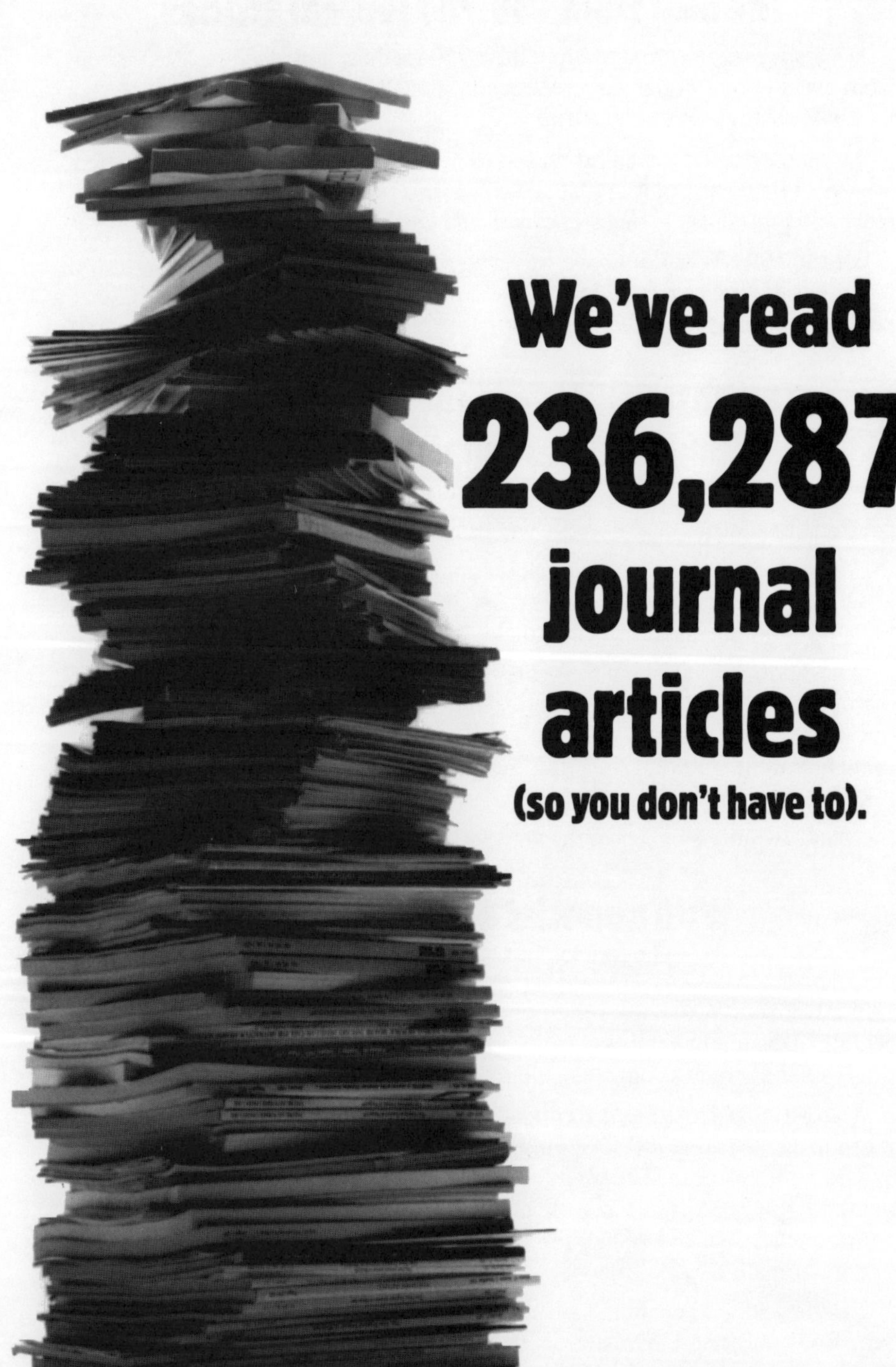
We've read
236,287
journal
articles
(so you don't have to).

The Year Books—
The best from 236,287 journal articles.

At Mosby, we subscribe to more than 950 medical and allied health journals from every corner of the globe. We read them all, tirelessly scanning for anything that relates to your field.

We send everything we find related to a given specialty to the distinguished editors of the **Year Book** in that area, and they pick out *the best*, the articles they feel *every practitioner in that specialty should be aware of.*

For the **1994 Year Books** we surveyed a total of 236,287 articles and found hundreds of articles related to your field. Our expert editors reviewed these and chose the developments you don't want to miss.

The best articles—condensed, organized, and with personal commentary.

Not only do you get the past year's most important articles in your field, you get them in a format that makes them easy to use.

Every article that the editors pick is condensed into a concise, outlined abstract, a summary of the article's most important points highlighted with bold paragraph headings. So you can quickly scan for exactly what you need.

In addition to identifying the year's best articles, the editors write concise commentaries following each article, telling whether or not the study in question is a reliable one, whether a new technique is effective, or whether a particular trend you've head about merits your immediate attention.

No other abstracting service offers this expert advice to help you decide how the year's advances will affect the way you practice.

With a special added benefit for Year Book subscribers.

In 1994, your **Year Book** subscription includes a new added benefit. Access to **MOSBY Document Express**, a rapid-response information retrieval service that puts copies of original source documents in your hands, in a little as a few hours.

With **MOSBY Document Express**, you have convenient, *around-the-clock-access to literally every article* upon which **Year Book** summaries are based. What's more, you can also order journal articles cited in references—or for that matter, virtually any medical or scientific article that can be located. Plus, at your direction, we will deliver the article(s) by FAX, overnight delivery service, or regular mail.

This new added benefit is just one of the enhanced services that makes your **Year Book** subscription an even better value—it's your key to the full breadth of health sciences information. For more details, see **MOSBY Document Express** instructions at the beginning of this book.